Urologic Surgery in the Digital Era

Domenico Veneziano • Emre Huri

Editors

Urologic Surgery in the Digital Era

Next Generation Surgery and Novel Pathways

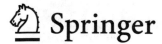 Springer

Editors
Domenico Veneziano
Grande Ospedale Metropolitano
Reggio Calabria
Italy

Emre Huri
Department of Urology
Hacettepe University
Ankara
Turkey

ISBN 978-3-030-63950-1   ISBN 978-3-030-63948-8   (eBook)
https://doi.org/10.1007/978-3-030-63948-8

This Springer imprint is published by the registered company Springer Nature Switzerland AG
The registered company address is: Gewerbestrasse 11, 6330 Cham, Switzerland

Foreword

The term "Endourology" embraces all closed controlled manipulation of the genito-urinary tract. This concept was created to encourage minimally invasive techniques. These procedures have exploded exponentially and this book shows the reader just how rapidly this field has developed. In the past, training residents to do open surgical procedures was a lengthy process, gradually allowing them to do more of the procedure until they were sufficiently competent to perform the entire operation under supervision and eventually without supervision. Welcome to the world of "Urologic Surgery in the Digital Era." The book clearly sets forth all the new approaches that have been developed to treat urologic pathology without the need for open surgery. Minimally invasive therapy has now progressed in certain circumstances to non-invasive therapy which may further decrease morbidity and benefit patients. I congratulate the editors and contributors on this significant contribution to our literature. I am certain that readers will benefit from this up-to-date text.

Endourological Society

A. Smith

Preface

The figure of the *surgeon* is historically surrounded by magic. Despite the ancient Greek word χειρουργία (pron. kheirurgia) being derived by "work with hands," surgeons have always taken advantage of a cutting-edge armamentarium, in comparison to the other contemporary practices. We are living today in the middle of a technological revolution, started when the integrated circuits were invented during the mid-twentieth century. Since then, computers started to aid humans in the development of novel technologies, thus exponentially accelerating the process in every single field. Despite this causing immediate and tangible consequences in our daily life, its results in the surgical field took some more time to become visible. Any invention or clever idea takes indeed a lot of time to reach the Operating Room, due to intricate pathways to be followed in order to obtain clearance by agencies like FDA (United States Food and Drug Administration). The convergence of different technologies and the demonetization of electronics recently contributed to increase reliability and to speed up the process with unprecedented results. Biomaterials, tridimensional visors, miniaturized microscopes, and a series of novel devices are guiding us to re-think almost every single surgical procedure, with a disruption that sometimes may redefine the old surgical dogmas. Understanding how technological progress is changing the urology of tomorrow is crucial today in order to move the right steps in the jungle of best practice. In this book, *Urologic Surgery in the Digital Era: next generation surgery and novel pathways,* we wanted to systematically review the application of the latest surgical techniques and potential future developments in urology, without leaving out innovative tools like artificial intelligence and social media. Thanks to the contribution of some of the most relevant names in the field, we hope that this volume will help the reader to open his mind toward a new era of exciting surgical innovation.

Reggio Calabria, Italy   Domenico Veneziano

Contents

Part I   Novel Pathways to Next Generation Surgery

Benign Prostatic Hyperplasia (BPH)............................. 3
Ioannis Giannakis, Thomas R. W. Herrmann, and Thorsten Bach

Bladder Cancer... 39
F. Pisano, J. M. Gaya, O. Rodriguez Faba, A. Breda, and J. Palou

Stone Treatment... 53
Luca Orecchia, Sara Anacleto, Stefano Germani, Roberto Miano,
and Estêvão Lima

3D Laparoscopy.. 69
Samson Yun-sang Chan, Steffi Kar-kei Yuen, and Eddie Shu-yin Chan

Kidney Transplantation..................................... 79
Angelo Territo, Iacopo Meneghetti, Julio Francisco Calderón Cortez,
Romain Boissier, and Alberto Breda

Sacral Neuromodulation..................................... 97
Marco Torella, Antonio Schiattarella, Nicola Colacurci, and A. Di Gesu

Injections and Biomaterials.................................. 111
Ömer Acar and Ervin Kocjancic

Robot-Assisted Surgery..................................... 129
P. Umari, E. Mazzone, R. De Groote, K. Maes, and A. Mottrie

Robot-Assisted Upper Tract Surgery.......................... 159
Jens Rassweiler, Marcel Fiedler, Remzi Saglam, and Jan-Thorsten Klein

Exoscope-Assisted 3D Open Surgery.......................... 177
Tahsin Batuhan Aydogan and Emre Huri

Confocal Laser Endomicroscopy...................................... 187
Alberto Breda, Salvatore Micali, Angelo Territo, Mino Rizzo,
Giulio Bevilacqua, Iacopo Meneghetti, Maria Chiara Sighinolfi,
Bernardo Rocco, and Giampaolo Bianchi

Live Surgery and Safety Standards............................... 203
Alessandro Tafuri, Giuseppe Carrieri, Angelo Porreca,
and Alessandro Antonelli

Part II   Future Perspectives

Artificial Intelligence 213
Hacı İsmail Aslan, Kadir Erdem Şahin, Mahdiyeh Nilgounbakht,
and Emre Huri

Social Media and E-Learning 221
Juan Gómez Rivas, Jeremy Yuen-Chun Teoh,
and Moises Rodriguez Socarrás

Aviation and Non-Technical Skills.................................. 239
Gianluigi Zanovello

Exponential Technologies and Future Scenarios 249
Nicola Marino, Giovanni Cacciamani, and Domenico Veneziano

Part I
Novel Pathways to Next Generation Surgery

Benign Prostatic Hyperplasia (BPH)

Ioannis Giannakis, Thomas R. W. Herrmann, and Thorsten Bach

1   The Beginning of Modern Endoscopic BPH Treatment

The first revolution in the treatment of benign prostate hyperplasia (BPH) began in New York in 1926 when Maximillian Stern designed the resectoscope with a wire loop that could be moved manually back and forth leading to removal of the obstructed prostate tissue. Stern's resectoscope was an excellent cutting tool but was deficient in coagulation. T.M. Davis developed a switch whereby two currents could be used, one undamped for cutting and one damped to perform hemostasis by induction of coagulation. He also enlarged the size of the loop and window to permit removal of larger pieces of tissue. Inspired by Davis, Joseph F. McCarthy of New York made significant improvements in the resectoscope. In 1932, McCarthy fashioned a lens system that widened the visual field, but most importantly he moved the wire loop and cutting window to the tip of the instrument. The Stern-McCarthy resectoscope, as it became known, was the first practical cutting-loop resectoscope, and TURP emerged as the dominant method used to treat the enlarged prostate for the next 70 years [1, 2].

I. Giannakis
Department of Urology, Kantonspital Frauenfeld, Kanton Thurgau, Switzerland

T. R. W. Herrmann
Department of Urology, Kantonspital Frauenfeld, Kanton Thurgau, Switzerland

European Association of Urology Section of Urotechnology (ESUT), Lower Tract Working Group, Arnhem, The Netherlands

T. Bach (✉)
European Association of Urology Section of Urotechnology (ESUT), Lower Tract Working Group, Arnhem, The Netherlands

Department of Urology, Asklepios Westklinikum Hamburg, Hamburg, Germany
e-mail: t.bach@asklepios.com

D. Veneziano, E. Huri (eds.), *Urologic Surgery in the Digital Era*,
https://doi.org/10.1007/978-3-030-63948-8_1

As operation time and complications seemed to be a direct function of surgical time the need for reduction of the operative time with simultaneously increase of the resected tissue volume was mandatory. Furthermore, other challenges like older patient age in ageing population and anticoagulatory or anti-platelet drugs complicating endoscopic surgery same into focus. Another factor arising was the call for less hospitalization time or ambulatory procedures in health care systems with growing pressure to limit expenses. All factors mentioned culminated into second revolution in the treatment of enlarged prostate glands with the development of various transurethral endoscopic enucleation techniques (EEP) and v to the vaporization-techniques using a great variety of sources in the last 2 decades to the vaporization-techniques.

The latest "revolution" in the past 7 years can be summarized in the introduction of novel mechanical devices (Urolift, iTind), novel ablative devices (Rezum) and the introduction of image guided transurethral resection/ablation (Aquaablation). All of the aforementioned devices focus on either meeting (relevant) secondary endpoints (Urolift, Rezum, Itind, Aquablation), or the fact that all these techniques need a low skill set to perform with high patient's intraoperative safety in the introducing studies. Furthermore, Urolift, iTind, and Rezum are marketed as ambulatory office-based procedures without general anesthesia.

2   The Second Revolution in BPH Surgery

Hiraoka described the blueprint of all transurethral anatomical enucleating techniques in 1983 using a prostate detachment technique along the false capsel of fibrous tissue between peripheral zone and adenoma [3]. In 2005, Frauendorfer and Gilling [4] developed and introduced Holmium-Laser and the HoLEP (Holmium-Laser Enucleation of Prostate) into the clinical praxis. However, despite excellent clinical results in randomized controlled trials HoLEP did not find wide acceptance among the urological community and HoLEP became a aspired technique mainly performed and demonstrated by key opinion leader centers around the globe.

After the introduction of Thulium YAG Laser in 2005, a number of transurethral techniques for the treatment of the prostate using the new energy source were subsequently introduced. Introducing vaporizing, incising, resecting and finally enucleating techniques the working groups virtually replicated the path that former Ho: YAG promoters had taken.

Vapoenucleation of the prostate focusing on the vapoincising capacity of the novel Thulium laser was published in 2009 by Thorsten Bach et al. (ThuVEP). The template removed resembled the transurethral enucleation appearance like demonstrated by the HoLEP community with the difference that incising and simultaneous sealing of the cutting plane did not match the expectation of the HoLEP market leaders. Out of the controversy whether enucleation can only be performed with Holmium laser and a discussion on the intraoperative anatomy and appearance of surgical planes. Herrmann et al. proposed a concept of anatomical widely blunt enucleation of the prostate using the Thulium laser energy only as *a* assisting tool for incising and coagulation only (ThuLEP).

Although bipolar enucleation of the prostate had been demonstrated equivalence in a randomized controlled trial of Neill et al. [5] it took a long way to get bipolar enucleation and therefore any transurethral anatomical enucleation on eye level with HoLEP until 2016.

Today, helpful bipolar tools like combined mechanical and vaporizing bipolar enucleation probes have entered the market offering mechanical detachment and at the same time an efficient hemostasis [6].

Since the 2016 update of the "EAU Guidelines on Management of Non-Neurogenic Male Lower Urinary Tract Symptoms (LUTS), including Benign Prostatic Obstruction (BPO)", Holmium laser enucleation of the prostate (HoLEP) and bipolar enucleation being summarized as anatomical enucleating techniques (AEEP) are proposed as first choice for the surgical management of BPO of large volume prostates.

Parallel to the AEEP, laser vaporization of the prostate with Holmium (Holmium Laser TUV-P), Thulium (Thulium Laser TUV-P), Diode-Laser or Green-Light Laser (first reported in 2003) offers a safe and effective treatment of BPH. All the above laser sources can be safely used for EEP also.

In this article each method will be analyzed with demonstration along with the most recently published studies, to provide a general icon of the most novel treatments in patients with LUTS because of BPH.

2.1 Laser's Characteristics

The basic principle of laser-using is the laser chromophore/tissue interaction, which set the properties of various laser sources leading to different therapeutic and thermal effects with reference to the content and stability of the chromophore in the prostatic tissue.

The different wavelengths from the lasers lead to different penetration depth and tissue absorption and consequently to different thermal effects. Briefly, thulium and holmium laser are absorbed mainly from their chromphore water and at a wavelength of 2000 nm and 2100 nm respectively. The tissuepenetration has been described at 0.2- and 0.4-mm. On the other hand Lithium Borat Lasers (LBO, Greenlinght R) has a wavelength of 532 nm. Its chromophore is the thermoinstable haemoglobin. In the highly perfused prostate the penetration depth of 0.8 mm is described. The various diode lasers have fundamental differences in their affinity to water as the absorption medium. The tissue penetration thereby widely differs and ranges from 5 mm to 7 mm to even deeper tissue penetrations (940–1470 nm)

Although, laser enucleation of the prostate was originally described with Holmium YAG laser, today mainly Thulium laser (ThuVEP [7], ThuLEP [8]) and

Greenlight R are in use [9], Diode laser (DiLEP, ELEP [10]) don't play a role anymore. However, Vaporization, called photoselective vaporization of the prostate is the mainstay of the so Greenlight R [11].

2.2 Enucleation/Vaporization

The EAU Guideline panel on Management of Non-Neurogenic Male Lower Urinary Tract Symptoms (LUTS), incl. Benign Prostatic Obstruction (BPO), introduced EEP (Endoscopic Enucleation of the Prostate) or AEEP (Anatomical Endoscopic Enucleation of the Prostate) to describe the transurethral enucleation of enlarged prostates in patients with LUTS. The interest of the novel methods woke up in the urological community in the last years after live operations and presentations in frame of international congresses and symposia such as European Section of Uro-Technology (ESUT). Nowadays, in the context of EEP open prostatectomy is no longer considered as first choice for the surgical management of large volume prostates in benign prostatic obstruction.

The honour for the historical achievement of exposing transurethral enucleation to a broader readership and surgical peers is due to Peter Gilling and Mark Fraundorfer [4] for their work and publication on "Holmium: YAG laser enucleation of the prostate combined with mechanical morcellation: preliminary results" in 1998. In the wake of HoLEP, transurethral plasmakinetic (i.e. bipolar) enucleation of the prostate (PkEP) followed in 2004. In the second half of the 2000s all other transurethral laser based enucleation techniques led by Tm: YAG Vapoenucleation (ThuVEP) and transurethral anatomical enucleation with Tm: YAG Support (ThuLEP), later diode laser enucleation of the prostate (DiLEP) and finally Lithium-Borate "Greenlight" enucleation of the prostate (GreenLEP) entered the endourological stage to finally replace open prostatectomy (OP) and TURP.

In principal, all enucleating techniques can be distinguished in two principles. "True" anatomical enucleation performed by mainly blunt dissection and thereby developing the surgical plane leaving the surface intact for visualization and orientation and on the other hand, vapo-enucleation uses the vaporizing identity of laser-sources to cut and seal the surface at the same time. Using vapo-enucleation cutting plane aims to reach the anatomical plane. In the best of circumstances these planes are identical as showed Kyriazis et al. (Fig. 1) [12], but a chance of extra-anatomical preparation with incomplete resection or excess of resection template with the chance of perforation of the capsule is possible as presented by Elshal et al. [13].

The transition from "anatomical" to "extraanatomical" is fluent (Fig. 2). In case of "vapo-enucleation" procedures some authors recommend to start with anatomical preparation.

A surrogate parameter for "complete resection" is the PSA-drop, postoperatively. Given the mainstay of enucleating techniques in total prostate volume larger than 80 ml, PSA-drop is expected to be around 80% for enucleation, 65% for TUR-P and 45% for vaporisation if of concomitant prostate cancer is absence (Table 1).

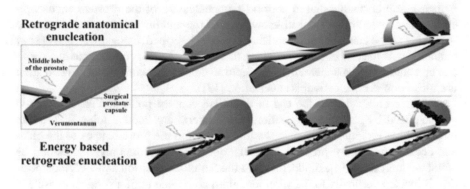

Fig. 1 Kyriazis I, Świniarski PP, Jutzi S, Wolters M, Netsch C, Transurethral anatomical enucleation of the prostate with Tm: YAG support (ThuLEP): review of the literature on a novel surgical approach in the management of benign prostatic enlargement. World J Urol. 2015 Apr; 33(4): 525–30. doi: https://doi.org/10.1007/s00345-015-1529-0. Epub 2015 Mar 15

Fig. 2 Gradual modification of enucleating techniques. From blunt anatomical to vapoenucleation (Herrmann TRW 2017)

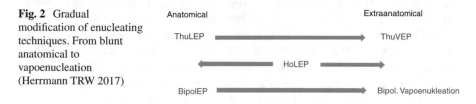

Table 1 PSA reduction after surgical intervention in (%)

Autor	Technik	PSA Reduktion/%
Timmouth 2005	HoLEP	81.7–86
Netsch 2015	ThuVEP	81–88
Herrmann 2010, Kim 2015	ThuLEP	83–93
Kim 2008	TmLRP-TT, Tangerine	82.5
Misrai 2016	GreenLEP	67
Liu 2010	Bipolare Enukleation (PkeP)	88.6
Thomas 2016 (Goliath)	TURP	58
Thomas 2016 (Goliath)	LBO—PVP 180 Watt	49
Lebdai 2016	Prostate embolization (PAE)	24

A crucial role for the development of the EEP played the improvement of the morcellator devices, which did not change the basic principle of the enucleating technique but helped to facilitate and potentially speed up the evacuation of the dissected tissue. However, by common consent the mechanical morcellation adds a further learning curve to the whole process of adapting EEP in daily practice [14]. However, enucleation techniques without morcellation to tissue removal (Thulium Laser Resection of the Prostate in Tangerine Technik (TmLR-TT) [15], Holmium laser enucleation of the prostate combined with electrocautery resection in mushroom technique were described [16].

It is comprehensible that to perform an enucleation of the prostate endoscopically is demanded distinguished knowledge of the anatomy of prostate. Since the beginning of the enucleation several methods are described, using difference energy modalities. At the end of the point, given that the procedure is carried out in a sensitive and anatomical manner, all AEEP seem to deliver the same result (Enucleation is enucleation is enucleation, is enucleation [17]).

Gilling's group first in the end of twentieth century published an enucleation characterized by separate enucleation of the lateral and medial lobes of prostate through three longitudinal excisions with origin from the prostate apex to the bladder neck followed by prostate morcellation. This is commonly understood as '3-lobe-enucleation' [4]. Bladder neck at the 5 o'clock position and 7 o'clock position is incised vertically to the verumontanum with deep until a surgical capsule is reached. Once the two incisions are joined just above the verumontanum to allow enucleation of the median lobe. As the tip of the laser moves side-to-side toward the bladder neck, the median lobe is dissected from the prostatic capsule and. Placed into the bladder for later morcellation. Next, both lateral lobes are enucleated; the medial edges of both lateral lobes are extended to the apex to more clearly define the apical anatomy. The enucleation of the left lateral lobe is proceeded by sweeping circumferentially until the 2 o'clock. A longitudinal incision should be made at the 12 o'clock position of the bladder neck, extended in the distal direction till the capsule layer. The space between the adenoma and the capsule is developed laterally and circumferentially with a sweeping motion. The enucleation from the upper and lower parts is connected to each other at the 2 o'clock position of the apex. After further enucleating the left lateral lobe, it is placed into the bladder, and the rightlateral lobe is enucleated similarly to the left lateral lobe. The method is recently in details prescribed and sketched from Kim et al. [18].

The Tokyo group (Endo et al.) in 2010 described am modification of the standard Gilling's method performing an anteroposterior enucleation of the prostate, in which surgical capsule of prostate is demonstrated after incision in the place of verumontanum directed to the lateral lobe. Afterwards, the mucosa in 12 o'clock is vaporized beginning from the sphincter directed to the bladder neck. The enucleation starts in the middle of the lateral lobe, dissecting the adenoma of the prostatic capsule after a towards manoeuvre of the lobe. The enucleation continues in anterior-downward trend to the 6 o'clock in the apical area of the prostate gland. The urethral mucosa is incised over the verumontarum until the surgical layer. The being left adenoma can be removed retrogradely [19].

To pass over situations such as remain prostate adenoma due to the dissimilar plane caused from the separate longitudinal incision as well as to avoid significant bleeding because of capsule perforation or incontinence due to sphincter traumatisation making the longitudinal incision at 12 o'clock a new en-bloc method was developed for the transurethral prostate enucleation.

En bloc AEEP/EEP like in open prostatectomy has been popularized mainly by third generation HoLEP promoters, and has gained momentum since. The overarching principle of all approaches using either Ho: YAG or Tm: YAG lasers is anatomical preparation, anterioposterior dissection, early release of the ventral mucosa and apical mucosa sparing incisions in order to reduce early postoperative incontinence [9, 20–24] and ease the learning curve by achieving several reproducible quality markers (Pentafecta) [25]. However, comparative assessment of effectivity remain inconclusive.

The Turin group (Scoffone CM, Cracco CM et al) introduced in 2010 an en-block no touch procedure, beginning the enucleation at the apex of prostate with an incision above verumontanum to the left lobe in order to identify the correct plane between prostatic capsule and adenoma. Further to this step an incision is made retrogradely between medial and left lateral lobe from the prostate apex to bladder neck at 5 o'clock. The anatomical structures can be so clearly identified. The left lobe can be further ascended dissected (from 5 o'clock completed to 12 o'clock). At this point the enucleation continues to the right lobe antegradely (from 12 o'clock to 9 o'clock). Returning to the start position, a horizontal incision above verumontarum to the right lobe allows the circumferentially joining with the proper incision, allowing the enucleation of the medial and right lobe, forming a horseshoe-formed enucleated prostate gland. The en-bloc enucleation will be completed with the incision of the anterior incision of adenoma parasphicterically with an incision at 10 o'clock and 2 o'clock as well as horizontally at 12 o'clock. The adenoma is placed intravesically to further morcellation [24].

Freiburg group (Miernik A, Schoeb DS) published in 2018 the 'three-horseshoes-like enucleation' in which the enucleation of prostate gland starts with an U-like incision in the apex of prostate over the verumontanum, letting the medial lobe be lifted and the appropriate surgical plane between adenoma and prostatic capsule be demonstrated. A second U-incision is made in the mucosa between the two lateral lobes and the external sphincter at 12 o'clock extended retrogradely to the bladder neck in the anterior commissure of prostate between 11 o'clock and 1 o'clock. The detachment of the lateral lobes is assessed with a third U-incision in the bladder neck. The lateral lobes are circularly mobilised and dissected and the whole adenoma is pushed in the bladder. The last place the adenoma is held between 4 o'clock and 8 o'clock will be lastly dissected and whole the adenoma is placed now intravesically to further morcellation [23] (Fig. 3).

The original concept of ThuLEP as *"transurethral anatomical prostatectomy with laser support"* was developed in 2009 and published in 2010 [8] has evolved to mainly 2 lobe technique [26]. Also, Thulium en bloc enucleation has been published [20] and gains momentum with the lately popularized Thulium fibre laser [27].

2 lobes for HoLEP has also been popularized [28, 29] as well as for bipolar enucleation using a dedicated combined mechanical and vaporizing probe (BipoLEP [26]) (Fig. 4). The incision begins with a horizontal incision proximal to the verumontanum followed by an incision of the mucosa laterally on the left and on the right lobe until the distal third of the verumontanum. To arise the surgical capsule, mechanical force is used. The tip of the resectoscopes sheath is placed proximal to the verumontanum moving steep down and towards to the left in a shearing movement to separate the apex of the transitional zone. The correct plane is demonstrated by mechanical and blunt disruption into the zone dorsally below the transitional zone. The correct surgical capsule can be easily identified by visualizing small

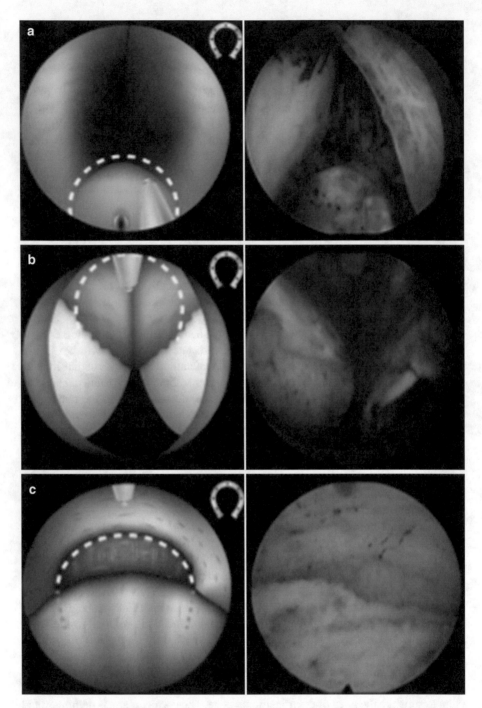

Fig. 3 Miernik A, Schoeb DS. "Three horse shoe-like incision" holmium laser enucleation of the prostate: first experience with a novel en bloc technique for anatomic transurethral prostatectomy. World J Urol 2019; 37: 523–8

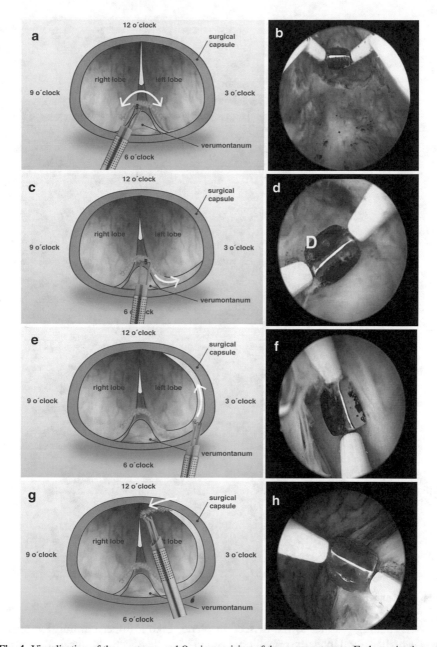

Fig. 4 Visualisation of the anatomy and Ω -circumcision of the verumontanum, Endoscopic view of Ω -circumcision (**c**) Exposure of the left dorsal surgical plane by mechanical shear around the apex of the transition zone (**d**) endoscopic view during (**c, e**) Apical loosing of the transitional zone by circulating around the adenoma. (**f**) endoscopic view during (**e, g**) Incision of broad mucosal band to maintain a ventral mucosal patch, (**h**) endoscopic view during (**g**). (**g**) Incision in at 5° clock position for medial disection of the left lobe, (**j**) endoscopic view during (**i, k**) Ascending mobilisation of the left lobe, (**l**) endoscopic vision during (**k, m**) Visualtiation of the left empty fossa, (**n**) mirror-wise shear to the right lobe, (**n**) Incision of the mucosal band on the right side, (**o**) the loosened adenoma of right and middle lobe is pushed through the intact bladder neck, (**p**) empty fossa with intact bladder neck

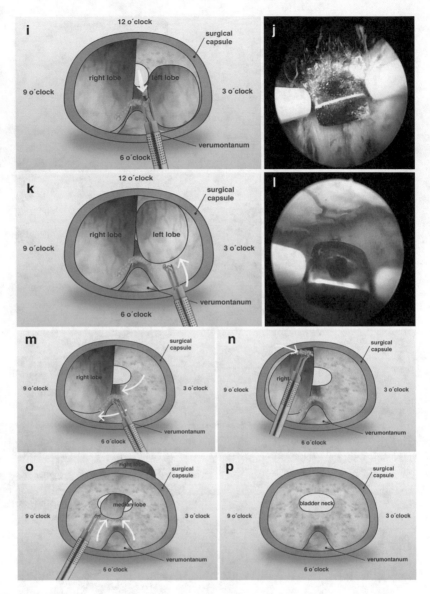

Fig. 4 (continued)

vessels running parallel to the dissection plane. Like a finger circling the apical edges of the lateral lobe, the transitional zone is detached from the surgical capsule. Additionally, the resectoscope is guided into the space between transitional and peripheral zone and the adenoma is loosened circumferentially with the top of the sheath of the resectoscope, after tissue detachment apically between 3 o'clock and 12'o clock position. After disconnection of the tissue between 3 o'clock and 12 o'clock, takes place the detachment of the remaining mucosa in the 12 o'clock position, which appeared as mucosal band After the dissection of the mucosal band, the resectoscope is moved towards over the midline and the tissue is dissected sloping downward from peripheral towards the lumen until the bladder neck becomes visible. Prior preparation of the adenoma from 6 o'clock to 3 o'clock position, the medial edge of the left lobe, is denoted by an incision from the bladder neck in the 5 o'clock position towards the apex of the prostate. To continue, the dorsal part of the left lobe has to be detached. Therefore, the left lobe is loaded up with the beak of the resectoscope and lifted, while the enucleation probe is advanced and pushed into the space between transitional and peripheral zone. The lobe is detached until the bladder neck and finally pushed into the bladder. The median and the right lobe are enucleated en bloc. The resectoscope is positioned at the 7 o'clock and performing blunt dissection with the resectoscopes sheath, the right lobe is loosened circumferentially from 7 o'clock to 12 o'clock position. The remaining mucosal band is cut like on the left side from peripheral towards the midline. The lobe is then detached using axial force and coagulation if necessary. Finally, the detached median and right lobe are pushed into the bladder and morcellation competes the procedure.

2.3   Enucleation VS Open Adenectomy (OP)

Kuntz et al. [30], showed in a RCT consisted of 120 patients, similar tissue removal, decrease of prostate volume as well as similar amelioration of maximal flow, IPSS-score and postvoiding residual urine in patients after HoLEP VS open adenectomy (OP). However, it was found a significant difference in mean procedure time (136 vs 91 min), mean bleeding rates with haemoglobin loss (1.9 vs 2.8 g/dL), median catheter time (1 day vs 6 days) and median hospital stay (2 days v 10 days) with superiority for the HoLEP-arm with follow up of 24 months [14]. Naspro et al. [31] prospectively analysing the postprocedural functional outcomes 2 years after HoLEP VS OP in enlarged (<70 g) prostates favoured HoLEP in terms of blood transfusion (0% VS 5%), catheterisation time (1.5 days VS 4.1 days, $p < 0.001$) and length of hospital stay (2.7 days VS 5.43 days, $p < 0.001$). The urodynamical outcomes showed a significant decrease of PdetQmax for both methods in comparison to the baseline values (HoLEP: from 80.6 cmH_2O to 30.6 cmH_2O. $p < 0.001$, OP: from 83.1 to 34.8 cm H2O, $p < 0.001$), while there was no difference in postoperative urge and stress incontinence, re-intervention rates and acute urine retention postprocedurally. The long-terms entanglements (dysuria and urethral/bladder neck structures) were complete identically for HoLEP and OP arms (2.8% VS 3.3% and 2.8% VS 3.3% respectively).

Li et al. [32] and Lin et al. [33] proved the efficiency the safety of the AEEP compared to OP published either a meta-analysis including 7 RCT's with 735 patients and 9 RCT's with 758 patients respectively. The comparable methods were mainly plasmakinetic enucleation (PkEP) and HoLEP VS OP. They mentioned to show clearly improvement of the functional parameters (IPSS, QoL, Qmax, PVE,

IIEF) in comparison to the baseline characteristics for both groups. This improvement was not significantly different between both groups. However, enucleation had numerically lower specimen weights compared with OP, while enucleation presented clearly superiority in terms of blood loss, blood transfusion, catheterization and hospitalisation time. No statistically significant difference was observed between the enucleation and OP groups with respect to re-catheterization, urinary tract infection, urinary incontinence, bladder-neck/urethral strictures or reintervention.

Elshal et al. [34] in a prospectively institutional matched pair data analysis based on the weight of the removal tissue, published similar results underlying superiority for HoLEP with reference to blood transfusion, catherization time hospital length of stay and overall costs. Post-procedurally, Qmax, IPSS, QoL, prostate adenoma removal (99.2 ± 34 and 103.7 ± 25, p = 0.31), Dindo complications Grade > 3 were similar in both groups. Using Holmium-Laser for the prostate enucleation ca. 10% of the whole prostate tissue will be vaporized, which should be considered by drawing the parallel between the two procedures regarding this point.

Recently, Misraï et al. [35] comparing GreenLEP VS OP in a retrospective single centre study managed to present non-inferior results from GreenLEP. Both methods had similar operating time (67 min VS 60 min) while GreenLEP showed significantly shorter catheterisation and hospitalization time. The specimen weight was similar (70 vs 60 g) and 6 months after the procedures Qmax, IPSS, QoL were comparable, PVR, whereas PSA reduction was identical and 3-and 6-months urinary incontinence-rate as well as urethral strictures rate were slightly more in the open group (1.9% VS 1.4% and 4.4% VS 1.4% respectively).

2.4   *Enucleation/Vaporenucleation VS TUR-P*

Compared to the 'gold' standard transurethral resection of the prostate transurethral enucleation of the prostate seems to have s severe superiority in an amount of perioperative and postoperative outcomes.

To begin with HoLEP VS TUR-P, Li et al. [36] performing an updated systematic review with meta-analysis and trial sequential analysis including 9 RCT's with follow up between 12 and 24 months (only one RCT with FU 9 months) demonstrated clearly favour of HoLEP-arm regarding Qmax, IPSS and PVR 1y postprocedural, while QoL and IIEF remained without significant difference in both groups. Moreover, perioperative data favoured HoLEP in regard to tissue removal, length of catheterization and hospital stay, whereas operative time favoured TUR-P above HoLEP. Early postoperative complications (urinary retention, urinary tract infection, transient haematuria) were more or less identical in both groups. The late complications (urethral stricture, urinary incontinence, re-treatment, bladder neck stenosis) showed a slightly not statistically relevant superiority of HoLEP-group. To the same outcomes leaded Yin et al. [37] as demonstrated in a meta-analysis from 6 RCT's with almost 250 patients.

Bipolar enucleation of the prostate (BEEP) is a wide category, including plasmakinetic enucleation of the prostate (PkEP), transurethral resection enucleation of the prostate (TUERP), bipolar plasma enucleation of the prostate (BPEP), transurethral vapor-enucleation resection of the prostate (TVERP), transurethral vapor-enucleation of the prostate (TVEP) and finally bipolar enucleation of the prostate BipoLEP). Chunxiao Liu et al. [38] published the effectiveness of the BEEP using the Plasmakinetic™ system, presenting in a series of 1.100 patients with a median follow up of ca. 4.5 years an indubitable Qmax elevation by 250% (21.7 ± 7.4 ml7/s at 6 years postop), PVR reduction by 90.8% (13.1 ± 6.4 ml), I-PSS reduction by 79.3% (4.9 ± 1.6) and finally QOL-score reduction by 67.4% (1.5 ± 0.3). The PSA-reduction 6 months postoperatively showed a decrease of 88.6%. Within the 6 year follow up postoperative complications included meatal stenosis in 9 cases, incontinence in 56, urethral stricture in 12 and bladder neck contracture in only 10 patients. In the same line Lingfeng Zhu et al. [39] demonstrated in a RCT with overall 80 patients comparing bipolar EEP vs. TURP, that bipolar EEP achieved greater resected prostate tissue, less blood, shorter catheterization time and postoperative hospital stay on favour of EEP. The postoperative improvement in IPSS, QoL, Qmax and PVR was similar in both groups at 1, 6, 12 and 24 months but significantly in favour of bipolar EEP at 36, 48 and 60 months. Recently, Aercaniolo et ESUT-Research Group [40], carried out e meta-analysis including 14 comparative studies (5 RCTs, 2 cohort prospective non-randomized, 1 propensity score-matched paired analysis and 6 cohort retrospective studies) with overall 2317 subjects (1178 patients for BEEP and 1139 for b-TURP). They achieved to make known the clearly superiority of BEEP as well in functional as in perioperative out-comes. There was no difference in terms of operative time, but there was a higher amount of resected tissue, shorter bladder irrigation and catheter time for BEEP. Lower haemoglobin drop was found in the BEEP, while post-operative complications (short and long-term complications) and transfusion rate were lower for BEEP. Long-term incontinence rate was not statistically different between the two groups. Furthermore, BEEP group had smaller residual prostate volume and post-operative PSA value translating into more "complete resection" compared to bTUR-P. There was no difference among the two procedures regarding urethral stricture rate, whereas re-intervention rate was higher in the b-TURP group.

Thulium-Laser can, amongst other things, be used either for the EEP enucleation of the prostate (ThuLEP) as firstly described by Bach et al. [41] and Herrmann et al. [8] or to perform a vapo-enucleation (ThuVEP) as firstly published by Bach [7, 28], proving that continuous wave lasers apart from their vaporizing/vapo-incising function may be used to enucleate. The vapo-incisions from ThuVEP into the prostate to cut out the sample incorporating the transitional zone were aiming at the level of the surgical capsule thereby emulating the template of conventional HoLEP. Both HoLEP and ThuVEP techniques alter the capsule either with boiling by the vapor bubble ("white"-HoLEP), or caramelizing in the vapoincision ("brown"-ThuLEP). Therefore, the surgical twins "ThuVEP" and "ThuLEP" demonstrated the whole spectrum of laser action in enucleating techniques. ThuVEP focusing vaporizing features during enucleation, ThuLEP focusing on almost blunt detachment and laser

Table 2 Thulium based approaches, modified from Bach et al. [41]

ThuVAP	ThuVARP	ThuVEP	ThuLEP	ThuLEP in Oyster technique
Thulium laser vaporisation of the prostate 2004 (Mattioli et al. 2008)	Thulium laser Vaporesection in Tangerine Technqiue TmLRP_TT 2005 (Xia 2009) Vaporesection 2006 (Bach et al. 2007)	Thulium laser vapoenucleation of the prostate 2008 (Bach et al. 2009)	ThuLEP Anatomical enucleation with Tm:YAG support ± mechanical tissue morcellator or mushroom 2009 (Herrmann TRW et al. 2010)	Tm:YAG Oyster Anatomical enucleation Oyster technique with Tm:YAG support and high power in situ vaporisation 2016 (Herrmann TRW 2016)

assistance. Currently, the maximum power of the laser has been improved to 120 W, and theoretically, a mean total of 1.08 g of tissue is vaporized/min. By combining resection, vaporization, and enucleation, the removal rate can be increased to approximately 2–3 g/min in trained hands (Table 2).

Iacono et al. [42] demonstrated functional outcomes of ThuLEP (120 W/40 W) in 148 patients in a retrospective study with FU of 12 months. Ending the FU-period the efficiency of ThuLEP was absolute clear: Qmax (8.23 ml/s to 28.67 ml/s), IPSS (21.10 to 3.9 points), QoL (4.38 to 0.94 points), PVR (146 ml to 12.89 ml), prostate volume (108 ml to 13.76 ml) and PSA (9.53 ng/ml to 0.93 ng/ml). Only 2.7% of the patients needed early postoperative blood transfusion due to persistent haematuria with continuous bladder irrigation and prolonged catheterization. 6.7% of patients had postoperative irritative symptoms with temporary urge incontinence and UTI occurred in 12.8% of patients. Only 2 patients developed urethral stricture during follow-up, they needed surgery with cold incision of the stricture part. Kyriazis and Swiniarski [43] making a review of literature including all studies with ThuLEP-procedures. He presented a mean operative time including morcellation ranged between 70 and 102 min. Blood loss as documented by haemoglobin decrease was minimum ranging between 0.5 and 1.27 g/dl. Catheterization time ranged between 2.1 and 2.4 days. PSA reduction as indicator of efficiency in adenoma resection varied between 30.4 and 90%. The clearly amelioration of IPSS, Qmax; QoL, PVR was also described.

Gross et al. [44], carried out a prospective study with 1080 patients underwent ThuVEP classifying the patients according to their prostate volume (<40 ml (median 30 ml)/40–79 ml (median 54 ml)/>80 ml (median 100 ml)). They managed to show an improvement of all functional outcomes in each subgroup with 45%, 58% and 63% tissue removal respectively. The most frequent early complications were urine retention (9%), re-intervention (re-morcellation, secondary apical resection, clot evacuation) in 4.7% of patients and bleeding requiring blood transfusion in 1.7%. The complications were prostate size-dependent and decreased significantly over time reflecting the learning curve the procedure. Netsch et al. [45] published the long-term results from a prospective analysis of 124 patients who underwent ThuVEP. At 12-month follow-up, IPSS, QoL, Qmax, and PVR improved significantly compared with preoperative assessment and continued to do so during follow-up. PSA decreased from 4.7 to 0.92 ng/ml corresponding to a PSA reduction of 83.6% at12-month follow-up. At 4 years postoperatively, Qmax (20 vs. 7.6 ml/s), PVR (25 vs. 107.5 ml), IPSS (4 vs. 21), and QoL (1 vs. 5) differed significantly from baseline. Major adverse requiring re-interventions within 4 weeks after surgery were necessary in 8.1% of the patients. About 6% had postoperative irritative symptoms, which required anticholinergic therapy with a median duration of 30 days, while 3.2% had postoperative mild urinary stress incontinence, which resolved in all within median 24.5 (15.8–97) days. Urinary tract infections occurred in 5.6% of patients and urethral stricture and bladder neck contracture each developed in 1% and 1.6% of the patients, respectively. Zhu et al. [46] in a systematic review and meta-analysis compared ThuVEP/ThuLEP (TmLRP) with TUR-P taking under consideration the data of seven studies (four RCTs and three non-RCTs). One year postoperatively the amelioration of Qmax and IPSS favoured ThuVEP/ThuLEP while PVR and QoL showed any significant difference, although the improvement was greater in the TmLRP group. The operation time of TmLRP was significantly longer than that of TURP, which seems to be associated with the learning curve. However, in patients with large prostates, TmLRP has an advantage on the operation duration over TURP. Furthermore, TmLRP offered the advantages over TURP in terms of serum sodium decreased, catheterization time, and hospital stay during the perioperative period.

2.5 ThuLEP VS HoLEP

Zhang et al. [47] tried to compare the clinical outcomes between ThuLEP (70 W) and HoLEP (90 W) in a prospective randomized trial with 133 patients 18 months of follow-up. The mushroom technique was used to fragment the enucleated lobes with the resection loop. ThuLEP required a longer operation time (72.4 vs 61.5 min) but resulted in less blood loss than HoLEP (130.0 vs 166.6 mL). Catheterization time was comparable. At the end of FU, IPSS decreased to 5.2 in the ThuLEP group and 6.2 in the HoLEP group. QoL and Qmax were similar between the 2 groups (1.3 vs 1.2 and 23.4 vs 24.2 mL/s) and PVR decreased by 82.50% and 81.73% in the ThuLEP and HoLEP groups, respectively. The mean PSA reduction after HoLEP and ThuLEP was 30.43% and 43.36%, respectively. No urethral or bladder neck stricture were found in either group. Obviously both methods relieve LUTS equally with high efficacy and safety. ThuLEP was statistically superior to HoLEP in blood loss and inferior to HoLEP in operation time, although the differences were clinically negligible.

Xiao et al. [48] accomplished a systematic review and metanalysis including 5 independent studies in a total of 1010 patients comparing ThuLEP VS HoLEP. The presented not statistically significant differences between the groups concerning operation time, nucleation time, morcellation time, catherization time and hospital stay. All the included studies recorded less haemoglobin drop in ThuLEP-arm; however, the difference was also not statistically significant. The high enucleation efficacy of the ThuLEP technique was reported in three included studies. This could be in debt of the wavelength of thulium laser, which is close to the water absorption peak, and water is the main absorbing substance which comprises about two-thirds of the prostate, thus results in a high energy absorption rate and therefore compared with the pulsed mode of the holmium:YAG laser, the continuous wave mode of the thulium:YAG laser might provide a faster enucleation. The difference in coagulation depth between thulium:YAG laser (2 mm) and holmium:YAG laser (4 mm) may be an explanation; for the final coagulation, more time may be required after ThuLEP compared with HoLEP. Both procedures provide satisfactory micturition improvement of LUTS symptoms, while they appear similar adverse events profile.

2.6   DiLEP VS HoLEP

The comparison between Diode (980 nm)-Laser Enucleatio of Prostate (DiLEP) and HoLEP detained He et al. [49], who randomised 126 patients and observed the functional outcomes and the adverse complications during 12 months follow up time. Qmax, PVR,IPSS, QoL were comparable between the 2 techniques as well as in case of operative time, resected tissue weight, catheter duration, and hospital stay, no significant difference was found between the two groups. However, the DiLEP group showed less blood loss and decrease in haemoglobin compared with the HoLEP group. The incidence of early or late complications was almost identical for both groups. To the same results leaded Das et al. [50], in a retrospective study with 50 subjects in each arm.

2.7   DiLEP VS BEEP

Continuing to the anatomical enucleation of the prostate with different laser sources, Zhihui Zou et al. [51] compares BEEP with DiLEP, founding non-inferiority of one method above the other. The functional outcomes were similar at the end of follow up (12 months) and significantly improved compared to the baseline characteristics. Parallel were found comparable operative time (41 min DiLEP VS 38 min BEEP), enucleation time (33 min DiLEP VS 37 min BEEP), enucleated prostate tissue (33 g DiLEP VS 37 g BEEP) with 71% tissue removal DiLEP, 74% BEEP, and haemoglobin drop 0.33 mg/L for DiLEP and 0.36 mg/L for BEEP.

2.8   Vaporization VS Open Appendectomy (OP)

Alivizatos et al. [52] comparing Greenlight-Vaporization with open prostatectomy in a prospective 1:1 randomized trial with 126 patients, presented at the end of follow up similar improvement of Qmax, IPSS, IIEF and PVW in both groups. Prostate size was significantly decreased after operation (−90% VS −40%) while PSA reduced 69% after the OP and 61% after vaporization. In the OP-arm 13% of patients needed to be transfuse intraoperatively, while any of GreenLight-arm needed blood products. Moreover, 17% of OP-patients re-catheterized because of obstructive LUTS while re-operation performed in 4.6% of Greenlight-group and 5% of OP-group. No patient in either group had urge or stress incontinence following the operation.

2.9   Vaporization VS TUR-P

GreenLight consist of a neodymium YAG: laser and kalium-titanyl-phosphate (KTP) or lithium triborate (LBO) and with a wavelength of 532 nm and penetration length 0.8- to 3-mm is absorbed mainly by haemoglobin, which explains his perfect haemostatic action. Firstly, a generator of 80 W (KTP) was developed, following from a 120 W-generator (2006) and finally from a 180 W-generator (2010). About the efficiency of the 80 W-Greenlight-Vaporization reported Ruszat et al. [53] studying the peri- and postoperative results in 500 patients and recording an overall improvement of Qmax by 108% at the end of 5y-follow-up time. IPSS and QoL improved by 58% and 65% respectively, whereas PSA reduced about 50%. Intraoperative bleeding referred in 3.6%, while regarding the early postoperative complications (<30 days) 15% of patients (especially patients with prostate volume > 80 ml) suffered under dysuria and 9.8% and 6.8% reported with macrohematuria. In regard to long term functional outcomes retreatment was necessary in about 7% of patients, bladder neck stricture was observed in 3.6% and urethral stricture in 4.4% respectively. Newly, Brunken et al. [54] performed a review including 10 studies to prove the efficacy of the 180 W generator in overall 1640 patients. Operation time varied between 40 and 60 min with laser time 22–45 min. All the functional outcomes found to be improved in contrast to the baseline characteristics in each study. Prostate volume reduced 24–61% and found to be gland size dependent, while PSA reduced 37–79%

Compared to the TUR-P, GOLIATH-study [55, 56] an open-label, multicentre, prospective, randomized, and controlled non-inferiority trial comparing GL-XPS and TURP with a 24-months follow-up performed in 291 patients, approved the durability, efficiency and non-inferiority of the vaporization, mentioned an equivalent amelioration of Qmax, IPSS, QoL and PVR between the 2 groups. Moreover, the prevalence and grade of urine incontinence at 24-mo were unchanged in both groups, while during the follow up period 83.6% of patients in GL-XPS group and 78.9% in TUR-P-arm stayed without complications. PSA reduced by 51% in GL-XPS VS 42% in TUR.P, whereas prostate volume reduced by 49% in the vaporization technique VS 48% in the TUR-P. The first 6 months postprocedurally irritative symptoms rates and dysuria were similar in both group and ending the follow-up period 9% of Greenlight patients and 7.6% respectively from TUR-patients underwent a retreatment because of recidivism of obstructive symptoms as a result of prostatic tissue re-growth or urethral/bladder neck strictures.

2.10 Greenlight-VAP VS DiVAP

Greenlight-Vaporisation and Diode-Vaporisation of prostate seems to have equivalent functional outcomes regarding Qmax, IPSS, QoL and PVR improvement as showed Chiang et al. [57] and Guo [58] underlying however that diode laser demonstrates superior haemostatic properties compared with the GreenLight HPS laser. Postoperative incontinence and postoperative irritative symptoms were more profound after diode laser prostatectomy with higher rates of dysuria with sloughing tissues and epididymitis [44] whereas Guo S reports significantly higher reoperation rate in the diode group (38% vs 9%), due to obstructive necrotic tissue (16% vs 0%), bladder neck stricture (16% vs 2%), and persisting or recurrent adenoma (5% vs 7%), respectively.

Facts from the third revolution technologies.

2.11 Aquablation

Based on the successful implementation of water-jet dissection in the enucleation of tumours in liver, lungs, bladder, kidneys, aquablation of prostate with high-velocity, heat-free waterjet is coming to form a safe and effective option in the treatment of patients with LUTS due to BPH.

The AquaBeam™ (PROCEPT BioRobotics, Redwood Shores, CA, USA) system is used for the surgical aquablation of the prostate utilizing the resected property of water administrated in near sound speed velocity. The procedure is guided robotically based upon surgeon planning and checked with real-time transrectal ultrasound. The patient is positioned in lithotomy place. Using a rigid cystoscope, the handpiece of Aquabeam can be inserted due to the sheath in the urethra. With the aid of transrectal ultrasound the surgeon is in a position to adjust the length of treatment, the sweep of angle as well as the depth of treatment under preservation of important for continence and ejaculation anatomical structures as external urethral sphincter and ejaculatory ducts. After completion of the planning of the resection contour follows the tissue-selective ablation of prostate between bladder neck and verumontanum. Once tissue removal is done, haemostasis may be performed if necessary and bladder neck traction is applied for the first postprocedural hours using a special catheter tensioning device. At this point the dual action of the aquablation of the prostate must be emphasized. During the resection phase saline (0.9%) is supplied at pressures ranging from 500 to 8000 pounds per square inch (PSI) in order to cut and dissect soft tissue according the targeted resection area. During the coagulation phase, saline is administrated at low pressure (5–15 PSI) while simultaneously the activation of 2 W green light laser (532 nm) allows tissue cauterization. At 2 W, the Aquabeam-system offers power density of 6366 W/cm^2, which is well within coagulation range. This lower power laser achieves an excellent superficial coagulation avoiding the unpleasure thermal effects of vaporisation.

This novel method was described for first time in the treatment of BPH in 2013 by Faber et Desai in canine models presenting efficiency and safety of the new treatment [59]. Gilling et al. in 2016 published the first results in a prospective, non-randomised, single-centre trial in men aged 50–80 years with moderate-to-severe LUTS with a mean prostate size from 56 ml (27–85 ml) and enlarges medial lobe in 40% of patients [60]. Especially, the mentioned to show a significantly improvement of IPSS, QoL and Qmax in comparison to the baseline characteristics of the patients at ending of a 6 months follow-up (IPSS: 23.1 VS 8.6 $p < 0.001$, QoL: 5.0 VS 2.5 $p < 0.001$, Qmax 8.6 VS 18.6 ml/s $p < 0.001$), while PVR decreased from a mean of 91 ml to a mean of 30 ml. Regarding the further functional outcomes PdetQmax failed from 66 cmH_2O to 45 cmH_2O ($p < 0.001$) while PSA decreased also from 3.2 to 2.6 ng/mL. The prostate volume measured by TRUS at a mean-value from 36 mL, translating into a 31% reduction in size vs baseline ($p < 0.001$). Regarding the postoperative adverse events temporarily transurethral catheterisation because of urine retention is mentioned in 5/15 patients, while all patients could avoid without problems. Self-limited dysuria and haematuria (Clavien-Dindo I) was described in only 3 patients. Incontinence, retrograde ejaculation, or erectile dysfunction reported in any of the patients. The same author presented exactly similar mid-term results in the same cohort of patients one year post-procedurally, underlying the safety and efficiency of the method [61].

Recently in 2019, Bach T et al. demonstrated a prospective study with the so far largest number of consecutive patients from a single-centre in real practise aiming to evaluate the effectualness of aquablation into the clinical routine in a non-selected patient collective [62]. The follow-up period was 3 months and 180 men with LUTS were included to this prospective trial. Mean age was 69 years with a prostate volume from 64.3 ml (range 20–154 ml), baseline IPSS 21.09 and QoL-score 4.56 points. Qmax was 10.75 (range 2.3–40) ml/sec and PVR ranged prior the Aquablation from 100 ml to 2500 ml with a mean value of 158.9 ± 282.9 ml. About 25% were on indwelling catheter consider before surgery due to recurrent urinary retention. Mean PSA was 4.3 µg/L. Mean operative time, defined as the time from TRUS placement until the final urinary catheter placement, was 20 (range 9–53) min. As an expression of the learning curve, the mean OR-time in case 1–50 was 24.2 min and dropped to a mean OR-time of 17 min after this, approving this way the short learning curve and the facility of the method. The catheterisation time was ca. 2.2 days, while over 95% of the patients discharged home free from catheter. Intraoperative electrocautery was used in four patients (3.4%), proving that Aquablation could took place completely athermal in over 96% of the cases. Haemoglobin levels dropped from a mean of 14.2 (range 9.2–17.6) g/dl at baseline to 12.42 (range 7.2–16.2, $p < 0.001$) g/dl postoperatively but only three patients (2.5%) requiring blood transfusion. Adverse events occurred in overall in 10 (8.5%) patients. These were Clavien–Dindo scale II (CD II: re-catheterisation, transfusion) while four patients (3.4%) underwent a secondary surgical intervention needing electrocautery due to delayed haematuria (CD IIIb). At the ending follow-up prostate-volume measured with TRUS decreased by 65% [22.44 (8.26, 8–40) ml]. About 75% of the patients with antegrade ejaculation prior procedure appeared persistent antegrade ejaculation after Aquablation treatment.

In terms of comparing Aquablation versus TUR-P, two randomised clinical trials (Water Ablation Therapy for Endoscopic Resection of prostate tissue trial, WATER and WATER II) took place. The WATER study (2018), a prospective, multicentre, double-blind, international trial compares Aquablation vs TUR-P in prostate adenomas 30–80 ml while WATER II a prospective, single-arm, multicentre, international study evaluates Aquablation in clearly enlarged prostates between 80 ml and 150 ml. WATER-study showed Aquablation to be non-inferior compared to TUR-P with both methods resulting into an improvement of IPSS, QoL, Qmax and PVR. Between the two groups the difference was not statistically significant at the end of follow-up (IPSS 14.5 points for TUR-P VS 13.8 points for Aquablation, QoL decrease 3.1 points VS 3.4 points, Qmax increase 11 ml/s VS 10 ml/s, PVR alleviation of 54 ml VS 39 ml respectively). Aquablation characterized by shorter resection time, while no difference was mentioned in mean operation time, in perioperative bleeding and in length of hospital stay. 30% of patients in Aquablation group and 23% of patients in TUR-P arm were discharged from hospital with catheter. One-year postprocedural PSA reduced in similar waxy in both groups (decrease 1.0 ng/ml and 0.7 ng/ml respectively). Overall clearly fewer patients in Aquablation arm experienced Clavien-Dindo I and II compared to TUR-P patients (20% VS 40%), including mainly sexual dysfunction. Any of patients suffered under incontinence postoperatively in both groups [63].

The WATER-II study (2018) focused on the treatment in clearly hypertrophic prostatic adenomas. The study includes 114 patients with a mean prostate volume of ca. 107 ml with 84% middle lobe enlargement. The mean operation time was 37 min with mean resection time from ca. 8 min, which rightfully explained due to the repeated passes because of the big tissue amount (single pass 33% of patients, 2 passes 56%, >2 passes 10% of patients). The mean length of hospital stay was 1.6 days, while over 60% of patients could be discharged home at 1 postoperative day with catheter, which could be removed in ambulant setting at 4 postprocedural day. Adverse events occurred in overall 55 patients, 30% of whom presented > Clavien Dindo II (CD II) complications. Significant bleeding postprocedural reported in 10% of patients while blood transfusion was mandatory in about 6% of patients [64].

Nguyen, Barber et al. [65] presented a head to head comparison of the results of the above-mentioned WATER studies. Generally, the operative time and the aquablation time seems to be directly independent from the prostate volume and the consecutive repeated handpiece-passes to reach to a complete anatomical removal of the prostatic tissue. On either study was described an amelioration of IPSS, QoL, Qmax and PVR compared with the baseline characteristics of each study, however this was in WATER-II study statistically significant and the end of one year follow up time. Between the studies these functional outcomes showed similar changes, although bigger changes were mentioned in the WATER-II study regarding IPSS, Qmax. and PVR. Referring to the intra- and postoperative complications, temporarily CD I adverse events reported similarly in both studies, whereas anejaculation was mostly referred in the WATER II study instead of WATER-study (18% VS 6%). Persistent adverse events translating into persistent sexual dysfunction and incontinence were referred in 6% of Water-study and about 18% of WATER-II study. > CD II complications were described in the WATER II trial with the majority of CD II entanglement to tally with infections and bladder irritation, which could be managed with drugs. Significant bleeding was statistically important In WATER II study, which is to expect due to the prostate volume. However, it must be emphasized that in WATER study additional haemostasis with electrocautery was performed in about 40% of the operations. On the other side WATER II study underwent completely athermal, which support the supportive use of electrocautery especially in big prostates.

There exists any direct prospective trial comparing Aquablation vs Enucleation VS Vaporisation yet. Reconstructed from the yet published data it could be said that Aquablation comprises a safe and efficacious and minimal invasive treatment of BPH with very promising results. To begin with operative time, this is compared with Laser-enucleation (HoLEP, ThuLEP, BipoLEP) as well as vaporisation (ThuVEP, Greenlight) plainly superior for Aquablation. The median operative time for enucleation/vaporization is estimated ca. 60–110 min especially for enlarged prostates >80 g [66–69]. According to the TRUS-measure and the pathological specimen the resection efficiency from enucleation calculated ca. 0.59 ml/min for vaporisation and 1.45 ml/min for enucleation, whereas at the same time resection efficiency from aquablation estimated at 5 ml/min. Continuing to the functional outcomes, GOLIATH study showed an improvement of IPSS, QoL, PVR and Qmax similar to Enucleation and similar to Aquablation.

In the same study about 34% of patients in Vaporisation-group and 30% in the TUR-P arm presented with CD I complications commonly with irritative voiding symptoms and bladder spasm. CD II complications were referred in 32/117 (22%) and 19/62 (14%) of all patients with adverse events in vaporisation- and TUR-P arm respectively. The most reported complication was UTI. Persistent moderate incontinence requiring intervention was reported in 4/16 patients (2%) suffered from urine loss, while no moderate incontinence rates were experienced in TUR-P arm. Mild temporarily incontinence occurred in 12/16 patients and in 4 patients in vaporisation and TUR-P group respectively. Comparing to the data from Aquablation studies, is concluded that Aquablation has slightly lower, however not statistically significant, complications rates especially in the treatment of prostate <50 g. The complications rates and especially the significant bleeding and the transfusion rates are increased in the treatment of big prostates with aquablation (ca. 14%) compared to enucleation (3–5%), vaporisation (ca. 4%). However, the above-mentioned dates are reconstructed from the WATER II study, which relief completely athermal without additional electrocautery, while other series (e.g. Bach T. et al) reported blood transfusion only in 2% of the patient. Holmiun enucleation and KPT vaporisation seems to have zero transfusions rates (0%) with late re-intervention rates (after post-procedural 90 days) because of urethral stricture, bleeding or bladder neck stricture about 4.4%, 0% and 1.2% respectively [42]. GOLIATH-study registered early necessary re-interventions in 3% of patient in vaporisation group and about in 10% in

TUR-P arm, while late re-intervention was needed in ca. 10% of vaporisation patients and 13% of patient after transurethral resection of prostate.

Regarding sexual function, in WATER study no patients were reported with erectile dysfunction while anejaculation was higher in TUR-P arm (45% VS 9% respectively). The WATER I and II trial reported retained antegrade ejaculation in 91% and 80% of the patients, which is clearly superior in comparison to enucleation (ca. 75%) and vaporisation (ca. 45%).

Moreover, Aquablation shows a decrease of PSA from a mean of 3.7 ng/ml to 2.7 ng/ml in the WATER study and from am mean of 7.1 ng/ml to 4.4 ng/ml at the end of follow-up in the WATER-II study. TRUS-volume was decreased from 54 ml to 37 ml (−31%) 3 months postprocedural in the WATER study and from 107 ml to 63 ml (−20%) in the same period in the WATER-II study. Bach et al. in a follow up from 3 months showed a TRUS-volume decrease by 65% (from 64.3 ml to 22.4 ml). Respectively, HoLEP enucleation decreases TRUS-volume by 50% and PSA by 61% as published by Gilling in a retrospective study from patients underwent HoLEP with follow-up time from 6 years [57]. Hospital length of stay is similar between all the transurethral procedures.

Furtherly, because of the under real-time controlled robotic nature of Aquablation, this technique appears to have a short learning curve (5–10 operations/surgeon) in comparison with enucleation and TUR-P (40–60 cases for the HoLEP and about 20 respectively) [70].

Concluded Aquablation seems to be as effective and safe as enucleation of the prostate with clearly superiority in terms of operative time, and shorter learning curve while offers a better QoL regarding the sexual life of the patients. The intermediate-terms functional outcomes of these novel treatment demonstrate its big potential. At the time is not strong-suggested in the EAU- and AUA- guidelines, however this will be probably change after the publication of the first long-term results from randomised clinical trials.

3   Urolift/iTIND

3.1   Urolift

Prostatic urethral lift (PUL) methods either with the permanent Urolift-device or with the temporarily iTIND are the alternative to resection/enucleation/vaporisation minimal invasive methods to treat patients with benign prostate hyperplasia. Both methods are possessed from the same principle, offering mechanically tissue remodelling of the bladder neck and prostatic urethra.

Urolift offers a mechanical dilatation of the prostatic urethra by creating a passage through the prostatic urethra beginning from bladder neck and ending distally to the verumontanum with implantation of permanent tissue-retracting sutures. The method allows the preservation of NVI and from plexus. Through a rigid cystoscope the Urolift delivery device is placed in the sheath and arriving into the prostatic urethra at the place in which the lateral lobes of the prostate are mostly prominent. At this place and about 1.5 cm distally from bladder neck, the sheath will be rotated to either 10 o'clock as well as 2 o'clock as a nonabsorbable polyethylene terephthalate (PET) monofilament suture is placed anterolaterally parallel to the bladder neck into the prostatic tissue to reach the extracapsular place. The suture is strained leading to elevation of the prostate lobe. Since the proximal prostatic fossa is expanded on each side implants should be placed distally of this point but proximately from verumontanum in case of enlarged prostates. Fluoroscopy or CT can be used to check the correct location of the Urolift-implants which after completion of the healing phase will be covered from urethral mucosa.

Perera et al. [71] in a meta-analyse in 2014 published the first reproducible data from 9 retrospective and prospective studies. The number of patients were recruited in the studies was between 4–140 and as a rule they had moderate to severe LUTS symptoms with IPSS>12 points, Qmax <12 ml/s and PVR <250 ml and prostate volume 30–80 ml. It must be underlined that patients with enlarged median prostatic lobe, PSA > 10 ng/ml, infection (prostatitis) or retention (6/8 studies) were excluded. The big majority of the studies had had a follow-up period from 12 months (except one study with FU-time of 24 months and 2 studies with end of follow up after 1 month post-procedurally). Doing a pooled analysis of the mainly functional parameters of the studies-data, IPSS showed a decrease at the ending of follow up of about 8 points (95%CI, −8.8 to −7.2) with QoL improvement of 2.2–2.4 points. Respectively, sexual scores consisted of IIEF-5, MSHQ, SHIM appeared a slightly improvement of 0–3 to 0.4 points. These parameters were characterized by high homogeneity rates in contrast to Qmax and PVR which presented high heterogeneity rates due to insufficient reporting. Qmax showed an improvement of 3.0–4.0 ml/s in the most heterogenous studies. The big majority of the procedures take place under local anaesthesia and the operative time varied between 19 and 66 min. With regard to the postoperative complications the most frequently adverse events were macroscopically urine bleeding (ca. 15–75%), irritative symptoms (ca. 25–55%), pelvic pain (ca. 4–20%) urine infection und temporal incontinence (3–10% and 2–15%, respectively). Moreover, ending the follow-up time about 2–16% of patients underwent a TUR-P because of persistent or failed improved symptoms, whereas about half of the inappropriate intravesical placed Urolift-implants (14/27) revealed encrustation, in whom two of these the removal was unavoidable.

Roehrborn et al. [72] presented the first long-term 5-years-results from a prospective, randomised, blinded, sham controlled study (L.I.F.T) valuating and proving the effectiveness and the durability of the technique. The included criteria were similar as above mentioned and totally 206 patients were randomized (2:1) with favour to Urolift-procedure (140 patients). Patients with obstructive medial lobe were excluded. After the close of the 60 months follow up, IPSS presented a decrease by 35% in comparison to the mean baseline IPSS points (from 22.3 to 14.4 points), whereas QoL decreased about 45% (from 4.62 to 2.54 points) and the maximal urine flow improved almost 50% (from7.88 ml/s to 11.08 ml/s). BPH Impact Index changed ca. 3.41 points (from 6.92 to 3.51). Inernational Index of Erectile Function (IIEF-5) and Male Sexual Health Questionnaire for Ejaculatory Dysfunction

(MSQH-EjD) appeared slightly amelioration (from 15.99 points to 16.69, change 18.5% and from 8.69 to 10.25 points) respectively. Surgical procedure due to persistent symptoms were mandatory in about 13.5% of the patients (ca. 4% became additional Urolift-implants and ca. 9.5% underwent transurethral resection or enucleation of the prostate). In about 30% of the patients a transurethral catheter was placed postoperatively because of failed voiding effort.

Comparing Urolift versus TUR-P, Gratzke et al. [73], showed comparable functional outcomes in a multicentre, prospective, randomized controlled study (BPH6 study) with 80 patients through 2-years follow-up time. Particularly, patients with LUTS and IPSS>12 points, Qmax<15 ml/s and prostate volume <60 ml were 1:1 randomized in the two study's arms. Primary outcome was the observation of current of the IPSS, QoL, Qmax, sexual function and the incontinence as well as the registration of the adverse events in a head to head comparison between these methods. At the end of study observation, TUR-P arm mentioned superiority against PUL regarding IPSS- and Qmax-improvement of −68% VS −43% change and +110% VS +65% (from a mean of 22.3 to 7.4 points VS from 21.4 to 12.2 points and from a mean of 9.6 ml/s to 25.5 ml/s VS from9.3 ml/s to 14.3 ml/s) respectively. Erectile function as presented from Sexual Health Inventory for Men (SHIM) questionnaire was similar in both groups (98% for Urolift VS 94% for TUR-P), whereas according to the Male Sexual Health Questionnaire for Ejaculatory Dysfunction (MSQH-EjD) protocol, ejaculatory function was significantly improved in the Urolift arm with all of the Urolift-patients to retain thein antegrade ejaculation in comparison with 66% of the subjects in the TUR-P arm. Incontinence rates, as assessed by Incontinence Severity Index-score, were similar in both groups with the TUR-P patients to show slightly higher rates of temporarily self-limited incontinence the first 2–3 months post-operatively. Over the follow up period 14% of PUL-patient and 6% of them in the TUR-P-arm needed a re-intervention because of symptoms persistence.

There is momently no head to head prospective randomised studies comparing Urolift and transurethral prostate enucleation/vaporisation or Aquablation. In conclusion, Urolift is a minimal invasive method, makeable under general anaesthesia which seems to be effective and safe in the treatment of middle-large prostates. However, the method cannot ne suggested in the treatment of prostates with enlarged medial lobe or in patients with significant bladder emptying storage and a big amount of post-voiding residual urine volume.

3.2   iTIND

iTIND, a nitinol-based non-permanent stent, is uniquely designed to mechanically induce tissue pressure causing ischemic necrosis and creates compression channels, leading to remodelling of the bladder neck and prostatic urethra. The device is inserted through a straightforward procedure, and, unlike currently available prostatic stents, is removed within 5–7 days of insertion, thereby reducing the risk of late-stage complications. The patient is placed in a lithotomy position. The bladder was transurethral accessed using a standard 19F–22F cystoscope, through which the iTind consisted of struts with nitinol wires shaped a "tulip"- form was advanced, and finally positioned within the bladder neck and the prostatic urethra, under direct vision urethroscopy. A device dislocation could be avoided due to a single nitinol leaflet placed direct cranially of the verumontanum. Finally, the bladder is emptied and the cystoscope is removed, leaving the polyester retrieval suture outside of the urethral meatus. No catheterisation is required. Patients were discharged home after device implantation. The removal took place also ambulant after 5 to 7 days through a Foley catheter using a dedicated retrieval system.

iTIND-treatment of BPH was initiated in 2015 when Porpiglia and co-workers treated the first patients in a single-arm, multicentre, prospective study included 32 patients with 1-year follow up period and reported the first functional outcomes of this novel treatment presenting a statistically significant amelioration of Qol such as IPSS and Qmax (45% and 67%, respectively) [74].

The same author (2018) in the same patient cohort reported at the end of a 3-years follow up a significant betterment of IPSS and Qmax compared to the baselines data with a median QoL about 2 points, 36 months after iTIND treatment [75].

In a prospective, multicentre study with 81 patients and 1 year of follow-up Propiglia et al. [76], using a second-generation of iTIND device (three double inter-twined instead of four single-layer struts, and intertwined wires fixated at the proximal end of the device VS the distal end aiming at to prevent injury to the bladder epithelium) cited also significant improvement of IPSS (22.2 to 8.78, p < 0.001), Qmax (7.28 ml/s to 14.1 ml/s, p < 0.001) and QoL (improvement >3 points, p < 0.001) [62]. Any of patients reported with sexual dysfunction or antegrade ejaculation. Regarding the procedure time, Porpigila et al. report a mean procedure time of 5.8 min.

Referring to adverse events, Porpiglia et al. reported moderate complications categorized maximally Clavien-Dindo II (CD II) including incontinence by device displacement, urine retention (9.9%), dysuria (7.4%), irritative symptoms (11%), self-limited macrohematuria (12%) and succeed treated infections (6.5%). Two patients underwent surgical procedure because of persistent symptoms.

When compared to TUR-P or TUIP, iTind induced only minimal surgical morbidity, and was associated with short-lived and self-resolving adverse effects. Routine postoperative catheterization was not required in any cases and there were no reports of retrograde ejaculation (TUR-P: 65%; TUI: 27%), erectile dysfunction (TUR-P: 10%; TUI:2%), or urinary incontinence (TUR-P: 3%; TUI: 2%).

The need for catheterization is an important factor affecting potential rates of infection. iTIND infections rates showing in line with results of PUL treatment (5–7%) and other minimally invasive therapies, including TUNA, TUMT and prostatic stents (6–10%).

iTind preserves sexual function and ejaculation, both well established and bothersome independent risk factors of BPH treatments. None of the patients who were previously sexually active reported a deterioration in sexual or ejaculatory abilities according to the proportional questionnaire during follow-up.

iTIND exists an effective non-invasive method in the interventional therapy of BPH, however like Urolif is not indicated for patients with enlarged medial lobe and save them, further prospective randomised studies with long-terms results have to be done in order to be considered as a standard method.

3.3   Transurethral Needle Ablation (TUNA) of Prostate

Transurethral needle ablation or TUNA primarily described in 1993 is developed as a minimal invasive technique in the treatment of BPH, causing a diminution of the prostate volume due to application of low dose of radiofrequency and consecutive tissue necrosis. Specially, TUNA system composed of a radiofrequency generator, a TUNA catheter with special needles at the top and a 0°-cystoscope. Overall 422 KHz are delivering to the prostate tissue through the 12–22 mm needles, which are inserting into the lateral lobes of the prostate transurethraly and according to the transverse diameter of the lobes as they are measured by the transrectal ultrasound. Inserting to the prostata the needle applicates radiofrequency leading to a overheat of the tissue over 110 °C, while urethral mucosa is protected due to retractable shield of the needles. The procedure can be done in multiple sites along the prostatic urethra beginning from bladder neck till 1 cm cranially from verumontanum. The urethra is irrigated continuously to avoid a thermal injury by temperatures over 43 °C.

Zlotta et al. [77], described the histopathological changes of this method examing 10 prostate specimens after open prostatectomy, 1–46 days after TUNA procedure, demonstrating the necrotic thermal injury of the tissue and the denervation of the peri-necrotic intraprostatic nerve fibres. These necrotic areas can meanly seize about 9% of the prostate volume as it was estimated in MRI-controlled trials after the procedure [78].

Zlotta et al. [79] published the long-term functional outcomes in 188 consecutive patients underwent TUNA. Mean Qmax increased from 8.6 ml/s to 12.1 ml/s (p < 0.01), IPSS and PVR decreased from 20.9 and 179 ml to 8.7 and 122 ml, respectively (p < 0.01). Overall 24% and 78% of patients improved by at least 50% their Qmax and IPSS compared to the baseline characteristics respectively. Mean prostate volume and PSA levels did not decreased significantly at the end of follow up (53.9 ml to. 53.8 ml and 3.3 ng/ml to 3.6 ng/ml, respectively). Overall 41 (23.3%) underwent additional treatment at 5 years follow-up following after the initial TUNA procedure. From these patients, 12 patients received additional medical support (alpha-blocker) because of persistence from LUTS, whereas 12 patients became a second TUNA operation and by 22/41 patients was a transurethral prostate resection obligated.

Haroun et al. [80], evaluated the 10-years efficacy of the method in a retrospective setting in 351 patients treated with TUNA between 2005 and 2014 (27–42 operations/year). In study included patients with prostate volume 40–70 ml, while patients with urethral strictures, enlarged medial lobe and neurogenic bladder dysfunction were excluded. The procedures were performed with local anaesthesia. Mean IPSS was decreased at 5 years after the procedure, showing a slightly increase at the end of follow up compared to the baseline characteristics (20.5 VS 13.6 VS 16.9 respectively). The similar occurred with the mean Qmax (8.4 ml/s VS 9.8 ml/s VS 9.3 ml/s). The intermediate complications (3- to 6-months postoperatively) existed mainly of macrohematuria (86%) followed by urine retention after catheter removal (15%) and urethral stricture (2%). Regarding the sexual function erectile malfunction was reported in ca. 7% of the patients, while any antegrade ejaculation was mentioned. Overall retreatment (re-TUNA, drop to other minimal invasive methods (TUR-P, Laser-enucleation) and supportive medical treatment (alpha-blockers, 5a-reductase inhibitors)) was observes at 18% of patients 5y postproce-dural and at 26% at the end of 10 years.

Several studies have made to compare TUNA with other transurethral minimal invasive techniques. The combined results of the studies [81–85] showed, that in comparison to standard TUR-P in a follow up period of 2–5 years, TUNA lead to similar amelioration of symptoms (IPSS and QoL) while presents clearly inferiority in terms of Qmax improvement, reduction of PVR as well as prostatic volume. Regarding the adverse events, irritative symptoms and dysuria such as urinary tract infections have similar rates in both groups, whereas urinary retention favoured clearly TUR-P. Retrograde ejaculation or anejaculation, urinary incontinence, bleeding, bladder neck stenosis, erectile disorders favoured TUNA against TUR-P.

Comparing to other transurethral techniques Schatzl et al. [86] and Minardi et al. [87] demonstrated superiority of TUNA in the subjective scores and functional out-comes compared to water induced thermotherapy and HIFU, while TUNA was infe-rior to transurethral electrovaporization of the prostate (TUVP) and visual Laser ablation of the prostate (VLAP).

3.4   ReZum

The Rezum system was firstly introduced to the clinical treatment of BPH in 2015 in the USA and in Europe. It utilizing radiofrequency to product thermal energy (up to 105 °C), which is convicted in form of water vapour energy transurethraly after injection in the prostatic tissue through a retractable needle of 10 mm under slightly surpa-interstitial pressure. The energy is applicated by repeated thermic bursts of 10 s length, which release about 540 cal/mL H_2O. Through the properties of water, the energy is applicated dispersed uniformly to the tissue leading to its overheating (up to 70 °C) and consecutively to cell necrosis by disrupting cellular membrane. Since water does not passes through the transitional zone of prostate because of the natural anatomical barrier, Rezum system allows an incisive, convictive, anatomical limited treatment of the prostate hyperplasia. The procedure is performed in similar way to TUNA with patients placed in lithotripsy position using a 30°-Optik cysto-scope, saline irrigation to cool the urethral mucosa and a specific needle with cir-cumferentially holes to homogenous water vapor application. Like TUMA the procedure begins with injection ca. 1 cm distally from bladder neck at 3′ and 9′ o'clock and additional injections are made every 5 mm until 1 cm above the verumontanum.

The mainly difference with TUNA rests in the transmission of the energy power. Rezum transmit the energy power with convection, whereas TUNA with conduction. The latest induces molecular agitation within the tissue after direct contact between two surfaces at different temperatures. The thermal gradient caused like this makes higher temperatures and longer periods of heating are necessary to assess a therapeutic temperature in the target tissue. Therefore, conduction causes bigger and extended thermal injuries.

The tissue necrosis after Rezum treatment can achieve up to 2 cm in the transition zone as identifies in a study with patients underwent open adenectomy after Rezum-procedure and examination of the prostate specimens [88]. Myndenrse et al. [89], controlling the postoperative effects of Rezum via 3D-MRI published a diminution of prostate size by 17% (61.2 ml at baseline to 43.5 ml 6 months post-procedurally) in 44 patients underwent Rezum water vapor treatment.

Mc Vary et al. [90] published the first intermediate-term outcomes in a 2:1for Rezum-operation randomised prospective clinical trial with follow up period of 4 years, including 197 patients with 132 patients undergo Rezum-procedure and the rest a sham rigid cystoscopy. In the study were enrolled patients with IPSS>13 points, Qmax <15 ml/s, PVR < 250 ml. Patients with urinary infection or PSA > 2.5 mg/ml (unless prostate cancer was with biopsy ruled out) were excluded from the study. IPSS was reduced by 47% (22.0 to 11.4 points) at the end of follow up, while QoL failed from a mean of 4.4 points to 2.3 points (−43%). Qmax improved from a mean of 9.9 ml/s to 13.7 l/s (+49%, p < 0.001), whereas PVR showed no statistically significant reduction (from a mean ca. 82 ml at baseline to 74 ml 4 years after procedure). Moreover, overactive bladder-score showed a significant amelioration ($\approx$ 39.6 points to 23.3 points, −30%). PSA reduced slightly (from about 2.1 ng/m to 1.9 ng7ml). Sexual function, as estimated with IIEF-5 and MSHQ questionnaire, and urine incontinence according to the international continence society score demonstrated not relevant changes and significant improvement respectively. 30% of the patients had enlarged medial lobe and appeared similar improvement and profit in terms of postprocedural functional outcomes. Concerning the side effects, the most common was dysuria (17%), followed by haematuria (12%) and irritative mictional storage (6%). Urinary retention and infection presented each in about 4% of the patients. Ending of follow up in 6/135 (4.5%) patients a secondary re-intervention was performed.

3.5   Prostatic Angioembolization (PAE)

Prostatic artery angioembolization (PAE) was primarily described in 2000 as minimal invasive therapeutic treatment in patients with BPH [91]. It is often a complicated procedure which requires excellent knowledge of pelvic blood supply and usage of advanced interventional radiology. The procedure begins with a Foley catheter inserted into the bladder and filled with a mixture of iodinated contrast medium and normal saline solution. This catheter is used as a landmark and provides good orientation to each prostate site providing a better understanding of the internal iliac artery branches and related structures. The patients placed in supine position. Pelvic angiography is performed to evaluate the iliacal vessels and the prostatic arteries. Afterwards, manual selective angiography with a 5F catheter takes place to exact evaluation of internal iliacal vessels bilaterally. Super selective embolization of the inferior vesical arteries is made with a microcatheter inside or ostial of the prostatic arteries. Recently, additional to the original PAE (oPAE) a new method called "PErFecTED Technique" (Proximal Embolization First, Then Embolize Distal for Benign Prostatic Hyperplasia) promises better results [92]. At this technique the embolization starts proximal when microcatheter cross any collateral branch to the bladder, rectum, corpus cavernosum, gonad, or penis and be placed distally into the prostatic artery before its branching to the central gland (urethral group of arteries) and peripheral zone (capsular group of arteries). Afterwards, the microcatheter should be advanced into the prostatic parenchyma branches for an intraprostatic embolization. Because BPH develops primarily in the periurethral region of the prostate, the urethral group of arteries are embolized first, while urethral and capsular intraprostatic groups of arteries should are embolized separately. The new method is believed to result in more extended areas of necrosis and therefore to bigger shrinkage of prostate gland.

Pisco et al. [93] published the first midterm (1–3 years) and long-term (>3.5–6 years) outcomes in 640 patients underwent PAE because of BPH. In the study recruited patients with moderate to severe LUTS symptoms (IPSS>18, QoL > 3, Qmax<12 ml/s and prostate volume > 30 g). All the procedures were made under local anaesthesia in ambulant setting, the main operative time was 77 min. Bilateral PAE was made in 92.6% of patients and unilateral in only 46 (7.4%) patients. He shows a statistically significant improvement of IPSS, QoL, Qmax and PVR. Prostate volume was reduced by a mean of 15% (mean of −16.85 ml) and PSA by 2.3 mg/ml. Major adverse events like bladder wall ischemia was reported in 0.2% while the majority of patients suffered under dysuria (24%) and urgency-frequency-symptomatic (23%). Obstipation observed in 13% of patients, while haematuria, haematospermia and rectal bleeding in 7.5%, 8& and 6% respectively.

In the same line, the same author [94] published in 2019 the results from a 1:1 randomised, single-blinded, sham controlled prospective study with follow up period of 6 months, in which patients with LUTS due to BPH became either PAE or sham procedure. Statistically significant amelioration presented in the IPSS, QoL and BPHII. PSA failed by a mean of 1.51 ng/ml and prostate volume by −17.6 ml. Qmax improved by about 6.8 ml/s and PVR waned ca. 60 ml, After PAE 35% of patients referred complications most frequent of them were urethral and perineal burning, dysuria, haematuria/haematospermia and inguinal haematoma [80].

Compared to TUR-P, Carnevale et al. [95] in a 1:1:1 randomised, prospective study evaluated TUR-P VS oPAE VS PErFecTED-PAE including 15 patients in each arm. He mentioned to show a betterment of Qmax/PVR/IPSS/QoL in all arms ending the follow up time 12 months postprocedural. Prostate volume was significantly lower among TURP patients than oPAE and PErFecTED patients. Among the patients after PAE (oPAE or PErFecTED), local pain, urethral burning and irritative symptoms were reported transiently for 3–4 day postprocedurally. Moreover, minimal rectal bleeding (1/15, 6.7% in each group), hematospermia (1/15, 6.7% in each group), and reduction in ejaculate volume (2/15, 13.3% in oPAE group, 1/15, 6.7% in PErFecTED group) was observed. On the other hand, TUR-P patients complained about urgency frequency symptoms and dysuria up to 2 weeks after the operation, whereas urinary incontinence was seen in 4/15 (26.7%), and retrograde ejaculation occurred in all (100%) patients.

Continuing, Abt et al. [96] compared PAE VS TUR-P in a randomised, open label, non-inferiority trial, with 51 PAE patients and 52 subjects in the TUR-P-arm through and follow-up of 3 months. Ending the follow up-period, the mean change in IPSS from baseline was −9.23 points after PAE and −10.77 points after TURP., whereas QoL improved by −2.33 points after PAE and − 2.69 points after TURP. The IIEF-5 changed by −0.98 points versus −1.84 points favour of PAE. By contrast, Qmax improved 5.19 mL/s VS 15.34 mL/s in favour of TURP and PVR decreased by −86.36 mL VS −199.98 mL in favour of TURP also. PSA reduced by 2.00 µg/L VS 3.11 µg/L favoured TURP. The mean change in prostate volume as measured by MRI was −12.17 mL VS −30.27 mL, showed clearly superiority for TUR-P Pressure flow studies showed significant disadvantages for PAE compared with TURP for the reduction of bladder outlet obstruction, indicated by a change in detrusor pressure at maximum urinary flow rate of −17.17 cm H2O for PAE versus −41.07 cm H_2O for TUR-P and a shift towards a less obstructive category in 56% of patients after PAE and 93% after TUR-P.

4 Conclusion

TUR-P procedure as an inside-out technique, in which during the progress of surgery no obvious anatomical layer reached and thermocoagulatoric effect the level of resection alters. However, TUR-P is the most widely accepted and performed treatment for benign prostatic obstruction (BPO) due to benign prostatic enlargement, and is set as the first choice for a subset of patients with prostate volumes in between 30 and 80 ml. Anatomical endoscopic enucleation of prostate seems to be the best option for treatment of BPH in larger and mid size prostates, allowing a complete and clear tissue removal along the surgical capsule/transitional zone of the prostate. These results into preservation of the integrity of transitional zone leading to minimal irritation, minimal change of erectile function, epithelialisation of the prostatic fossa and rapid disappear of the stress urinary incontinence.

Regarding the source can be used to perform an anatomical endoscopic enucleation of prostate, bipolar enucleation of the prostate (BipoLEP) performs safe and efficient mechanical enucleation of the prostate offering at the same time an excellent coagulation and is as effective as Holmium-/Thulium-/Diode-Laser, leading to result that to perform an enucleation todays does not need necessarily lasers.

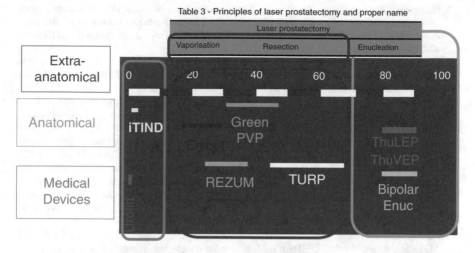

Fig. 5 Principles of laser prostatectomy and proper name. Source: Herrmann TRW 2019

Vaporization of the prostate should be suggested in patients with obligated anti-coagulant therapy. Aquaablation has the potential to deliver a highly uniform and standardized outcome due to the image guided ablation process, while iTING, Urolift, Rezum and in some patients angioembolisation can be an option for patients interested in either secondary endpoints like antegrade ejaculation or in the subset of patients unfit for invasive treatment under general or spinal anesthesia. The future course of these later technologies is determined as to what extend they are able to deliver the described benefits in extended use and long-term efficacy (Fig. 5).

References

1. Stern M. Resection of obstruction at the vesical orifice; new instruments resectotherm; resectoscope and new method. JAMA. 1926;87:1726–30.
2. McCarthy JF. A new apparatus for endoscopic plastic surgery of the prostate, diathermia and excision of vesical growths. J Urol. 1931;26:695–9.
3. Hiraoka Y. A new method of prostatectomy, transurethral detachment and resection of benign prostatic hyperplasia. Nihon Ika Daiqaku Zasshi. 1983;50(6):896–8.
4. Fraundorfer MR, Gilling PJ. Holmium:YAG laser enucleation of the prostate combined with mechanical morcellation: preliminary results. Eur Urol. 1998;33:69–72.
5. Neill MG, Gilling PJ, et al. Randomized trial comparing holmium laser enucleation of prostate with plasmakinetic enucleation of prostate for treatment of benign prostatic hyperplasia. Urology. 2006;68(5):1020–4.
6. Wolters M, Herrmann TRW et al, Anatomical enucleation of the prostate with the novel combined mechanical and bipolar vaporization probe in ejaculation sparing and two-lobe manner. Videourology;30(6). Published Online: 15 Dec 2016. doi:https://doi.org/10.1089/vid.2016.0028
7. Bach T, Wendt-Nordahl G. Feasibility and efficacy of Thulium:YAG laser enucleation (VapoEnucleation) of the prostate. World J Urol. 2009;27(4):541–5. https://doi.org/10.1007/s00345-008-0370-0.

8. Herrmann TR, Bach T, et al. Thulium laser enucleation of the prostate (ThuLEP): transurethral anatomical prostatectomy with laser support. Introduction of a novel technique for the treatment of benign prostatic obstruction. World J Urol. 2010;28(1):45–51. https://doi.org/10.1007/s00345-009-0503-0.

9. Gomez Sancha F, Rivera VC, et al. Common trend: move to enucleation-Is there a case for GreenLight enucleation? Development and description of the technique. World J Urol. 2015;33(4):539–47. https://doi.org/10.1007/s00345-014-1339-9.

10. Lusuardi L, Myatt A, et al. Safety and efficacy of Eraser laser enucleation of the prostate: preliminary report. J Urol. 2011;186(5):1967–71. https://doi.org/10.1016/j.juro.2011.07.026.

11. Bachmann A, Tubaro A, Barber N, et al. 180-W XPS GreenLight laser vaporisation versus transurethral resection of the prostate for the treatment of benign prostatic obstruction: 6-month safety and efficacy results of a European Multicentre Randomised Trial—The GOLIATH study. Eur Urol J Urol. 2015;193(2):570–8. https://doi.org/10.1016/j.juro.2014.09.001.

12. Kyriazis I, Świniarski PP, Jutzi S, Wolters M, Netsch C. Transurethral anatomical enucleation of the prostate with Tm:YAG support (ThuLEP): review of the literature on a novel surgical approach in the management of benign prostatic enlargement. World J Urol. 2015 Apr;33(4):525–30. https://doi.org/10.1007/s00345-015-1529-0.

13. Elshal AM, Elkoushy MA, El-Nahas AR, Shoma AM, Nabeeh A, Carrier S, Elhilali MM. GreenLight™ laser (XPS) photoselective vapo-enucleation versus holmium laser enucleation of the prostate for the treatment of symptomatic benign prostatic hyperplasia: a randomized controlled study. J Urol. 2015;193(3):927–34. https://doi.org/10.1016/j.juro.2014.09.097.

14. Bae J, Oh SJ, Paick JS. The learning curve for holmium laser enucleation of the prostate: a single-center experience. Korean J Urol. 2010;51(10):688–93.

15. Xia SJ. Two-micron (thulium) laser resection of the prostate-tangerine technique: a new method for BPH treatment. Asian J Androl. 2009;11(3):277–81. https://doi.org/10.1038/aja.2009.17.

16. Hochreiter WW, Thalmann GN, Burkhard FC, Studer UE. Holmium laser enucleation of the prostate combined with electrocautery resection: the mushroom technique. J Urol. 2002;168(4 Pt 1):1470–4.

17. Herrmann TR. Enucleation is enucleation is enucleation is enucleation. World J Urol. 2016;34(10):1353–5. https://doi.org/10.1007/s00345-016-1922-3.

18. Kim M, Lee HE, Oh SJ. Technical aspects of holmium laser enucleation of the prostate for benign prostatic hyperplasia. Korean J Urol. 2013;54:570–9.

19. Endo F, Shiga Y, Minagawa S, Iwabuchi T, Fujisaki A, Yashi M, et al. Anteroposterior dissection HoLEP: a modification to prevent transient stress urinary incontinence. Urology. 2010;76:1451–5.

20. Kim M, Piao S, Lee HE, et al. Efficacy and safety of holmium laser enucleation of the prostate for extremely large prostatic adenoma in patients with benign prostatic hyperplasia. Korean J Urol. 2015;56(3):218–26. https://doi.org/10.4111/kju.2015.56.3.218.

21. Minagawa S, Okada S, et al. En-Bloc technique with anteroposterior dissection holmium laser enucleation of the prostate allows a short operative time and acceptable outcomes. Urology. 2015;86(3):628–33. https://doi.org/10.1016/j.urology.2015.06.009.

22. Saitta G, Becerra JEA, et al. 'En Bloc' HoLEP with early apical release in men with benign prostatic hyperplasia. World J Urol. 2019;37(11):2451–8. https://doi.org/10.1007/s00345-019-02671-4.

23. Miernik A, Schoeb DS. "Three horse shoe-like incision" holmium laser enucleation of the prostate: first experience with a novel en bloc technique for anatomic transurethral prostatectomy. World J Urol. 2019;37(3):523–8. https://doi.org/10.1007/s00345-018-2418-0.

24. Scoffone CM, Cracco CM. The en-bloc no-touch holmium laser enucleation of the prostate (HoLEP) technique. World J Urol. 2016;34(8):1175–81. https://doi.org/10.1007/s00345-015-1741-y.

25. Peyronnet B, Robert G. Learning curves and perioperative outcomes after endoscopic enucleation of the prostate: a comparison between GreenLight 532-nm and holmium lasers. World J Urol. 2017;35(6):973–83. https://doi.org/10.1007/s00345-016-1957-5.

26. Wolters M, Huusmann S, Oelke M, Kuczyk MA, Herrmann TRW. Anatomical enucleation of the prostate with the novel combined mechanical and bipolar vaporization probe in ejaculation sparing and two-lobe manner. Videourology. 2016;30(6)

27. Becker B, Enikeev D, Glybochko P, et al. Effect of optical fiber diameter and laser emission mode (cw vs pulse) on tissue damage profile using 1.94 μm Tm:fiber lasers in a porcine kidney model. World J Urol. 2020;38(6):1563–8. https://doi.org/10.1007/s00345-019-02944-y.

28. Dusing MW, Krambeck AE, et al. Holmium laser enucleation of the prostate: efficiency gained by experience and operative technique. J Urol. 2010;184(2):635–40. https://doi.org/10.1016/j.juro.2010.03.130.

29. Baazeem AS, Elmansy HM, Elhilali MM. Holmium laser enucleation of the prostate: modified technical aspects. BJU Int. 2010;105(5):584–5. https://doi.org/10.1111/j.1464-410X.2009.09111.x.

30. Kuntz RM, Lehrich K, Ahyai S. Transurethral holmium laser enucleation of the prostate compared with transvesical open prostatectomy: 18-month follow-up of a randomized trial. J Endourol. 2004;18(2):189–91.

31. Naspro R, Suardi N, et al. Holmium laser enucleation of the prostate versus open prostatectomy for prostates >70 g: 24-month follow-up. Eur Urol. 2006;50(3):563–8.

32. Li M, Qiu J, Hou Q, Wang D, Huang W, Hu C, Li K, Gao X. Endoscopic enucleation versus open prostatectomy for treating large benign prostatic hyperplasia: a meta-analysis of randomized controlled trials. PLoS One. 2015;10(3):e0121265. https://doi.org/10.1371/journal.pone.0121265. eCollection 2015

33. Lin Y, Wu X, Xu A, Ren R, Zhou X, Wen Y, Zou Y, Gong M, Liu C, Su Z, Herrmann TR. Transurethral enucleation of the prostate versus transvesical open prostatectomy for large benign prostatic hyperplasia: a systematic review and meta-analysis of randomized controlled trials. World J Urol. 2016;34(9):1207–19. https://doi.org/10.1007/s00345-015-1735-9.

34. Elshal AM, et al. Holmium laser enucleation of the prostate for treatment for large-sized benign prostate hyperplasia; is it a realistic endourologic alternative in developing country? World J Urol. 2016;34:399–405.

35. Misraï V, Pasquie M, Bordier B. Comparison between open simple prostatectomy and green laser enucleation of the prostate for treating large benign prostatic hyperplasia: a single-centre experience. World J Urol. 2018;36(5):793–9. https://doi.org/10.1007/s00345-018-2192-z.

36. Li S, Zeng XT. Holmium laser enucleation versus transurethral resection in patients with benign prostate hyperplasia: an updated systematic review with meta-analysis and trial sequential analysis. PLoS One. 2014;9(7):e101615. https://doi.org/10.1371/journal.pone.0101615. eCollection 2014

37. Yin L, Teng J, et al. Holmium laser enucleation of the prostate versus transurethral resection of the prostate: a systematic review and meta-analysis of randomized controlled trials. J Endourol. 2013;27(5):604–11. https://doi.org/10.1089/end.2012.0505.

38. Liu C, Zheng S, Li H, Xu K. Transurethral enucleation and resection of prostate in patients with benign prostatic hyperplasia by plasma kinetics. J Urol. 2010;184(6):2440–5. https://doi.org/10.1016/j.juro.2010.08.037.

39. Zhu L, Chen S, Yang S, Wu M, Ge R, Wu W, Liao L, Tan J. Electrosurgical enucleation versus bipolar transurethral resection for prostates larger than 70 ml: a prospective, randomized trial with 5-year follow up. J Urol. 2013;189(4):1427–31. https://doi.org/10.1016/j.juro.2012.10.117.

40. Arcaniolo D, Manfredi C, et al. Bipolar endoscopic enucleation versus bipolar transurethral resection of the prostate: an ESUT systematic review and cumulative analysis. World J Urol. 2020;38(5):1177–86. https://doi.org/10.1007/s00345-019-02890-9.

41. Bach T, Xia SJ, Yang Y, et al. Thulium:YAG 2 mum cw laser prostatectomy: where do we stand? World J Urol. 2010;28(2):163–8. https://doi.org/10.1007/s00345-010-0522-x.

42. Iacono F, Prezioso D. Efficacy and safety profile of a novel technique, ThuLEP (Thulium laser enucleation of the prostate) for the treatment of benign prostate hypertrophy. Our experience on 148 patients. BMC Surg. 2012;12(Suppl 1):S21. https://doi.org/10.1186/1471-2482-12-S1-S21.

43. Kyriazis I, Swiniarski PP. Transurethral anatomical enucleation of the prostate with Tm:YAG support (ThuLEP): review of the literature on a novel surgical approach in the management of benign prostatic enlargement. World J Urol. 2015;33:525–30. https://doi.org/10.1007/s00345-015-1529-0.

44. Gross AJ, Netsch C. Complications and early postoperative outcome in 1080 patients after thulium vapoenucleation of the prostate: results at a single institution. Eur Urol. 2013;63(5):859–67. https://doi.org/10.1016/j.eururo.2012.11.048.

45. Netsch C, Engbert A, Bach T, Gross AJ. Long-term outcome following Thulium VapoEnucleation of the prostate. World J Urol. 2014;32:1551–8. https://doi.org/10.1007/s00345-014-1260-2.

46. Zhu Y, Zhuo J, et al. Thulium laser versus standard transurethral resection of the prostate for benign prostatic obstruction: a systematic review and meta-analysis. World J Urol. 2015;33:509–15. https://doi.org/10.1007/s00345-014-1410-6.

47. Zhang F, Shao Q, Herrmann TR. Thulium laser versus holmium laser transurethral enucleation of the prostate: 18-month follow-up data of a single center. Urology. 2012;79(4):869–74. https://doi.org/10.1016/j.urology.2011.12.018.

48. Xiao KW, et al. Enucleation of the prostate for benign prostatic hyperplasia thulium laser versus holmium laser: a systematic review and meta-analysis. Lasers Med Sci. 2019;34(4):815–26. https://doi.org/10.1007/s10103-018-02697-x.

49. He G, Shu Y, Wang B, Du C, et al. Comparison of diode laser (980 nm) enucleation vs holmium laser enucleation of the prostate for the treatment of benign prostatic hyperplasia: a randomized controlled trial with 12-month follow-up. J Endourol. 2019;33(10):843–9. https://doi.org/10.1089/end.2019.0341.

50. Das AK, Teplitsky S, Uhr A, Leong JY. A retrospective comparison of diode to holmium for laser enucleation of the prostate. Can J Urol. 2019;26(4):9836–42.

51. Zou Z, Xu A, Zheng S, Chen B, et al. Dual-centre randomized-controlled trial comparing transurethral endoscopic enucleation of the prostate using diode laser vs. bipolar plasmakinetic for the treatment of LUTS secondary of benign prostate obstruction: 1-year follow-up results. World J Urol. 2018;36:1117–26.

52. Alivizatos G, Skolarikos A, Chalikopoulos D. Transurethral photoselective vaporization versus transvesical open enucleation for prostatic adenomas >80ml: 12-mo results of a randomized prospective study. Eur Urol. 2008;54(2):427–37.

53. Ruszat R, Seitz M, Wyler SF, et al. GreenLight laser vaporization of the prostate: single-center experience and long-term results after 500 procedure. Eur Urol. 2008;54(4):893–901.

54. Brunken C, Seitz C, Woo HH. A systematic review of experience of 180-W XPS GreenLight laser vaporisation of the prostate in 1640 men. BJU Int. 2015;116(4):531–7. https://doi.org/10.1111/bju.12955.

55. Thomas JA, Tubaro A, et al. A multicenter randomized noninferiority trial comparing GreenLight-XPS laser vaporization of the prostate and transurethral resection of the prostate for the treatment of benign prostatic obstruction: two-yr outcomes of the GOLIATH study. Eur Urol Eur Urol. 2016;69(1):94–102. https://doi.org/10.1016/j.eururo.2015.07.054.

56. Bachmann A, Tubaro A. 180-W XPS GreenLight laser vaporisation versus transurethral resection of the prostate for the treatment of benign prostatic obstruction: 6-month safety and efficacy results of a European Multicentre Randomised Trial--the GOLIATH study. Eur Urol. 2014;65(5):931–42.

57. Chiang PH, Chen CH. GreenLight HPS laser 120-W versus diode laser 200-W vaporization of the prostate: comparative clinical experience. Lasers Surg Med. 2010;42(7):624–9. https://doi.org/10.1002/lsm.20940.

58. Guo S, Müller G. GreenLight laser vs diode laser vaporization of the prostate: 3-year results of a prospective nonrandomized study. J Endourol. 2015;29(4):449–54. https://doi.org/10.1089/end.2014.0572.

59. Faber K. Image-guided robot-assisted prostate ablation using water jet-hydrodissection: initial study of a novel technology for benign prostatic hyperplasia. J Endourol. 2015;29(1):63–9. https://doi.org/10.1089/end.2014.0304.

60. Gilling P, Reuther R, Kahokehr A, Fraundorfer M. Aquablation - image-guided robot-assisted waterjet ablation of the prostate: initial clinical experience. BJU Int. 2016;117(6):923–9. https://doi.org/10.1111/bju.13358.
61. Gilling P, Anderson P, et al. Aquablation of the prostate for symptomatic benign prostatic hyperplasia: 1-year results. J Urol. 2017;197:1565–72.
62. Bach T, Giannakis I, et al. Aquablation of the prostate: single-center results of a non-selected, consecutive patient cohort. World J Urol. 2019;37(7):1369–75. https://doi.org/10.1007/s00345-018-2509-y.
63. Gilling P, Barber N, et al. WATER: a double-blind, randomized, controlled trial of Aquablation® vs transurethral resection of the prostate in benign prostatic hyperplasia. J Urol. 2018;199(5):1252–61. https://doi.org/10.1016/j.juro.2017.12.065.
64. Desai M, Bidair M. WATER II (80-150 mL) procedural outcomes. BJU Int. 2019;123(1):106–12. https://doi.org/10.1111/bju.14360.
65. Nguyen DD, Barber N. Waterjet Ablation Therapy for Endoscopic Resection of prostate tissue trial (WATER) vs WATER II: comparing Aquablation therapy for benign prostatic hyperplasia in 30-80 and 80-150-mL prostates. BJU Int. 2019; https://doi.org/10.1111/bju.14917.
66. Zhang J, Ou Z, et al. Holmium laser enucleation of the prostate versus thulium laser enucleation of the prostate for the treatment of large-volume prostates > 80 ml: 18-month follow-up results. World J Urol. 2020;38(6):1555–62. https://doi.org/10.1007/s00345-019-02945-x.
67. Netsch C, Becker C, et al. A prospective, randomized trial comparing thulium vapoenucleation with holmium laser enucleation of the prostate for the treatment of symptomatic benign prostatic obstruction: perioperative safety and efficacy. World J Urol. 2017;35(12):1913–21.
68. Krambeck AE, et al. Experience with more than 1,000 holmium laser prostate enucleations for benign prostatic hyperplasia. J Urol. 2010;183(3):1105–9. https://doi.org/10.1016/j.juro.2009.11.034.
69. Gilling P, et al. Holmium laser enucleation of the prostate: results at 6 years. Eur Urol. 2008;53(4):744–9.
70. Marra G, Sturch P, et al. Systematic review of lower urinary tract symptoms/benign prostatic hyperplasia surgical treatments on men's ejaculatory function: time for a bespoke approach? Int J Urol. 2016;23(1):22–35. https://doi.org/10.1111/iju.12866.
71. Perera M, Roberts MJ. Prostatic urethral lift improves urinary symptoms and flow while preserving sexual function for men with benign prostatic hyperplasia: a systematic review and meta-analysis. Eur Urol. 2015;67(4):704–13. https://doi.org/10.1016/j.eururo.2014.10.031.
72. Roehrborn CG, Barkin J, et al. Five years results of the prospective randomized controlled prostatic urethral L.I.F.T. study. Can J Urol. 2017;24(3):8802–13.
73. Gratzke C, Barber N, et al. Prostatic urethral lift vs transurethral resection of the prostate: 2-year results of the BPH6 prospective, multicentre, randomized study. BJU Int. 2017;119(5):767–75. https://doi.org/10.1111/bju.13714.
74. Porpiglia F, Fiori C, Bertolo R, Garrou D, Cattaneo G, Amparore D. Temporary implantable nitinol device (TIND): a novel, minimally invasive treatment for relief of lower urinary tract symptoms (LUTS) related to benign prostatic hyperplasia (BPH): feasibility, safety and functional results at 1 year of follow-up. BJU Int. 2015;116(2):278–87.
75. Porpiglia F, Fiori C, Bertolo R, et al. 3-year follow-up of temporary implantable nitinol device implantation for the treatment of benign prostatic obstruction. BJU Int. 2018;122(1):106–12.
76. Porpiglia F, Fiori C, et al. Second-generation of temporary implantable nitinol device for the relief of lower urinary tract symptoms due to benign prostatic hyperplasia: results of a prospective, multicentre study at 1 year of follow-up. BJU Int. 2018; https://doi.org/10.1111/bju.14608.
77. Zlotta AR, Raviv G. Possible mechanisms of action of transurethral needle ablation of the prostate on benign prostatic hyperplasia symptoms: a neurohistochemical study. J Urol. 1997;157(3):894–9.
78. Mynderse LA, Larson B. Characterizing TUNA ablative treatments of the prostate for benign hyperplasia with gadolinium-enhanced magnetic resonance imaging. J Endourol. 2007;21(11):1361–6.

79. Zlotta AR, et al. Long-term evaluation of transurethral needle ablation of the prostate (TUNA) for treatment of symptomatic benign prostatic hyperplasia: clinical outcome up to five years from three centers. Eur Urol. 2003;44(1):89–93.
80. Haroun H, Eltatawy H. Evaluation of outcome of transurethral needle ablation for treating symptomatic benign prostatic hyperplasia: a 10-year experience. Urol Ann. 2019;11(2):198–203. https://doi.org/10.4103/UA.UA_99_18.
81. Roehrborn C, Burkhard FC. The effects of transurethral needle ablation and resection of the prostate on pressure flow urodynamic parameters: analysis of the United States randomized study. J Urol. 1999;162(1):92–7.
82. Cimentepe E, Unsal A, et al. Randomized clinical trial comparing transurethral needle ablation with transurethral resection of the prostate for the treatment of benign prostatic hyperplasia: results at 18 months. J Endourol. 2003;17(2):103–7.
83. Arai Y, Aoki Y. Impact of interventional therapy for benign prostatic hyperplasia on quality of life and sexual function: a prospective study. J Urol. 2000;164(4):1206–11.
84. Hill B, Belville W, Bruskewitz R, Issa M, Perez Marrero R, Roehrborn C, Terris M, Naslund M. Transurethral needle ablation versus transurethral resection of the prostate for the treatment of symptomatic benign prostatic hyperplasia: 5-year results of a prospective, randomized, multicenter clinical trial. J Urol. 2004;171:2336–40.
85. Schatzl G, Madersbacher S, Lang T, Marberger M. The early postoperative morbidity of Transurethral resection of the prostate and of 4 minimally invasive treatment alternatives. J Urol. 1997;158:105–11.
86. Schatzl G, Madersbacher S. Two-year results of transurethral resection of the prostate versus four 'less invasive' treatment options. Eur Urol. 2000;37(6):695–701.
87. Minardi D, Galosi AB. Transurethral resection versus minimally invasive treatments of benign prostatic hyperplasia: results of treatments. Our experience. Arch Ital Urol Androl. 2004;76(1):11–8.
88. Dixon CM, Cedano ER. Transurethral convective water vapor as a treatment for lower urinary tract symptomatology due to benign prostatic hyperplasia using the Rezūm system: evaluation of acute ablative capabilities in the human prostate. Res Rep Urol. 2015;7:13–8.
89. Mynderse LA, Hanson D, et al. Rezūm system water vapor treatment for lower urinary tract symptoms/benign prostatic hyperplasia: validation of convective thermal energy transfer and characterization with magnetic resonance imaging and 3-dimensional renderings. Urology. 2015;86(1):122–7.
90. McVary KT, Rogers T, Roehrborn CG. Rezūm water vapor thermal therapy for lower urinary tract symptoms associated with benign prostatic hyperplasia: 4-year results from randomized controlled study. Urology. 2019;126:171–9. https://doi.org/10.1016/j.urology.2018.12.041.
91. DeMeritt JS, Elmasri FF. Relief of benign prostatic hyperplasia-related bladder outlet obstruction after transarterial polyvinyl alcohol prostate embolization. J Vasc Interv Radiol. 2000;11(6):767–70.
92. Carnevale FC, Moreira AM, Antune AA. The "PErFecTED technique": proximal embolization first, then embolize distal for benign prostatic hyperplasia. Cardiovasc Intervent Radiol. 2014;37:1602–5.
93. Pisco JM, Bilhim T. Medium- and long-term outcome of prostate artery embolization for patients with benign prostatic hyperplasia: results in 630 patients. J Vasc Interv Radiol. 2016;27(8):1115–22. https://doi.org/10.1016/j.jvir.2016.04.001.
94. Pisco JM, Bilhim T, Costa NV, Torres D, Pisco J, Pinheiro LC, Oliveira AG. Randomised clinical trial of prostatic artery embolisation versus a sham procedure for benign prostatic hyperplasia. Eur Urol. 2020;77(3):354–62.
95. Carnevale FC, Iscaife A, et al. Transurethral resection of the prostate (TURP) versus original and PErFecTED prostate artery embolization (PAE) due to benign prostatic hyperplasia (BPH): preliminary results of a single center, prospective, urodynamic-controlled analysis. Cardiovasc Intervent Radiol. 2016;39:44–52.
96. Abt D, Hechelhammer L, Müllhaupt G, et al. Comparison of prostatic artery embolisation (PAE) versus transurethral resection of the prostate (TURP) for benign prostatic hyperplasia: randomised, open label, non-inferiority trial. BMJ. 2018;361:k2338.

Bladder Cancer

F. Pisano, J. M. Gaya, O. Rodriguez Faba, A. Breda, and J. Palou

1 Background

Bladder cancer (BC) is the sixth leading cause of cancer in the EU, with 124,000 people diagnosed and >40,000 people dying from the disease each year. Despite major advances in other cancers, the diagnostic and therapeutic approach in BC remained largely unchanged for more than 30 years. Nevertheless, in the last decade, technology has revolutionized the study of cancer biology, providing diagnostic, prognostic, and treatment strategies.

The aim of this chapter is to present the new technologies available in the diagnosis and treatment of BC.

2 Diagnosys and Staging

2.1 New Frontiers in Uro Radiology

Scientific investigation in bladder cancer (BC) research is focused on finding a patient-tailored diagnostic and therapeutic approach. New technologies allow to reduce the need of invasive diagnostic procedures and, consequently, to reduce morbidity. Ultrasound (US) represents quite often the first diagnosis approach to bladder cancer [1]. By the way neither traditional US nor white light cystoscopy improve the oncological staging of the patients [2]. The main limit of traditional US is the measurement of mechanical contrast only which determines a low accuracy in

F. Pisano (✉) · J. M. Gaya · O. Rodriguez Faba · A. Breda · J. Palou
Department of Urology, Fundacion Puigvert, Autonomous University of Barcelona,
Barcelona, Spain

© The Author(s), under exclusive license to Springer Nature
Switzerland AG 2021
D. Veneziano, E. Huri (eds.), *Urologic Surgery in the Digital Era*,
https://doi.org/10.1007/978-3-030-63948-8_2

detecting small foci. In order to improve the diagnostic accuracy of non invasive procedures such as bladder US, a number of imaging techniques are currently under evaluation.

The concept of micro ultrasound (micro US) has been recently introduced in urology. Lughezzani et al. compared a 29-MHz micro US techonology with magnetic resonance imaging (MRI) in the diagnosis of prostate cancer [3]. Micro US was able to identify clinically significant prostate cancers with high sensitivity and a high negative predictive value (NPV), suggesting that it could be a valid and less expensive alternative to MRI. A similar technology has been applied in bladder cancer by the same group of authors. The aim of the study was to test the ability of micro US in differentiating between non muscle invasive and muscle invasive bladder cancer (NMIBC and MIBC respectively) [4]. This observational prospective study evaluated 23 patients with bladder cancer. Micro US was able to differentiate between the bladder wall layers and to identify BC stage. Pathological findings confirmed all the 14 NMIBC patients while 2 cases of MIBC were downstaged. The main drawback of this technology was the size of the lesion, since micro US failed to detect lesions smaller than 5 mm.

During the last years, MRI has been introduced in BC management. Expecially, T2-weighted and dynamic contrast-enhanced MRI is currently considered the gold standard for MIBC diagnosis [5]. A meta-analisys of 17 studies showed a 91% sensitivity and 96% specificity for 3.0-T MRI combined with diffusion-weighted imaging (DWI) to differentiate $\leq$ T1 tumours from $\geq$ T2 tumours before surgery [6]. Unfortunately, one of the potential limits of this diagnostic approach is the lack of a validated score able to better define the lesion. Trying to exceed this limit, Panebianco et al. had recently developed the Vesical Imaging Reporting and Data System (VI-RADS) score [7]. Despite the growing interest and the promising preliminary results, the absence of a strong evidence makes BC staging with MRI recommendable only in case of contraindications to perform a CT.

2.2   High Tech Endoscopy: A Step Toward the Future

Cistoscopy with trans urethral resection of the bladder (TURB) represents the gold standard diagnostic and staging procedure for BC. The goal of this procedure is to completely remove all visible lesions. Routinely, TURB is performed using white light (WL), by the way this technique can lead to missing lesions that are present but not visible. In particular, the detection reliability for smaller tumours or carcinoma in situ (CIS) is poor, with up to 30% of patients having a tumour identified at the first-check cystoscopy at 3 months and 50% of patients developing tumours within 12 months [8]. In order to improve the detection rate of this procedure, a number of new technologies have been designed.

Photodynamic diagnosis (PDD) uses violet light after intravesical instillation of 5-aminolaevulinic acid (ALA) or hexaminolaevulinic acid (HAL). HAL, the lipophilic hexylester of 5-ALA, has been commercially available since 2006 and has been established as the preferred intravesical agent to detect NMIBC. According the current evidence, the effect of 5-ALA-induced fluorescence on tumour detection in the urinary bladder improves bladder cancer detection during, especially CIS and flat lesions [9]. A meta-analysis compared blue light and with light cystoscopy in the diagnosis of BC, found a 21% increase in tumour detection with PDD [10]. According to these authors, PDD technology resulted in fewer residual tumors at check cystoscopy (relative risk [RR], 0.37, 95% CI, 0.20–0.69) and longer recurrence-free survival (RR, 1.37, 95% CI, 1.18–1.59), compared with white cystoscopy. Another meta-analysis reached similar results in 2019, confirming that PDD had higher sensitivity than white light endoscopy in the pooled estimates for analyses at both the patient-level (92% vs. 71%) and biopsy-level (93% vs. 65%) [11]. Despite these nice perspectives, PDD had lower specificity than white-light endoscopy (63% vs. 81%) and a quite high false positive rate [10]. Both recent TURB and BCG induced inflammation can increase the risk of false positive.

Narrow band imaging (NBI) is a new image processing modality that filters white light down to two narrow band widths of 415 and 540 nm, with advantage of avoiding the need for intravesical contrast administration. Haemoglobin absorbs these wavelengths preferentially, resulting in dark neovascularised bladder cancer appearing very different from the light background of the normal mucosa [12]. Kim et al. demonstrated in a randomized prospective study on 198 patients treated with TURB that NBI had benefits for detecting tumors overlooked by WLC. According to their results, the probability of diagnosing cancer was 80.9% and 85.5% in WL and NBI respectively. Moreover, after switching from WLC to NBI for second-look cystoscopy in the NBI group, NBI was shown to detect additional tumors with a detection rate of 35.1% [13]. The diagnostic accuracy of NBI has been confirmed by several studies, even in the diagnosis of CIS and flat dysplasia [14]. Despite these good results, NBI presents some limitations too. According to Dalgaard et al., a detection rate improvement of 22% was associated to a higher percentage (35%) of false positive if compared to WL [15].

Storz S-Technology is another example of enhanced endoscopy in bladder cancer. S-technology combines WL cystoscopy with an innovative software-based visualization mode [16]. More in detail, this system uses the following modalities: Spectra A and B by colour spectral separation using different colour filter settings that allow better contrast between tissues, Clara: by manipulating the image brightness to achieve better views of dark spots, Chroma by increasing color contrast and Clara+Chroma by combining both [17]. These systems allow to better identify the boundaries of the lesions and additional suspicious areas. Emiliani et al. evaluated the image quality of flexible cystoscopy with S-Technology and confirmed its superiority compared to WL cystoscopy [16].

Optical Coherence Tomography (OCT) is a high resolution imaging technique that applies infrared light to measure texture and elasticity of the tissue. OCT currently works with a 2.7 mm probe that can be passed through a standard cystoscope [18]. Schmidbauer et al analyzed the diagnostic performance of OCT combined with fluorescence cystoscopy and confirmed that OCT reduced the need for unnecessary biopsies. In this prospective study the per-lesion sensitivity and specificity of OCT were 97.5% and 97.9% respectively [19].

Confocal laser endomicrosopcy (CLE) is a high-resolution optical imaging technique that uses fiber-optic cables to transmit 488-nm wavelength laser light to tissues that have been exposed to fluorescent dyes. It allows optical sectioning of tissue and visualisation of the cellular microarchitecture during endoscopy. [20]. The aim of this technology is to provide "optical biopsies" of the tissue. The first ex vivo and in vivo CLE imaging of the urinary tract was performed by Son et al. [21, 22]. According to these authors, the concordance between CLE and histopathology was 70% and 76% for high and low grade lesions, respectively. Currently, there are 2 ongoing prospective trials trying to assess the accuracy of CLE in urothelial cancer diagnosis [23].

2.3   Precision Medicine in Bladder Cancer Diagnosis

Precision medicine is a modern concept that combines genomic sequencing, proteomics technology, bioinformatics and big data analysis. It aims to investigate ethiological factors and therapeutic targets in order to personalize medicine [24].

2.3.1   Advances in Uro-Radiology

Innovations in radiology during the last years dramatically improved the accuracy in the diagnosis of BC. In this field virtual reality imaging has been developed using computer assisted rapid image acquisition and three-dimensional image reconstruction. This technology has been applied to many organs including the colon, stomach, and bronchus [25]. Thanks to commercially available softwares, also an invasive procedure like cystoscopy can be replaced by virtual endoscopy [26]. The diagnostic power of virtual cystoscopy has been tested by Abrol S et al. in a population of 50 patients with history and investigations suggestive of urothelial cancer. Virtual cystoscopy detected 23 out of 25 patients with bladder tumor, while were falsely detected as negative. The sensitivity, specificity, positive predictive value, and negative predictive value of virtual cystoscopy were 92% each. Similar results had already been reached by Kim JK et al. in 2002 [27]. Seventy-three consecutive patients who had gross hematuria were prospectively evaluated with virtual cystoscpy. In this population, the agreement between the findings of virtual and conventional cystoscopy was promising, with only 3 false negative. Moreover, vistual cistoscopy was able to detect 88% of lesions smaller than 0.5 cm [Kim JK, Ahn JH, Park T et al. Virtual cystoscopy of the contrast material-filled bladder in patients with gross hematuria. AJR Am J Roentgenol. 2002;179(3):763–8].

The use of contrast in radiology has improved also the diagnostic accuracy. Both CT and MRI are accurate techniques for bladder cancer detection when they are performed with the injection of intravascular contrast agents. The introduction of microbubble contrast agents and the development of contrast-specific software have increased the value of ultrasound [28]. Contrast enhanced US (CEUS) allows the assessment of the macrovasculature and microvasculature in different parenchymas and the quantification of organ perfusion by the quantitative analysis of the echo-signal intensity [28]. This technology has been tested in bladder cancer by Nicolau et al. According to these authors CEUS provided higher accuracy than baseline ultrasound for bladder cancer detection, with 88.37% of BC correctly detected, compared to a 72% of detection rate for conventional ultrasound [29].

Photoacustic (PA) imaging technique is based on the use of contrast agents able to amplify the acoustic signal of tumour lesions. PA effect generates an acoustic wave through the transient thermoelastic expansion of optical excitation [30]. A number of materials have been proposed as contrast agents of PA imaging, all of them are characterized by a relatively high ability to absorb the energy of near infra-red light and convert it into heat. Di et al. synthesized a signal self-amplifiable PA liposomal nanoprobe composed by ammonium hydrogen carbonate and aggregated purpurin-18 (P18) [31]. The authors tested this probe in vivo using female BALB/c nude mice and confirmed its ability to individuate small tumour lesions <5 mm. According to these results PA imaging improves the diagnostic accuracy in BC lesions compared to conventional US [31].

2.3.2 Deep Learning in Bladder Cancer Diagnosis

Deep learning is an artificial intelligence function that imitates the workings of the human brain in processing data. Acting as a subset of machine learning in artificial intelligence, it has networks capable of learning unsupervised from data that is unstructured or unlabeled. In the last years, deep learning-based approaches have emerged as powerful techniques in medical image areas [32]. In this framework, Shkolyar E et al. developed in 2019 CystoNet, an image analysis platform based on convolutional neural networks, for automated bladder tumours detection [33]. The aim of CystoNet was to improve the diagnostic power of cystoscopy and the efficacy of TURB. In a population of 54 patients undergoing TURB, CystoNET demonstrated a per-frame sensitivity and specificity of 90.9% and 98.6%. Moreover, this system was able to identify three cases of CIS, suggesting the presence of detectable features for all BC types [33].

Recently, a tumour classifier based on a convolutional neural network (CNN) has been developed [34]. A population of 109 patients was evaluated. The tumour classifier demonstrated sensitivity and specificity of 89.7% and 94.0% respectively. In the test data 20 false positive, and 9 were negative were detected. Notably, among the 9 false negative, 6 early 5 raised lesions that included Ta tumours. This study confirmed that artificial intelligence can help in BC diagnostic process by classifying tumor lesions and normality with high accuracy [34].

3   Treatment Strategies

3.1   New Technologies for Intravesical Chemotherapy: Where We Are?

Electromotive drug administration (EMDA) and chemo-hyperthermia (C-HT) are minimally invasive device-assisted methods for enhanced intravesical administration of therapeutic agents such as mitomycin C (MMC). Both EMDA and C-HT aim to increase the tissue uptake of MMC. The electromotive administration is realized thanks to a controlled electric current of 0–30 mA/0–55 V direct current delivered by a battery powered current generator. This electric current produces several electro-molecular interactions (iontophoresis, electroosmosis, electroporation) that finally enhance the transport of drug molecules through biological membranes and into the underlying tissue. C-HT produces a similar effect by using intravesical microwave applicator that delivers hyperthermia directly to the bladder wall. Has been demonstrated that the combination of local hyperthermia with selected cytostatic agents enhances the efficacy of the drug. As previously explained, EMDA is defined as intravesical administration of a drug accompanied by electrical current, designed to enhance transepithelial drug uptake. According to a recent Cochrane review [35], three RCT including 672 patients with NMIBC were conducted to evaluate the efficacy of EMDA. According to these RCT, the use of an electric current to give a dose of MMC before TURB and the use of MMC with EMDA prior to BCG induction and long-maintenance regime, may delay the time to recurrence in selected populations (HR 0.47; 95% CI, 0.32–0.69 and HR 0.40; 95% CI, 0.28–0.57, respectively). These results present some limitations. First, the benefit on time to progression was uncertain in all the RCT included; moreover, an evaluation of serious adverse events was unclear because of study limitations and imprecision. Hyperthermia is a cytotoxic treatment used to attack directly the tumoral cells and the vascular supply to the tumor and also to trigger an immune response. Moreover, the temperature rise allows vasodilation which increases drug (such as MMC) delivery, having a synergistic effect. The treatment approach has been investigated as an alternative to those patients with high-risk tumors who do not respond to standard therapy [36]. Synergo SB-TS 101 system (Medical Enterprises, Amsterdam, the Netherlands) is an FDA-approved device, which induces chemo-HT with radiofrequency using a bladder catheter inserted through the urethra with a safety-cooling system. Synergo is the most widely used system for chemo-HT treatment [37]. In a systematic review of chemo-HT with radiofrequency, tumor recurrence was seen 59% less than after MMC alone in adjuvant clinical setting with an overall bladder preservation rate after c-HT of 85%. Based on a single comparative multicentric study, the efficacy was proved to be comparable to BCG. Because of short follow-up, no conclusions can be drawn about time to recurrence and progression rate [36]. According to a recent review analyzing tolerance and security of chemoHT with MMC using different devices, it seems to be a well tolerated technique, with adverse effects being mainly grade 1–2 (pain, bladder spasms, and hematuria). The reported adverse effects presented different profiles related to the device used (Synergo, Combat BRS, or Unithermia). C-HT treatments analyzed did not increase the incidence of adverse effect if compared to instillations of MMC alone and presented a better toxicity profile than those reflected in the literature with respect to the treatment with BCG alone [38]. Definitely, C-HT is considered a promising alternative treatment in case of failure of BCG. Nevertheless, a recent trial comparing C-HT with a second course of BCG failed to find a significant difference in the overall disease-free survival between the two groups. On the contrary, the subgroup of patients with CIS (primary or concomitant) treated with CHT had a lower disease-free survival if compared with repeated BCG. Based on these results, the authors suggested C-HT as second-line therapy in non-CIS recurrence following BCG failure [39].

3.2   New Delivery Drug Systems for Intravesical Terapy (Polymer Hydrogel, etc.)

According to its 'urine storage' function, the bladder has relatively waterproof walls to prevent absorption of the waste products. This relative impermeability minimizes the absorption of the drugs and consequently reduces both therapeutic and side effects. In order to overcome this limitations, new technologies to increase drug exposure and absorption has been studied. WGA-PGA-Doxo is a novel drug delivery system made of wheat germ agglutinin as targeter, poly-lglutamic acid as backbone that utilizes doxorubicin as active pharmaceutical ingredient (API). It has been developed by Apfelthaler et al. These authors demonstrated in an in-vitro study that WGA-PGADoxo can be internalized into urothelial cells and inhibit cell viability up to 99%. Moreover, this delivery system revealed a higher affinity to malignant than to healthy urothelial cells and its cytotoxic potential could improve efficacy of intravesical chemotherapy [40]. Bioadhesive microspheres have been recently studied as delivery system for gemcitabine, to prolong residence time in bladder and to enhance its efficiency. Thanks to invivo studies using bladder-tumor-induced rats these microspheres were found to be an effective and promising alternative for NMIBC intravesical therapy [41]. Nanotechnology is fascinating world that could help to improve treatment efficacy for bladder cancer. In this field of research a number of transporters have been developed, including metals, proteins, lipids, and polymers. Liposomes are spherical vesicles made of phospholipids with a water body; they have been studied for their ability to increase the stability and solubility of drugs in the urine. GuhaSarkar et al. published the results of a combination of gel and liposomes (LP-Gel System). Although the gel promotes adhesion to the urothelium, the liposomes helps the incorporation of the drug to the cell. Instillations of paclitaxel through this gel showed drug retention for at least 7 days, substantially higher than free drug and without an increase of systemic levels [42]. A different paclitaxel transporter has been recently proposed by Hu et al. [43]. These authors developed a lumbrokinas/paclitaxel nanocarrier that has been tested in rat bladder cancer model with promising results. Another interesting research area is represented by mucoadhesive molecules and nanogel. Mucoadhesive polymers have been widely developed as innovative nanoscopic drug delivery systems. They are characterized by colloidal stability, sustained drug delivery ability and the capability to improve tissue mucoadhesiveness and permeability. Guo et al. developed a disulfide-crosslinked polypeptide nanogel of poly(llysine)–poly(l-phenylalanine-co-l-cystine) to deliver 10-hydroxycamptothecin for the treatment of bladder cancer. This nanogel was able to rapidly deliver the drug inside bladder cancer cells; moreover, it inhibited proliferation of human bladder cancer cells in vitro [44].

3.3 Viral Gene Therapy and Cancer Vaccines

To find alternative treatment options for nonresponder patients with BCG, new fields are under investigation. Gene therapy is a promising and attractive strategy for cancer biotherapy and some authors have already pointed out the potential antitumor effect exerted by the intravesical application of onco-viruses. In 2012, the intravesical viral therapy was applied in humans for the first time [45]. In this phase I clinical trial, a mutated oncolytic adenovirus was used (GC0070). The most interesting characteristic of this virus is its interaction with retinoblastoma pathway that is frequently deregulated in bladder cancer. Thirty-five BCG refractory patients were treated with intravesical administration of single or multidose adenovirus. The overall response rate (defined as the absence of recurrence at cystoscopy with or without a pathology report) was 48.6%, with better result in patients treated with the lowest dose [46]. Another recent phase II trial confirmed the efficacy of CG0070 in the treatment of BCG failure [47]. Forty-five patients with high-risk BCG failure NMIBC were treated with intravesical CG0070. At 6 months follow up, the overall recurrence rate was 47%. Reaching a 50% in patients with CIS. The IFN adenoviral vector rAd–IFNa/Syn3 demonstrated a promising clinical results in NMIBC. According to a recent published randomized phase II trial, intravesical treatment with this adenoviral vector is a valuable alternative to radical cystectomy in BCG failure patients. rAd–IFNa/Syn3 in 75 ml was administered intravesically in 43 patients with high grade (HG) BCG-refractory or relapsed NMIBC. The 12 months recurrence-free survival was 35% and median time to HG recurrence or death was 6.5 months (90% CI, 3.52–12.78 months). Overall, 39 patients experienced at least one adverse event but only 22% (19%) reported a grade 3 complication [48]. Vicinium currently represents one of the new frontiers in conservative treatment for NMIBC. Vicinium is a single-chain anti- epithelial cell adhesion molecule (EpCAM) antibody fragment fused with a truncated fragment of Pseudomonas exotoxin A. Vicinium specifically targets and induces apoptosis in EpCAM-positive tumors. Twenty-free BCG-refractory or intolerant patients with CIS received Vicinium weekly for 6 weeks. Efficacy data showed a complete response in 9 of 23 patients at 3 months [49]. The intravesical targeted gene therapy approach has been proposed also for low-grade NMIBC. In this subgroup of NMIBC, intravesical ade-norviral and retroviral mediated gene therapy has been demonstrated to be effective and well tolerated.

3.4 Surgery in the Era of Minimally Invasive Approach

3.4.1 Endoscopic Resection of Bladder Tumor

TURB is the first diagnostic approach in BC. The goal of TURB is to make the correct diagnosis and completely remove all visible lesions. The principal limitation of conventional or fractioned TURB is the fragmentation of the tissue that leads to a poor specimen quality. In order to ameliorate the quality of resection, and consequently the accuracy of diagnosis and staging, a novel surgical approach has been proposed. En bloc resection of bladder tumor (ERBT) represents an alternative technique for resection of intravesical tumors in one piece [50]. Various studies over the last two decades have demonstrated that the method is safe and feasible [51]. ERBT can be performed using monopolar or bipolar current, Thulium-YAG or Holmium-YAG laser. Regardless the technique, the main advantage deriving from ERBT is the improvement of the quality of tumor specimens. According to available literature, more than 90% of the cases have muscularis propria and apparently a lower recurrence rate, if compared to conventional TURB [52, 53]. There is no trial showing an oncological benefit (differences in recurrence or progression), a recent meatanalisys revealed that hospitalization time and catheterization time is superior in patients treated with ERBT than conventional TURB, and ERBT patients also have a lower complication rate [54].

In the era of precision medicine, a group of Authors proposed to combine ERBT with near-infrared (NIR) imaging technique [55]. NIR technology uses the combination of a molecular targeted drug, AntiCD47-Alexa Fluor 790, with CD47 antibody with Alexa Fluor 790. This combination can be activated by near-infrared light. A group of 26 patients newly diagnosed with single NMIBC received ERBT with monopolar current. After surgery, the fresh specimen was incubated with antiCD47-Alexa Fluor 790, and then imaged under NIR imaging technique [55]. In this population, a significantly higher mean fuorescence intensity (MFI) signals in tumor tissue compared to adjacent normal background tissue has been detected. Moreover, the higher MFI signals in surgical margin was a predictive factor for residual tumor [55].

3.4.2 Innovations in Radical Surgery

Radical cystectomy with pelvic lymph node dissection is the gold standard treatment for organ-confined MIBC, and it is also a valid option for selected patients with high-grade NMIBC. This is a complex procedure that involves simultaneous surgery on the urinary and gastrointestinal tracts, and is associated with a high rate of complications. In order to reduce the morbidity, the idea of replacing bladder with a synthetic prosthesis or engineered neobladders has always been attractive and the source of investigation [56]. A number of materials have been proposed to realize a synthetic neobladder. Unfortunately, in the most of the cases these synthetic reservoirs were not successful. According to Cosentino et al., the principal limitations of these models were deposition of connective tissue, encrustations, infections, hydroureteronephrosis, leakages of urine from urethral or ureteral anastomosis, and problems related to biocompatibility [56].

Atala et al. in 2006 used engineered bladder constructs to perform cystoplasty in a group of 7 patients with myelomeningocele [57]. The engineered neobladders were constructed by using urothelial and muscle cells taken with a bladder biopsy from each patient. These cells were grown in culture, and seeded on a biodegradable bladder-shaped scaffold made of collagen, or a composite of collagen and polyglycolic acid. According to these Authors, engineered neobladders recovered an adequate function promptly after surgery and a biopsy confirmed an adequate structural architecture and phenotype [57]. Recently, Shen et al. proposed an animal model of bladder reconstruction [58]. Transplantation of autologous peritoneum for bladder reconstruction operation was carried out in 6 female porcines by transplanting the peritoneum into an ileum segment which mucosa and submucosa had been removed. These flaps were used to mend and reconstruct the neobladder. According to the Authors, no complication occurred, the Voiding behavior was normal and reconstructed bladders were healthy at the autopsy [58].

References

1. Stamatiou K, Papadoliopoulos I, Dahanis S, Zafiropoulos G, Polizois K. The accuracy of ultrasonography in the diagnosis of superficial bladder tumors in patients presenting with hematuria. Ann Saudi Med. 2009;29:134–7.
2. Palou J, Granados EA, de la Torre P, Vicente J. Evaluation of tumor staging using echography in bladder tumors. Actas Urol Esp. 1991;15(6):544–7.
3. Lughezzani G, Saita A, Lazzeri M, et al. Comparison of the diagnostic accuracy of micro-ultrasound and magnetic resonance imaging/ultrasound fusion targeted biopsies for the diagnosis of clinically significant prostate cancer. Eur Urol Oncol. 2019;2(3):329–32.
4. Saita A, Lughezzani G, Buffi NA, et al. Assessing feasibility and accuracy of high resolution microultrasound imaging for baldder cancer detection and staging. Eur Urol. 2019;77(6):727–32.
5. Lee M, Shin SJ, Oh YT, et al. Non-contrast magnetic resonance imaging for bladder cancer on predicting response and survival after neoadjuvant chemotherapy. Eur Urol. 2017;72:544–54.
6. Huang, L., Kong Q, Liu Z et al The diagnostic value of MR imaging in differentiating T staging of bladder cancer: a meta-analysis radiology, 2018. 286: 502.
7. Panebianco V, Narumi Y, Altun E, et al. Multiparametric magnetic resonance imaging for bladder cancer: development of VI-RADS (Vesical reporting Imaging and Data System). Eur Urol. 2018;74:294–306.
8. Schwaibold HE, Sivalingam S, May F, et al. The value of a second transurethral resection for T1 bladder cancer. BJU Int. 2006;97:1199–201.

9. Daniltchenko DI, Riedl CR, Sachs MD, et al. Long-term benefit of 5-aminolevulinic acid fluorescence assisted transurethral resection of superficial bladder cancer: 5-year results of a prospective randomized study. J Urol. 2005;174:2129–33.

10. Moat G, N'Dow J, Vale L, et al. Photodynamic diagnosis of bladder cancer compared with white light cystoscopy: systematic review and meta-analysis. Int J Technol Assess Health Care. 2011;27:3–10.

11. Chen C, Huang H, Zhao Y, et al. Diagnostic performance of image technique based transurethral resection for non-muscle invasive bladder cancer: systematic review and diagnostic metaanalysis. BMJ Open. 2019;9:e028173.

12. Bryan RT, Shah ZH, Collins SI, et al. Narrow-band imaging flexible cystoscopy: a new user's experience. J Endourol. 2010;24:1339–43.

13. Kim SB, Yoon SG, Tae J, et al. Detection and recurrence rate of transurethral resection of bladder tumors by narrow-band imaging: prospective, randomized comparison with white light cystoscopy. Investig Clin Urol. 2018;59(2):98–105.

14. Drejer D, Béji S, Oezeke R, et al. Comparison of white light, photodynamic diagnosis and narrow band imaging in detection of carcinoma in situ or flat dysplasia in transurethral resection of the bladder: the DaBlaCa-8 study. Urology. 2017;102:138–42.

15. Dalgaard LP, Zare R, Gaya JM, et al. Prospective evaluation of the performances of narrow-band imaging flexible videoscopy relative to white-light imaging flexible videoscopy, in patients scheduled for transurethral resection of a primary NMIBC. World J Urol. 2019;37(8):1615–21.

16. Emiliani E, Talso M, Baghdadi M, et al. Evaluation of the spies TM modalities image quality. Int Braz J Urol Off J Braz Soc Urol. 2017;43(3):476–80.

17. Bus MT, de Bruin DM, Faber DJ, et al. Optical diagnostics for upper urinary tract urothelial cancer: technology, thresholds, and clinical applications. J Endourol. 2015;29:113–23.

18. Pearace S, Daneshmand S. Enhanced endoscopy in bladder cancer. Curr Urol Rep. 2018;19:84.

19. Schmidbauer J, Remzi M, Klatte T, et al. Fluorescence cystoscopy with high-resolution optical coherence tomography imaging as an adjunct reduces false-positive findings in the diagnosis of urothelial carcinoma of the bladder. Euro Urol. 2009;56(6):914–9.

20. Lerner SP, Goh A. Novel endoscopic diagnosis for bladder cancer. Cancer. 2015;121(2):169–78.

21. Sonn GA, Mach KE, Jensen K, et al. Fibered confocal microscopy of bladder tumors: an ex vivo study. J Endourol. 2009;23:197–201.

22. Sonn GA, Jones S-NE, Tarin TV, et al. Optical biopsy of human bladder neoplasia with in vivo confocal laser endomicroscopy. J Urol. 2009;182:1299–305.

23. Liem EI, Freund JE, Baard J, de Bruin DM, Laguna Pes MP, SavciHeijink CD, et al. Confocal laser endomicroscopy for the diagnosis of urothelial carcinoma in the bladder and the upper urinary tract: protocols for two prospective explorative studies. JMIR Res Protoc. 2018;7(2):e34.

24. Hongwei S, Haitao J, Tao T, et al. Hope and challange: precision medicine in bladder cancer. Cancer Med. 2019;8:1806–16.

25. Abrol S, Jairath A, Ganpule S, et al. Can CT virtual cystoscopy replace conventional cystoscopy in early detection of bladder cancer? Adv Urol. 2015;2015:926590.

26. Yadav R, Kumar R. Virtual versus real cystoscopy. Indian J Urol. 2007;23(1):85–6.

27. Kim JK, Ahn JH, Park T, et al. Virtual cystoscopy of the contrast material-filled bladder in patients with gross hematuria. Am J Roentgenol. 2002;179(3):763–8.

28. Quaia E. Microbubble ultrasound contrast agents: an update. Eur Radiol. 2007;17:1995–2008.

29. Nicolau C, Bunesch L, Peri L, et al. Accuracy of contrast-enhanced ultrasound in the detection of bladder cáncer. Br J Radiol. 2011;84:1091–9.

30. Huynh E, Jf L, Helfield BL, et al. Porphyrin shell microbubbles with intrinsic ultrasound and photoacoustic properties. J Am Chem Soc. 2012;134:16464–7.

31. Di Z, Ziqui W, Lu W, et al. High-performance identification of human bladder cancer using a signal sel-amplifiable photoacoustica nanoprobe. ACS Appl Mater Interfaces. 2018;10:28331–9.

32. Ma J, Song Y, Tian X, et al. Survey on deep learning imaging for pulmonary medical imaging. Front Med. 2019;14(4):450–69. https://doi.org/10.1007/s11684-019-0726-4.

33. Shkolyar E, Jia X, Chang TC, et al. Augmented bladder tumor detection using deep learning. Euro Urol. 2019;76:714–8.
34. Ikeda A, Nosato H, Kochi Y, et al. Support system of cystoscopic diagnosis for bladder cancer based on artificial intelligence. J Endourol. 2020;34(3):352–8. https://doi.org/10.1089/end.2019.0509.
35. Jung JH, Gudeloglu A, Kiziloz H, et al. Intravesical electromotive drug administration for nonmuscle invasive bladder cancer. Cochrane Database Syst Rev. 2017;9:CD011864.
36. Soria F, Milla P, Fiorito C, et al. Efficacy and safety of a new device for intravesical thermochemotherapy in nongrade 3 BCG recurrent NMIBC: a phase I-II study. World J Urol. 2016;34:189–95.
37. Coenen JJMJH, van Valenberg FJP, Arends TJH, Witjes JA. Chemohyperthermia using MMC in nonmuscle-invasive bladder cancer: current status and future perspectives. Arch Esp Urol. 2018;71:400–8.
38. León-Mata J, Domínguez JL, Redorta JP, et al. Analysis of tolerance and security of chemo hyperthermia with Mitomycin C for the treatment of nonmuscle invasive bladder cancer. Arch Esp Urol. 2018;71:426–37.
39. Tan WS, Panchal A, Buckley L, et al. Radiofrequency-induced thermochemotherapy effect versus a second course of Bacillus Calmette-Guerin or institutional standard in patients with recurrence of nonmuscle-invasive bladder cancer following induction or maintenance Bacillus Calmette-Guerin Therapy (HYMN): a phase III, open-label, randomised controlled trial. Eur Urol. 2019;75:63–7.
40. Apfelthaler C, Skoll K, Ciola R. A doxorubicin loaded colloidal delivery system for the intravesical therapy of nonmuscle invasive bladder cancer using wheat germ agglutinin as targeter. Eur J Pharm Biopharm. 2018;130:177–84.
41. Karavana SY, Şenyiğit ZA, Çalışkan Ç. Gemcitabine hydrochloride microspheres used for intravesical treatment of superficial bladder cancer: a comprehensive in vitro/ex vivo/in vivo evaluation. Drug Des Devel Ther. 2018;12:1959–75.
42. GuhaSarkar S, More P, Banerjee R. Urothelium- adherent, ion-triggered liposome-in-gel system as a platform for intravesical drug delivery. J Control Release. 2017;245:147–56.
43. Hu B, Yan Y, Tong F. Lumbrokinase/paclitaxel nanoparticle complex: potential therapeutic applications in bladder cancer. Int J Nanomedicine. 2018;13:3625–40.
44. Guo H, Li F, Xu W, et al. Mucoadhesive cationic polypeptide nanogel with enhanced penetration for efficient intravesical chemotherapy of bladder cancer. Adv Sci (Weinh). 2018;5:1800004.
45. Camargo JA, Passos GR, Ferrari KL, et al. Intravesical immunomodulatory imiquimod enhances Bacillus Calmette-Guerin downregulation of nonmuscleinvasive bladder cancer. Clin Genitourin Cancer. 2018;16:587–93.
46. Laudano MA, Barlow LJ, Murphy AM, et al. Long-term clinical outcomes of a phase I trial of intravesical docetaxel in the management of nonmuscleinvasive bladder cancer refractory to standard intravesical therapy. Urology. 2010;75:134–7.
47. Packiam VT, Lamm DL, Barocas DA, et al. An open label, single arm, phase II multicenter study of the safety and efficacy of CG0070 oncolytic vector regimen in patients with BCG unresponsive non muscle invasive bladder cancer: interim results. Urol Oncol. 2018;36:440–7.
48. Shore ND, Boorjian Stephen A, et al. Intravesical rAd–IFNa/Syn3 for patients with high-grade, Bacillus Calmette-Guerin– refractory or relapsed non–muscle-invasive bladder cancer: a phase II randomized study. J Clin Oncol. 2017;35:3410–6.
49. Kowalski M, Jones N, Jewett MAS, et al. Treatment with intravesical Vicinium. Results in durable responses in patients with carcinoma in situ (CIS) previously treated with BCG. Paper presented at the 30th Congress of the Societe Internationale d'Urologie; November 1–5; Shanghai, China; 2009.
50. Kramer MW, Wolters M, Herrmann TRW. En bloc resection of bladder tumors: ready for prime time? Eur Urol. 2016;69:967–70.
51. Herrmanna TRW, Woltersa M, Kramerb MW. Transurethral en bloc resection of nonmuscle invasive bladder cancer: trend or hype. Curr Opin Urol. 2017;27(2):182–90.

52. Kramer MW, Rassweiler JJ, Klein J, et al. En bloc resection of urothelium carcinoma of the bladder (EBRUC): a European multicenter study to compare safety, efficacy, and outcome of laser and electrical en bloc transurethral resection of bladder tumor. World J Urol. 2015;33(12):1937–43.

53. Hurle R, Lazzeri M, Colombo P, et al. EN bloc resection of nonmuscle invasive bladder cancer: a prospective single-center study. Urology. 2016;90:126–30.

54. Yang H, Lin J, Gao P, et al. Is the En bloc transurethral resection more effective than conventional transurethral resection for non-muscle-invasive bladder cancer? A systematic review and meta-analysis. Urol Int. 2020;7:1–8. https://doi.org/10.1159/000503734.

55. Yang Y, Yang X, Liu C, Li J. Preliminary study on the application of en bloc resection combined with near-infrared molecular imaging technique in the diagnosis and treatment of bladder cáncer. World J Urol. 2020;38(12):3169–76. https://doi.org/10.1007/s00345-020-03143-w.

56. Cosentino M, Gaya JM, Breda A, et al. Alloplastic bladder substitution: are we making progress? Int Urol Nephrol. 2012;44:1295–303.

57. Atala A, Bauer SB, Soker S, Yoo JJ. Tissue-engineered autologous bladders for patients needing cystoplasty. Lancet. 2006;367(9518):1241–6.

58. Shen J, Wu JF, Zhang J, et al. An animal model of bladder reconstruction by autologous peritoneum transplantation. Zhonghua Wai Ke Za Zhi. 2019;57(11):853–9.

Stone Treatment

Luca Orecchia, Sara Anacleto, Stefano Germani, Roberto Miano, and Estêvão Lima

Urolithiasis is a common urologic problem and its prevalence and incidence are rising around the world, constituting a significant burden on health care systems [1]. In fact, urolithiasis is now the second most expensive urological disease [1]. Therefore, safe, efficacious and affordable treatment modalities are required to better deal with this prevalent disease.

Shock wave lithotripsy (SWL), retrograde intra-renal surgery (RIRS) and percutaneous nephrolithotomy (PCNL) are the most common procedures used to treat upper urinary tract stones. PCNL is the gold standard for large kidney stones, being recommended as the first line treatment for kidney stones ≥2 cm by the European Urology Association [2].

PCNL is a complex surgery with some critical steps, including the percutaneous puncture of a renal calyx, tract dilatation, nephroscopy, stone fragmentation and removal and renal drainage.

Obtaining a safe percutaneous renal access is crucial for a good PCNL [3]. Ultrasound and fluoroscopy are generally used to guide the percutaneous access. However, there is a steep learning curve to perform these techniques correctly [4].

Ultrasound has the advantage of providing real –time visualization of the collecting system, as well as nearby structures. However, it only allows two dimensional

L. Orecchia (✉) · S. Germani
Urology Unit, Policlinico Tor Vergata Foundation, Rome, Italy

S. Anacleto
Urology Department, Hospital de Braga, Braga, Portugal

R. Miano
Department of Surgical Sciences, University of Rome Tor Vergata, Rome, Italy

E. Lima
Urology and Uro-Oncology Coordinator - CUF Hospitals, Lisboa, Portugal

School of Medicine, University of Minho, Braga, Portugal

© The Author(s), under exclusive license to Springer Nature Switzerland AG 2021
D. Veneziano, E. Huri (eds.), *Urologic Surgery in the Digital Era*,
https://doi.org/10.1007/978-3-030-63948-8_3

53

images and is extremely operator-dependent. Fluoroscopy is less operator-dependent but implies exposition of the patient and health care staff to ionizing radiation. The combination of both techniques allows safe and successful punctures but does require ionizing radiation and may be time-consuming.

To overcome these problems and improve the quality and safety of the procedure, alternative puncture techniques have been explored.

The ideal renal drainage approach after PCNL has also been questioned during last years and tubeless and totally tubeless modalities are becoming more popular [5–7]. In addition, new biodegradable ureteral stents (BUS) are emerging as a convenient option, allowing for stone clearance while avoiding the need for a second manipulation to remove the stent [8].

In this chapter, we will focus in new techniques in percutaneous access and renal drainage after PCNL.

1 Improvements in Percutaneous Access

The search for the perfect access approach has stimulated PCNL technique improvements. Developments in surgery planning, sheaths size and puncture techniques are making PCNL easier and safer [3].

Small caliber nephroscopes have been tested to try to reduce access-related complications and morbidity related to the size of the tract.

Mini-PCNL can be performed with sheath sizes of 15, 18, 19.5, or 24Fr [9]. This procedure enables the use flexible nephroscopy and might be associated with less bleeding, complications and analgesic use [3]. Lower stone free rates and longer operative times are the drawbacks though [10].

Ultramini-PCNL uses 3.5Fr nephroscope through a 13Fr outer sheath and a 6Fr inner sheath. Stones are fragmented with laser and a side channel is used for irrigation. Experience with this technique is limited [11].

Micro-PCNL is performed through a 4.85Fr tract using a micro-optical needle as a camera without dilatation [12].

Ultramini and micro-PCNL are mainly investigative techniques and currently do not overtake RIRS, which is less invasive and does not need percutaneous access [3]. They might be useful for 1- to 1.5-cm lower pole stones that are inaccessible to RIRS but not big enough for standard PCNL [3].

A systematic review in tract sizes in miniaturized PCNL concluded that procedures performed with small instruments tended to be associated with less blood loss but required longer surgical times [13]. Other complications were not different between PCNL types [13].

Besides miniaturization, new kidney puncture techniques have been developed in order to facilitate PCNL.

Endoscopic guided access (EGA) uses the ureterorenoscope (URS) to confirm the caliceal puncture [14]. When utilizing a ureteral access sheath and flexible URS, it enables direct visualization and selection of the calyx while an ultrasound serve as guide for the needle insertion [15].

The concept of EGA was broadened beyond guiding the puncture to actually performing combined RIRS with PCNL [16]. This technique improves stone clearance and avoids a second puncture in cases where stones in parallel calices are amenable to RIRS [17]. Larger stones may also be relocated with the URS, allowing fragmentation and removal with the nephroscope, a maneuver known as *pass the ball* [18].

Other approach incorporates an optical system in the puncture needle enabling a real-time visualization of the collecting system and avoiding the use of fluoroscopy [19]. The needle positioning in the renal collecting system can be identified immediately after entry. However, the use of ultrasound is still needed, it is not possible to redirect the needle in case of error and the technique is highly operator-dependent. The success rate for puncture at the first attempt was 73.3%.

An iPad-assisted technique for kidney puncture has also been described [20]. Before surgery, computed tomography (CT) is performed and the images are analyzed to obtain a 3D reconstruction. With the patient already under general anesthesia, the iPad camera is used to take the images that are subsequently merged with the virtual CT images. Puncture is performed according to the virtual 3D image and a digital fluoroscopy real-time image. In one study of iPad-assisted puncture, the success rate for puncture at the first attempt was 68.4%.

This technique does not allow needle repositioning during the procedure and the patient must be in the same position of preoperative CT, which may lead to some errors. In addition, it requires the use of ionizing radiation and needs longer puncture time for experienced surgeons. On the other hand, it facilitates puncture, enables better anatomical knowledge of adjacent structures and provides shorter time to puncture for training surgeons.

The Uro-Dyna-CT is a modified angiography unit that allows the rotation of the fluoroscopic unit around the patient, creating images similar to CT [21]. The puncture site and path may be observed in 3D multiplanar reconstructions of the collecting system. The needle position may be confirmed with conventional fluoroscopy and corrected if necessary. The success rate for puncture at the first attempt was 58.3% and the average puncture time was 60 s.

This technique is fast, provides a 3D anatomical image and allows adjustment of needle trajectory during procedure. However, it is extremely influenced by renal movement, requires higher ionizing radiation doses and has a steep learning curve and high costs.

The Guidance positioning system (SonixGPS) is a new real- time ultrasound-guided needle tracking system [22]. In this technique, the catheter is inserted in the pyelocaliceal system and saline is instilled. A global positioning system (GPS) electromagnetic transducer is placed near the patient and a SonixGPS ultrasound probe is used to identify the ideal needle position during puncture. This system provides the current and predicted needle tip position on the ultrasound screen in real time and allows the adjustment of the needle position if necessary. The success rate was 100% at the first attempt and the average puncture time was 5.5 min.

Another promising puncture technique involves the use of electromagentic sensors (6). The electromagnetic tracking sensors were tested initially in *ex vivo* [23] and *in vivo* animal models [24].

A flexible URS is used to identify the best calyx for puncture and to place the catheter. Electromagnetic sensors are incorporated in the catheter and in the tip of the puncture needle and an electromagnetic field generator is placed nearby to create a real time visual path of the relative position of the devices. The surgeon observes the 3D visual trajectory and confirms the correct alignment of the needle and catheter. If necessary, the needle can be replaced and a new virtual path would be calculated and showed.

The animal experiment was performed in six female pigs placed in supine position. Two surgeons made four punctures in each animal: one in the kidney and one in the ureter in both sides. The number of attempts and the time for evaluation of the visual path and puncture were assessed. All 24 punctures (12 in the middle ureter and 12 in the renal calyces) were successful. It took on average 15 s to assess the visual path in the ureter and 13 s in the kidney (mean 14 s). The average time for puncture was 19 s in the kidney and 51 s in the ureter.

This technique was also experimented in humans in the IDEAL trial stage 1 [25]. In this study, PCNL was performed in 10 patients. Similarly to the *in vivo* study, patients were placed in the supine position and flexible URS was used to select the ideal calyx for the access. An electromagnetic field generator was placed nearby the patient and a ureteral catheter with electromagnetic sensor was inserted through the working channel. Ultrasound was used to confirm that the path between the skin and the calyx was free of unintended adjacent structures. After that, a 18G needle with an electromagnetic sensor on the tip punctured the calyx guided by real-time 3D images observed on a monitor (Fig. 1).

After this step, the technique proceeds as usual, with the dilation of the puncture tract, placement of Amplatz sheath and use of nephroscope through the sheath.

This new navigation system consists of the following components: (1) a software for surgical guidance, which gathers and processes information from different devices; (2) an electromagnetic field generator; (3) a 18G needle and a ureteral catheter, both with an electromagnetic sensor on the tip; (4) a monitor with a four-view 3D representation of the trajectory and position of the needle and catheter and (5) a monitor displaying the URS video image (Fig. 2).

In this study, all stones were in the renal pelvis and median stone size was 2.13 cm (1.5–2.5 cm). The success rate was 100% in the first attempt and fluoroscopy was not necessary. The median time from insertion of the needle to puncture was 20 s (range 15–35) and no complications were reported.

This technique allows real-time positioning with 3D images of the needle trajectory, avoids the use of ionizing radiation, has a quick learning curve, is fast, enables permanent monitoring through the electromagnetic sensors and endoscopic view and may be performed in supine position. In addition, it does not depend entirely on ultrasound, being helpful in obese patients and for surgeons with limited ultrasound skills.

The disadvantages are the possible difficulties in placing the ureteral catheter when the calyx is fully occupied with calculus and the lack of visualization of nearby anatomical structures. The latter is common to most puncture techniques tough.

Comparing the new puncture techniques, efficacy, applicability and safety should be considered.

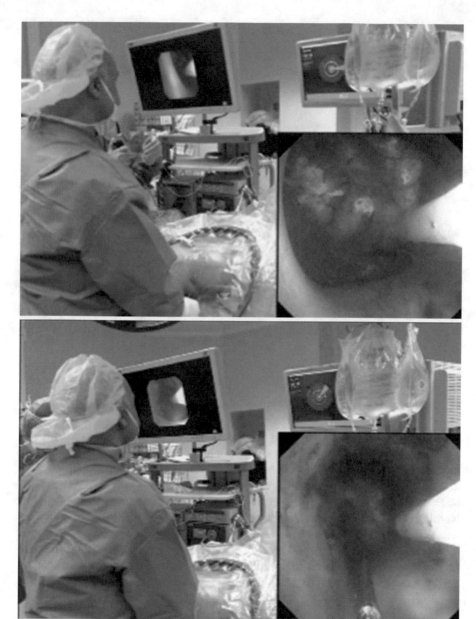

Fig. 1 Using the electromagnetic system, puncture is guided by the 3D navigation software system on the monitor and simultaneously confirmed with the ureterorenoscope image

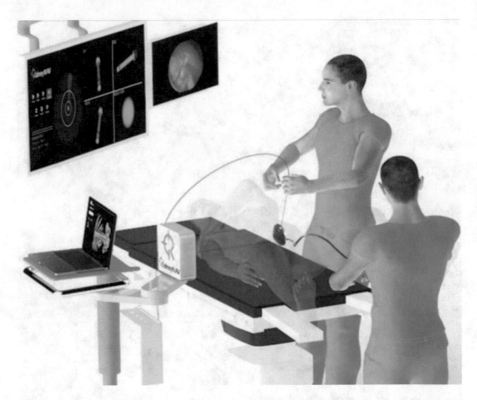

Fig. 2 Surgical set-up for puncture of the renal collecting system using electromagnetic sensors

Electromagnetic sensors and the SonixGPS navigation system have the highest success rates at first attempt (100% success in both) [22, 25]. The high success rate might be explained by ability of the two systems to monitor the needle position throughout the procedure, allowing adjustment of the needle path in real time [25].

Puncture techniques guided by electromagnetic systems seem to have shorter learning curves than standard techniques [24]. Similarly, SonixGPS navigation system seems to facilitate renal puncture, since needle position can be controlled throughout the procedure [22]. The optical system incorporated in the needle only improves visualization when the needle is already in the collecting system and so does not facilitate the puncture [19]. The iPad guided approach [20] and the Uro-Dyna-CT [21] are more difficult to perform and apply in clinical practice.

Regarding safety issues, the optical, SonixGPS and the electromagnetic system minimize risks since they do not need fluoroscopy for needle guidance. On the other hand, the iPad-assisted puncture system and the Uro-Dyna-CT require ionizing radiation, with higher radiation doses than conventional fluoroscopy [21].

Thus, the electromagnetic system and SonixGPS system seem to be the most promising techniques for assist renal puncture in PCNL.

However, these techniques were tested in few and selected patients and it is necessary broaden the scope of research to more challenging cases, such as patients with obesity or larger stone burden [25]. Moreover, cost effectiveness assessment should also be carried out.

2 Improvements in Renal Drainage

The ideal renal drainage approach after PCNL is not clear and the decision to leave a nephrostomy tube and a stent is sometimes difficult to take.

Multiple studies have shown that in selected cases outcomes are similar if patients are managed with a ureteral stent and no nephrostomy tube (tubeless), or even without [5, 6] a stent or nephrostomy tube (totally tubeless) [7].

Stents may assure stone clearance and ureter permeability but can also produce significant symptoms, like infection, encrustation and patient discomfort [26]. Moreover, a second procedure is required for stent removal and not rarely the so-called "forgotten stent syndrome" can lead to kidney loss or even death [26].

Hence biodegradable materials have been investigated in order to minimize stent-related morbidity and to avoid the need of stent removal [27].

Many BUS have been developed, but most of them have failed due to problems in biocompatibility and degradation [28, 29]. In fact, fragments from stent degradation can act as a nucleation point for bacterial adhesion and encrustation leading to further complications and are the main reason why BUS are not available yet [8].

A BUS produced with natural-based polymers was recently described and showed to have good properties and results [8, 30].

In the study [8], 10 domestic pigs were used to compare BUS with standard stents. After 10 days, animals were killed and necropsy was performed. BUS were only visualized on X-ray during the first 24 h and were completely degraded in urine after 10 days in all cases. BUS showed homogeneous degradation and good urine drainage and were associated with less hydronephrosis and better biocompatibility.

However, investigation to improve radiopacity and lengthen BUS indwelling time is still needed before testing its use in humans [8].

3 Use of 3D Printing for Kidney Stones Treatment

3.1 Introduction

Learning the surgical techniques for the endoscopic/percutaneous treatment of kidney stones might represent a challenging task for the urologists in training due to several reasons: the complexity of the access, the narrowness of the operating field, the variety of the upper urinary tract anatomy, the high fragility of the flexible instruments and the potential life-threatening complications. In order to reach adequate surgical expertise while training in a risk-free environment, several authors advocate for the practice of the surgical steps outside of the operating room [31–33].

Therefore, next to the traditional surgical apprenticeship model (Halsted's model of "see one, do one, teach one"), based on acquiring increasing amounts of responsibility that culminate in near-independence [34], there is a constant ongoing research on the development of reliable surgical simulation models. Simulation allows to "play out a wide variety of scenarios and error-prone situations and to reflect on performance without jeopardizing a patient's safety, while providing a controlled setting in which rigorous skill assessment and feedback occur to help trainees to develop clinical competence" [35]. Simulation-based medical education with deliberate practice was found to be superior to the traditional clinical medical education in achieving specific clinical skill acquisition goals [36].

Several surgical simulation models for training on upper urinary tract endoscopic surgery are described in the literature. While the animal model still represents an option and historically was the first accepted surrogate, it carries several complications in terms of ethics, costs, need for fresh organs, dedicated facilities, a disposal service and only partial resemblance to the urinary tract of the human [32]. Endourological training programs on cadaveric fresh-frozen and embalmed models have been described [37], while the almost complete resemblance to the living human tissue is the advantage of this model, its widespread diffusion might be hindered by very low reusability rates and the need of a close collaboration between the Anatomy and Urology departments for the supply of cadavers. Synthetical organ models produced using endocasts, moulds or hybrid techniques were described and proved to be valuable as anatomical tools for preoperative studies. Digital virtual trainers are another training option which is nonetheless characterized by very high costs [32].

In recent times, the production technique known as three-dimensional (3D) printing gained a predominant role in the medical world and is currently representing the most promising alternative for simulation training in terms of cost-effectiveness and applications. Thanks to decisive technological advancements, urologists and engineers have been able to work conjunctly to design and print several anatomical prototypes.

3D printing plays a significant role in Urology and has four main applications [38]:

1. Preoperative surgical planning
2. Surgical training in order to improve technical skills
3. Validation of new techniques or devices
4. Patients counselling

3.2   How 3D Printing Works

3D printing is an additive manufacturing process in which an object is built by overlaying slices of production materials (plastics, resins, metal etc.). In order to print a 3D anatomical model multiple steps are required. Data must be obtained from medical imaging (usually CT or MRI scans) through dedicated software and algorithms capable of interpreting DICOM files. High resolution images such as the ones

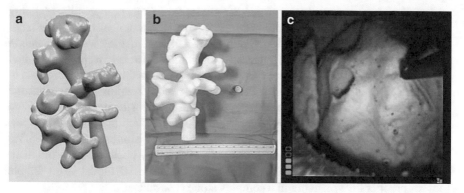

Fig. 3 Example of an experimental 3D printed model for the simulation of flexible ureterorenoscopy and lithotripsy: (**a**) Digital reconstruction of the upper urinary tract, (**b**) 3D printed simulation model and stone, (**c**) Endoscopic view during the simulation

deriving from multiple slice CT scans and contrast enhanced sequences are indicated for better digital 3D reconstruction. The process of transformation of a 2D image of a region of interest (ROI) in a 3D mesh is known as segmentation. The mesh can be further modelled using a dedicated software by a bioengineer expert in the relevant anatomical features of interest to obtain the most accurate and educationally valid final model. Once the design phase is completed the 3D project can be converted in a stereolithography (.stl) format which is recognized by a slicing software. Using this software printing parameters are defined and sent to the printer as G-code file. Several type of filaments and extrusion techniques can be used for printing the finalized model (Fig. 3). The costs of consumables for 3D printing is usually low, while the printers price still ranges up to several thousand euros. Printer rental or off-sourcing of the printing process are options which can mitigate the costs of the whole process.

3.3 3D Printing for Percutaneous Nephrolithotomy

In percutaneous nephrolithotomy (PCNL) the main challenges are represented by the achievement of a stone free state and the access to the collecting system [39, 40]; the use of 2D images to guide the puncture of the selected calyx proves to be a technically challenging phase of the procedure [31, 41, 42]. There is no definitive data on the case load needed for a urologist to be proficient in PCNL, but there is widespread agreement on the steepness of its learning curve, with studies reporting 24–60 procedures needed to achieve competence [32, 39]. Therefore, PCNL may benefit from training models and preoperative thorough anatomical studies, especially during the learning phase or if a complex anatomy is expected [40]. For the purpose of achieving proficiency in every aspect of PCNL, several models developed through 3D printing techniques have been reported in literature.

In 2012 Li et al. described a virtual 3D model for PCNL preoperative planning [42]. Although the authors did not print any physical anatomical model, the technique and software used for the segmentation of medical imaging were the same in use for 3D printing. Using a 3D virtual model reconstructed from four-channel multi-detector CT scans of 15 complex kidney stone cases the authors were able to simulate the optimal orientation of the puncture needle keeping into account the anatomical relationships of the kidney vasculature, the surrounding bones and organs together with the position of the stones in the collecting system. After performing the 15 PNCLs, the authors reported a one-stage stone-free rate of 93.3% with no intraoperative complications and pain as the only postoperative complication observed in one case only. The authors described the 3D model as a valuable tool for preoperative planning in a complex stone case scenario.

In 2014 Turney described a 3D printed simulator for caliceal access during PCNL [31]. A kidney model was printed from CT scans with a water soluble polyvinyl acetate (PVA) filament and then embedded in a silicone cast. After dissolution of the 3D model, the resulting cast was filled with contrast media and waterproofed in order to obtain a reusable simulator for fluoroscopy-guided caliceal puncture. The author reported low material costs (€70), the reusability of the model for up to 20 punctures and the possibility of printing model of increasing anatomical complexity with embedded stones for the development of a training program.

In 2016 Antonelli et al. reported the use of a 3D printed model of the human collecting system to test a polyethylene sack (PercSac) developed to capture a stone and contain fragments during PCNL [43]. The model was designed in 3D and allowed the validation of the device during a PCNL simulation. In this study simulation stones were made using a mixture of water and BegoStone Plus (BEGO USA, Lincoln, RI).

Between 2016 and 2017 Atalay et al. published two studies on Urology residents' understanding of the pelvicalyceal anatomy and PCNL patients' preoperative counselling using 3D printed models [40, 44]. In the study published in 2016, 10 Urology residents completed a questionnaire about 5 patients with complex renal stones eligible for PCNL. The questionnaire evaluated if residents were able to assess the number of posterior and anterior calyces, stone location and the best puncture site for PCNL using computerized tomography urography (CTU) scans. Subsequently five anatomically accurate models which were 3D printed from the CTU of the selected patients were given to the residents for further evaluation and the same questionnaire was administered again. The authors reported a statistically significant improvement in all the domains evaluated by the questionnaire thanks to the use of the 3D printed model: 86–88% in differentiating anterior from posterior calyces, 60% in understanding stone location and 64% in choosing the best puncture site. The reported costs of 3D printing totalled around $100 per model. In the 2017 study the authors describe the use of the five 3D-printed models for preoperative case discussion with the patients. Dedicated questionnaires were administered to the patients with the same modality as the previous study, the results showed a statistically significant improvement in patients' understanding of kidney anatomy (60%), stone position (50%), percutaneous procedure (60%) and its related complications (50%). This study validated the 3D printed models as a useful educational tool for the patients.

A study from 2017 by Ghazi et al. described and validated a 3D printed, single use, model for a complete PCNL simulation [32]. A digital model of pelvicalyceal system with staghorn stone was designed using multiple images from real cases and then 3D printed and assembled in a complete anatomical system including a stented ureter, dorsal spine with 11th and 12th ribs, adipose tissue and posterior abdominal wall layers in order to obtain a realistic and complete simulation of prone fluoro-scopic-guided PCNL. The model was then validated against cadaveric tissue for the accuracy of the resistance to the needle exerted by the tissues with results falling within one standard deviation. Five experts (four urologists and one interventional radiologist) and ten novices (eight urologists and two interventional radiologists) tested the model. The radiologist performed only calyceal access and dilation while the urologist performed a complete PCNL. A Likert scale questionnaire was admin-istered at the end of the procedures and the model received high ratings for its accu-racy, use as a teaching tool and the realism of each surgical step. A statistically significant difference in expert versus novices performance was observed. The authors also described reusability for percutaneous renal access and stone clearance training. The costs of the model were not reported.

3.4 3D Printing for Ureterorenoscopy

As per PCNL, there is no published study clearly defining the learning curve of ureterorenoscopy (URS). Few retrospective case-series studies on individual sur-geons' learning curves for flexible URS (fURS) have been published, while evi-dence on semirigid URS is still lacking [45]. Therefore, equally to PCNL, Objective Structured Assessment of Technical Skills (OSATS) based surrogate markers have been identified to assess proficiency with URS, including: operating and fluoros-copy times, stone free rate, radiation doses, tissue and instrument handling/damage, intra- and postoperative complications. According to several studies and interna-tional Urology curriculums, 40–60 URS should be performed by the training urolo-gist to obtain proficiency during the residency period, but concern has been expressed on the effective possibility to achieve the required case load during the training years [46]. Consequently, different printed training models for URS have been developed aiming at shortening the learning curve of the different URS tech-niques. Some non 3D printed bench models for fURS have been developed includ-ing the low-fidelity K-Box (K-BOX®, Porgès-Coloplast, France), validated for navigation and relocation [47] and the Advanced Scope Trainer (Mediskills, Northampton, UK), validated for navigation, relocation, lithotripsy and basketing [48]. The published material on 3D printed training models for URS is still scarce.

A study from 2015 by Blankestein et al. validated a URS part-task model built by Cook Medical (Bloomington, IN, USA) [33]. The model consisted of a 3D printed complete bladder, ureter and left kidney system, a dual calyceal system and a tortuous ureter. The three anatomical structures were positioned in a plastic box and submerged in water. The model also included a filling and drainage tubing system. For the valida-tion process, 15 Urology residents with different level of expertise were required to

perform a flexible URS and lower pole renal stone relocation exercise; expert endourologists evaluated the performance of the participants. The authors reported statistically significant improvements in all the assessed technical domains thanks to the use
of the simulation model, a direct correlation between previous URS experience and
performance during the simulation and positive feedback from novices and experts in
terms of usefulness as a training device. Manufacture reported cost was $650.

A study from 2016 by Adams et al. validated a 3D printed kidney model for flexible URS [49]. The authors created ten different models in three different polymers:
silicone elastomer, agarose gel and transparent polydimethylsiloxane (PDMS). The
CT scans for segmentation were obtained from three different kidneys extracted and
scanned during autopsies. The model was obtained by 3D printing a soluble inner
mold of the pelvicalyceal system which was first covered by the liquid polymer
poured in 3D printed casts and then dissolved. The dimensions of the resulting models proved to have a mean error of 1% (0.6 mm) when compared to the real organs.
The models were validated for ultrasound scans (agarose gel) and proved to be visu-
ally identical in URS. The PDMS model was the most promising for URS due to its
transparency which allowed a complete external visualization of the pelvicalyceal
system and the flexible instrument during the simulation suggesting possible further
applications in training.

Recently, Orecchia et al. described different 3D printed pelvicalyceal system
training models completed with different type of stones to simulate an entire retrograde intrarenal surgery (RIRS) [50]. Strengths of the models are the high fidelity of
the simulation, the high variety in anatomical complexity, the usage of radiotrans-
parent polymers for the upper urinary tract to allow positioning of a stent, the radi-
opaque mixtures for the stones, the several different options in stone size, shape or
positioning into the pelvicalyceal system, the different response of stones to holmium laser allowing fragmentation or dusting and the virtually endless reusability.
All these features could enable the design of a standardized modular training program for RIRS in a completely risk-free environment.

3.5 Conclusion

The definitive 3D printed model for training in URS/PCNL and lithotripsy is yet
to be described, every developed model has its hindrances and there are no comparative studies available at the moment. No 3D printed model capable of simulat-
ing a complete fURS and lithotripsy had been described yet and the absence of
reproduction of respiratory movements and tissue bleeding still represents an obsta-
cle to the development of a fully advanced surgical simulation. Despite this, 3D
printing represents a real breakthrough in Urology. Its applicability to virtually any
field of surgical simulation and the ever-growing panorama of reported uses might
represent an invaluable asset in surgical training and patient counselling. The widespread use of 3D printing in training might allow the new generation of Urologist to

shorten their learning curve for the most complex surgical techniques, achieving proficiency faster while ensuring higher patient safety.

References

1. Raheem OA, Khandwala YS, Sur RL, Ghani KR, Denstedt JD. Burden of urolithiasis: trends in prevalence, treatments, and costs. Eur Urol Focus. 2017;3:18–26.
2. Turk C, Skolarikos A, Neisius A, et al. Guidelines on urolithiasis 2019. European Association of Urology. https://uroweb.org/guideline/urolithiasis/
3. Ghani KR, Andonian S, Bultitude M, Desai M, Giusti G, Okhunov Z, Preminger GM, de la Rosette J. Percutaneous nephrolithotomy: update, trends, and future directions. Eur Urol. 2016;70:382–96.
4. Kalogeropoulou C, Kallidonis P, Liatsikos EN. Imaging in percutaneous nephrolithotomy. J Endourol. 2009;23:1571–7.
5. Marchant F, Recabal P, Fernández MI, Osorio F, Benavides J. Postoperative morbidity of tubeless versus conventional percutaneous nephrolithotomy: a prospective comparative study. Urol Res. 2011;39:477–81.
6. Kara C, Resorlu B, Bayindir M, Unsal A. A randomized comparison of totally tubeless and standard percutaneous nephrolithotomy in elderly patients. Urology. 2010;76:289–93.
7. Istanbulluoglu MO, Cicek T, Ozturk B, Gonen M, Ozkardes H. Percutaneous nephrolithotomy: nephrostomy or tubeless or totally tubeless? Urology. 2010;75:1043–6.
8. Barros AA, Oliveira C, Ribeiro AJ, Autorino R, Reis RL, Duarte ARC, Lima E. In vivo assessment of a novel biodegradable ureteral stent. World J Urol. 2018;36:277–83.
9. Ganpule AP, Bhattu AS, Desai M. PCNL in the twenty-first century: role of microperc, miniperc, and ultraminiperc. World J Urol. 2015;33:235–40.
10. Giusti G, Piccinelli A, Taverna G, Benetti A, Pasini L, Corinti M, Teppa A, Zandegiacomo de Zorzi S, Graziotti P. Miniperc? No, Thank You! Eur Urol. 2007;51:810–5.
11. Desai J, Solanki R. Ultra-mini percutaneous nephrolithotomy (UMP): one more armamentarium. BJU Int. 2013;112:1046–9.
12. Desai MR, Sharma R, Mishra S, Sabnis RB, Stief C, Bader M. Single-step percutaneous nephrolithotomy (microperc): the initial clinical report. J Urol. 2011;186:140–5.
13. Ruhayel Y, Tepeler A, Dabestani S, et al. Tract sizes in miniaturized percutaneous nephrolithotomy: a systematic review from the european association of urology urolithiasis guidelines panel [Figure presented]. Eur Urol. 2017;72:220–35.
14. Kidd CF, Conlin MJ. Ureteroscopically assisted percutaneousrenal access. Urology. 2003;61:1244–5.
15. Khan F, Borin JF, Pearle MS, McDougall EM, Clayman RV. Endoscopically guided percutaneous renal access: "seeing is believing". J Endourol. 2006;20:451–5.
16. Scoffone CM, Cracco CM, Cossu M, Grande S, Poggio M, Scarpa RM. Endoscopic combined intrarenal surgery in galdakao-modified supine valdivia position: a new standard for percutaneous nephrolithotomy? Eur Urol. 2008;54:1393–403.
17. Knoll T, Wezel F, Michel MS, Honeck P, Wendt-Nordahl G. Do patients benefit from miniaturized tubeless percutaneous nephrolithotomy? A comparative prospective study. J Endourol. 2010;24:1075–9.
18. Undre S, Olsen S, Mustafa N, Patel A. "Pass the ball!" Simultaneous flexible nephroscopy and retrograde intrarenal surgery for large residual upper-pole staghorn stone. J Endourol. 2004;18:844–7.
19. Bader MJ, Gratzke C, Seitz M, Sharma R, Stief CG, Desai M. The "all-seeing needle": initial results of an optical puncture system confirming access in percutaneous nephrolithotomy. Eur Urol. 2011;59:1054–9.

20. Rassweiler JJ, Müller M, Fangerau M, Klein J, Goezen AS, Pereira P, Meinzer H-P, Teber D. iPad-assisted percutaneous access to the kidney using marker-based navigation: initial clinical experience. Eur Urol. 2012;61:628–31.
21. Ritter M, Rassweiler M-C, Michel MS. The uro dyna-CT enables three-dimensional planned laser-guided complex punctures. Eur Urol. 2015;68:880–4.
22. Li X, Long Q, Chen X, Dalin H, He H. Real-time ultrasound-guided PCNL using a novel SonixGPS needle tracking system. Urolithiasis. 2014;42:341–6.
23. Slater RC, Ost M. Percutaneous stone removal: new approaches to access and imaging. Curr Urol Rep. 2015;16:29.
24. Rodrigues PL, Vilaça JL, Oliveira C, Cicione A, Rassweiler J, Fonseca J, Rodrigues NF, Correia-Pinto J, Lima E. Collecting system percutaneous access using real-time tracking sensors: first pig model in vivo experience. J Urol. 2013;190:1932–7.
25. Lima E, Rodrigues PL, Mota P, Carvalho N, Dias E, Correia-Pinto J, Autorino R, Vilaça JL. Ureteroscopy-assisted percutaneous kidney access made easy: first clinical experience with a novel navigation system using electromagnetic guidance (IDEAL stage 1). Eur Urol. 2017;72:610–6.
26. Damiano R, Oliva A, Esposito C, De Sio M, Autorino R, D'Armiento M. Early and late complications of double pigtail ureteral stent. Urol Int. 2002;69:136–40.
27. Chew BH, Lange D. Advances in ureteral stent development. Curr Opin Urol. 2016;26:277–82.
28. Chew BH, Paterson RF, Clinkscales KW, Levine BS, Shalaby SW, Lange D. In vivo evaluation of the third generation biodegradable stent: a novel approach to avoiding the forgotten stent syndrome. J Urol. 2013;189:719–25.
29. Olweny EO, Landman J, Andreoni C, Collyer W, Kerbl K, Onciu M, Välimaa T, Clayman RV. Evaluation of the use of a biodegradable ureteral stent after retrograde endopyelotomy in a porcine model. J Urol. 2002;167:2198–202.
30. Barros AA, Rita A, Duarte ARC, Pires RA, Sampaio-Marques B, Ludovico P, Lima E, Mano JF, Reis RL. Bioresorbable ureteral stents from natural origin polymers. J Biomed Mater Res Part B Appl Biomater. 2015;103:608–17.
31. Turney BW. A new model with an anatomically accurate human renal collecting system for training in fluoroscopy-guided percutaneous nephrolithotomy access. J Endourol. 2014;28:360–3. https://doi.org/10.1089/end.2013.0616.
32. Ghazi A, Campbell T, Melnyk R, et al. Validation of a full-immersion simulation platform for percutaneous nephrolithotomy using three-dimensional printing technology. J Endourol. 31:1314–20. https://doi.org/10.1089/end.2017.0809.
33. Blankstein U, Lantz AG, D'A Honey RJ, et al. Simulation-based flexible ureteroscopy training using a novel ureteroscopy part-task trainer. Can Urol Assoc J. 2015;9:331–5. https://doi.org/10.5489/cuaj.2811.
34. Cameron JL. William Stewart Halsted: our surgical heritage. Ann Surg. 1997;225:445–58. https://doi.org/10.1097/00000658-199705000-00002.
35. Barry Issenberg S, Mcgaghie WC, Petrusa ER, et al. Features and uses of high-fidelity medical simulations that lead to effective learning: a BEME systematic review. Med Teach. 2005;27:10–28. https://doi.org/10.1080/01421590500046924.
36. McGaghie WC, Issenberg SB, Cohen ER, et al. Does simulation-based medical education with deliberate practice yield better results than traditional clinical education? A meta-analytic comparative review of the evidence. Acad Med. 2011;86:706–11. https://doi.org/10.1097/ACM.0b013e318217e119.
37. Huri E, Skolarikos A, Tatar İ, et al. Simulation of RIRS in soft cadavers: a novel training model by the Cadaveric Research On Endourology Training (CRET) Study Group. World J Urol. 2016;34:741–6. https://doi.org/10.1007/s00345-015-1676-3.
38. Cacciamani GE, Okhunov Z, Meneses AD, et al. Impact of three-dimensional printing in urology: state of the art and future perspectives. A systematic review by ESUT-YAUWP Group. Eur Urol. 2019;76:209–21. https://doi.org/10.1016/j.eururo.2019.04.044.

39. de la Rosette JJMCH, Laguna MP, Rassweiler JJ, Conort P. Training in percutaneous nephrolithotomy—a critical review. Eur Urol. 2008;54:994–1003. https://doi.org/10.1016/j.eururo.2008.03.052.

40. Atalay HA, Volkan Ü, Iter A, et al. Impact of three-dimensional printed pelvicaliceal system models on residents' understanding of pelvicaliceal system anatomy before percutaneous nephrolithotripsy surgery: a pilot study. J Endourol. 30:1132–7. https://doi.org/10.1089/end.2016.0307.

41. Baumhauer M, Feuerstein M, Meinzer H-P, Rassweiler J. Navigation in endoscopic soft tissue surgery: perspectives and limitations. J Endourol. 2008;22:751–66. https://doi.org/10.1089/end.2007.9827.

42. Li H, Chen Y, Liu C, et al. Construction of a three-dimensional model of renal stones: comprehensive planning for percutaneous nephrolithotomy and assistance in surgery. World J Urol. 2013;31:1587–92. https://doi.org/10.1007/s00345-012-0998-7.

43. Antonelli JA, Beardsley H, Faddegon S, et al. A novel device to prevent stone fragment migration during percutaneous lithotripsy: results from an in-vitro kidney model. J Endourol. 30:1239–43. https://doi.org/10.1089/end.2016.0466.

44. Atalay HA, Canat HL, Ülker V, et al. Impact of personalized three-dimensional (3D) printed pelvicalyceal system models on patient information in percutaneous nephrolithotripsy surgery: a pilot study. Int Braz J Urol. 2017;43:470–5. https://doi.org/10.1590/s1677-5538.ibju.2016.0441.

45. Quirke K, Abdullatif A, Brunckhorst O, et al. Learning curves in urolithiasis surgery: a systematic review. J Endourol. 32:1008–20. https://doi.org/10.1089/end.2018.0425.

46. Skolarikos A, Gravas S, Laguna MP, et al. Training in ureteroscopy: a critical appraisal of the literature: *TRAINING IN URETEROSCOPY*. BJU Int. 2011;108:798–805. https://doi.org/10.1111/j.1464-410X.2011.10337.x.

47. Villa L, Emre Şener T, Somani BK, et al. Initial content validation results of a new simulation model for flexible ureteroscopy: the key-box. J Endourol. 31:72–7. https://doi.org/10.1089/end.2016.0677.

48. Al-Jabir A, Abdullatif A, Takashige A, et al. Validation of the advanced scope trainer for flexible ureterorenoscopy training. Urology. 110:45–50. https://doi.org/10.1016/j.urology.2017.07.047.

49. Adams F, Qiu T, Mark A, et al. Soft 3D-printed phantom of the human kidney with collecting system. Ann Biomed Eng. 2017;45:963–72. https://doi.org/10.1007/s10439-016-1757-5.

50. Orecchia L, Manfrin D, Germani S, Del Fabbro D, Asimakopoulos AD, Finazzi Agrò E, Miano R. Introducing 3D printed models of the upper urinary tract for high-fidelity simulation of retrograde intrarenal surgery. 3D Print Med. 2021;7(1):15. https://doi.org/10.1186/s41205-021-00105-9.

3D Laparoscopy

Samson Yun-sang Chan, Steffi Kar-kei Yuen, and Eddie Shu-yin Chan

1 Introduction

Laparoscopic surgery has become the gold standard for most surgeries since its development in the 1980s. It has been proven that laparoscopic surgery can reduce perioperative morbidity, intraoperative blood loss and post-operative pain, shorter hospital stay and better cosmetic outcomes [1, 2]. Despite its advantages, the two-dimensional (2D) vision provides limited degrees of instrumental freedom and steeper learning curves leave huge room for improvement in laparoscopic surgery. Although with technological advancements and development of high definition cameras, the limitations of 2D laparoscopy including the lack of depth perception and loss of spatial orientation still have yet to be compensated.

Three-dimensional (3D) camera system was invented in the early 1990s using the Shutter Glass technique [3] but they were not popularized due to its poor image resolution and requirement of expensive instruments. With technological improvements using the Film-type Patterned Retarder 3D laparoscope [4], high definition and stable images can be generated. More recently, the industry has developed novel 3D systems where the imaging closely approximates the stereoscopic vision, where depth perception is brought about by different unique images received by each eye. This gives possible edge during laparoscopic performances.

Current evidence on 2D versus 3D laparoscopic surgeries on training model, cadaveric and animal models and clinical trials shows benefits of 3D over conventional 2D laparoscopic systems. In this chapter, we will visit the history, developments and benefits of 3D laparoscopic surgery in urology.

S. Y.-s. Chan · S. K.-k. Yuen · E. S.-y. Chan (✉)
Division of Urology, Department of Surgery, The Chinese University of Hong Kong,
Shatin, NT, Hong Kong
e-mail: eddie@surgery.cuhk.edu.hk

© The Author(s), under exclusive license to Springer Nature
Switzerland AG 2021
D. Veneziano, E. Huri (eds.), *Urologic Surgery in the Digital Era*,
https://doi.org/10.1007/978-3-030-63948-8_4

1.1   History of 3D Image in Surgery

The first binocular microscopes were first used by Gunnar Holmgren in otolaryngology in 1922 [5] to overcome the lack of depth perception associated with monocular operating microscopes. In the 1980s, Gerhard Buess used the first stereo-endoscope with two optical channels in Transanal Endoscopic Microsurgery (TEMS) [6], he viewed the 3D image through binocular eyepieces. In 1992, his team adopted the first prototype laparoscopic stereo-endoscope in animal studies and later laparoscopic cholecystectomies [7]. They concluded the property of stereopsis facilitated complex laparoscopy.

The initial video system prototype employed 3D monitors with standard resolution and low visual ergonomics and single-channelled laparoscope. The heavy weighted active shutter glasses contribute to inferior image qualities, leading to surgeon ocular fatigue, nausea, tiredness and headache. Thanks to technological improvements, Film-type Patterned Retarder 3D laparoscopes were subsequently introduced. Those produced more stable high definition stable images, alleviating the stress on the surgeon's eyes. Over the years, the quality of images progressively improved from dual-channel video, to dual chip-on-the-tip, to deflectable tip laparoscope, to autostereoscopic displays incorporating liquid crystal display (LCD) technology.

1.2   Technology and Principles in 3D Laparoscopy

1.2.1   Depth Perception

Before understanding the principles of creating 3D images, one has to comprehend how humans perceive depth by naked eyes. The human eye cannot naturally perceive depth information when the 3D image projects onto a 2D retina. The human brain has to combine various monocular and binocular cues received from the retinas to recover the depth, spatial relationship and three dimensional images of objects.

One of the most important cues of depth perception is 'stereopsis'—a process which causes each eye to have a slightly different view of the same scene due to anatomical separation between the two eyes. The visual cortex will then analyse and combine the received information of the binocular disparities derived from both retinas. Therefore, stereoscopy or 3D imaging is a technique for creating the illusion of depth in an image by means of stereopsis in binocular vision.

1.2.2   Image Acquisition in Laparoscopy

There are generally two methods of capturing images of the operative field during surgery. A traditional rod-lens laparoscope can be used to transmit the light from the image to outside of the patient. A video camera then captures the image and sends it as an electrical signal to an image processor. With technological advancement, rod-lens technology is now being replaced by digital laparoscope utilizing small camera chips to capture the image at the tip of the laparoscope. The electrical signal is transmitted along the laparoscope to an image processor.

1.2.3   Laparoscope

Single and dual channel systems were able to extract 3D images and transmit to the video system. Single channel system works by splitting the image either with a prism or filter in order to extract two perspectives of the operative field from a single point. However, by doing so, this does not results in a true binocular image. Dual channel systems captures two horizontally separated images from the operative fields and produce two different perspectives to create a true binocular image.

1.2.4   3D Projection System

Shutter Glass

Shutter Glass (SG) technique works by presenting the image intended for the left eye while blocking the right eye's view, then presenting the right-eye image while blocking the left eye. This process is repeated so rapidly that the interruptions do not interfere with the perceived fusion of the two images into a single 3D image. Operator wears active shuttering glasses so that each eye receives only the corresponding right or left eye image.

Film-type Patterned Retarder

Film-type Patterned Retarder (FPR) is a technology based on circular polarization and is commonly used nowadays. It shows left and right images through different patterns in a circular polarizer which allows the left and right images to be seen by the left and right eyes separately. FPR technology uses the precise film which polarizes different pixels differently to show a different image for each eye. Operators wears lightweight polarizing glasses to separate the correct image to each eye.

When compared to Shutter Glass (SG) technique, flickering was markedly reduced to improve eye fatigue and picture quality. SG technique prevents photo-sensitive epilepsy. FPR panels also provide brighter 3D images. In addition, the FPR glasses are passive and do not use electricity as does SG (which require connection to the video system). They are cheaper and lighter in weight.

Da Vinci Surgical System & Head Mounted Display

Da Vinci robotic systems use a fixed viewing environment like microscope. The console surgeon has a separate image displayed to each eye. Head Mounted Displays also provide independent images to each eye with its own screen to achieve stereopsis.

1.2.5   3D Laparoscopy

Nowadays, dual channel 3D laparoscopic system consists of two adjacent cameras which simulate the stereoscopic view of human eyes. The parallax images will be fused into a single 3D image with depth perception. The camera can be a built-in or clip-on system. Conventional system which consists of special endoscope and a 3D camera head can be used (e.g. Aesculap Einstein Vision® 3D camera system or da Vinci® system). The photon-receptive component, charge-coupled device (CCD) can also be mounted at the very tip of the laparoscope for the ease of setup (e.g. Olympus® EndoEye Flex 3D or Storz IMAGE 1S™ 3D).

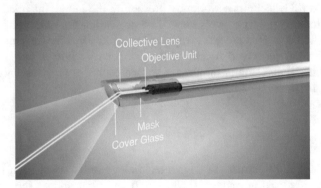

1.2.6   Advances in 3D Laparoscopy

In the era of high image resolution, the 3D laparoscopy are mostly in high definition (HD). Equipped with more pixels, HD system can deliver clearer view during surgery and makes digital magnification possible without the sacrifice of details [8]. Due to the intrinsic limitation of forming 3D images, camera rotation while maintaining horizontal orientation is only possible recently (Olympus EndoEye 3D). This is overcome by using a set of prisms to maintain the correct orientation while changing of viewing angle.

There are manufacturers developing systems to incorporate augmented reality into 3D laparoscopy. This technology allows to superimpose patient anatomy (data from CT or MRI images) to the surgical field. This enhances the accuracy and precision on minimal invasive surgery. Computer-assisted surgery (CAS) [9], a concept that use computer technology in surgical planning, guiding and performing operations. A sophisticated 3D optical system is essential for CAS in mapping of anatomy and registering soft tissue movement.

1.3 Potential Benefits and Pitfalls of 3D Laparoscopy

1.3.1 Benefits to Training

Training is always the first step to skills and experience acquisition. It can be taken place in the form of laparoscopic box trainer and animal model. Numerous studies have shown the usage of 3D monitors can improve accuracy and speed in performing phantom tasks. The subjects comprise of laparoscopic naive medical students, trainees or experienced surgeons. Poudel et al. [10]. showed that 3D environment helped shorten the training time of basic laparoscopic skills to novices. Patel et al. [11] has shown the benefits also extend to experienced laparoscopic surgeons. With these data, it showed 3D laparoscopic not only benefits the novices in skills training, but also further enhance the seasoned ones.

From a systematic review by Arezzo et al. [12], amongst the 33 identified randomised controlled trials, 3D imaging was associated with a significant reduction in task completion time, reduced errors and higher task specific scores. Major limitations include most studies were single centre, only 36% used validated tasks and the majority (94.4%) used in box trainer simulators. Whether these data can be extrapolated to clinical benefits still remains questionable.

1.3.2 Benefits on Operative Outcomes

It has been suggested that 3D laparoscopy shortens operative time across all surgical specialties, in particular general surgery, urology and gynaecology. In a meta-analysis [12] pooling data from 18 studies, it showed 3D laparoscopic surgery significantly reduced operative time (mean difference −11 min), in particular for procedures involving suturing (mean difference −15 min). When subdividing surgery on solid or hollow organ, there was a mean difference of 21.7 min on solid organ surgery, whilst no significant difference was found on hollow organ surgery.

For urological procedure involving intracorporeal suturing (radical prostatectomy, pyeloplasty and partial nephrectomy), meta-analysis [12] found there was no difference in operative time between 2D and 3D laparoscopic surgery. However, when specific analysis focusing solely on radical prostatectomy, the operative time significantly favoured 3D approach (mean difference −35 min) [13]. In addition, the cumulative analysis of the above procedures showed a significant reduction of blood loss and shorter hospital stay favouring 3D laparoscopic surgery (mean difference −21.6 ml & −0.6 days).

Furthermore, the pooled data from different settings suggest a lower overall complication rates for 3D laparoscopy in procedures involving suturing. In Arezzo's meta-analysis [12], 3D laparoscopy in procedures involving laparoscopic suturing showed significant reduction in complication rate (RR 0.57) but not general surgical procedure. When performing a subgroup analysis with only the RCTs and prospective trials, the RR further reduced to 0.5.

1.3.3   Urological Procedures

Reviewing current literature on 3D laparoscopy on urological procedures, a recent meta-analysis by Dirie et al. [14] included 13 studies (3 randomised and 10 observational studies) comparing 2D to 3D systems during urological laparoscopic surgeries. In that meta-analysis, they mainly compared partial nephrectomy, pyeloplasty and radical prostatectomy. The main benefits were seen in reducing warm ischemic time in partial nephrectomies and estimated blood loss in radical prostatectomies.

1.3.4   Partial Nephrectomy

Partial nephrectomy has nowadays become the standard treatment for cT1 renal tumor and is strongly recommended by international guidelines. With the advancement in surgical technologies, minimally invasive approach had become the more popular means of technique.

Studies by Komatsuda et al. [15] and Ruan et al. [16] comparing 2D to 3D laparoscopic partial nephrectomies showed no significant difference in operating time, dissection time and complication rates. The only improved factor is the reduction in warm ischemic time in the 3D laparoscopy image system group. It was a surprise that no study show improvement in operating and dissection time as studies in training model showed improvement in task completion time with 3D system. Multiple factors including the renal nephrometry scores could have an impact on the outcome. With the limited high quality studies on this forefront, one cannot exclude the potential benefits of 3D laparoscopy brings.

1.3.5 Pyeloplasty

Laparoscopic or robotic pyeloplasty are commonly performed procedures for treatment of pelviureteric junction (PUJ) obstruction. Two studies [17, 18] looking into 2D versus 3D laparoscopic pyeloplasty showed significantly shorter operating time, favouring the 3D system with similar complication rates. However, only retrospective studies were available in this context with a small case number, no conclusive benefits can be drawn.

1.3.6 Radical Prostatectomy

With longer life expectancy in men, improving prostate cancer diagnostics and screening programmes, more prostate cancer was diagnosed, rendering the need for treatment. According to Centres for Disease Control and Prevention of the United States, prostate cancer has become the number one incidence of all malignancies at 23%. Laparoscopic or robotic radical prostatectomy have gained increasing favour amongst centres all over the world. Better visualization of surgical anatomy can provide a better platform to ensure smoother surgery with negative surgical margin, preservation of continence and erectile function. As a result, more robotic prostatectomy was performed than laparoscopic approach because of the superiority of 3D vision and dexterity of robotic arm. Despite all its pros, the robotic system comes at a high cost, too high for some healthcare systems. This brings up the next inevitable question—can 3D laparoscopy really improve the surgery?

Many urologists would agree on the fact that performing the urethro-vesical anastomosis is one major hurdle in laparoscopic prostatectomy. Two prospective trials [19, 20] did show 3D laparoscopic surgery can help shorten the anastomosis time and improve the surgical outcomes. For postoperative continence recovery, meta-analysis [14] showed the 3D laparoscopy group had quicker recovery at 3 months with HR 0.4. Limited studies comparing 3D to 2D laparoscopic radical prostatectomy showed hastened erection recovery. Bove et al. [20] showed a trend of improved outcome with 3D system at 63% compared to 58% with 2D.

1.3.7 Pitfalls of 3D Laparoscopy

3D laparoscopy has always been criticised for causing visual fatigue and headaches of the operators, especially when the setups were suboptimal. Although with technological advancement and the use of lightweight polarizing glasses, Zhou et al. [21] still showed higher incidence of blurred vision, irritated and dry eyes, headache and eyestrain. However, the objective visual functional parameters such as distance/ near exophoria, distance/near esophoria, fusion range, accommodative convergence/accommodation and tear film breakup time had no significant difference between the two groups. Kinoshita et al. [22] carried out a subjective evaluation by surgeons using a validated questionnaire, showing 3D laparoscopy was superior and did not increase fatigue.

1.3.8 Cost Effectiveness

There were no prospective trials directly investigating the cost effectiveness of 3D laparoscopic training or surgery. However, the average cost of a robotic unit is approximately 2 millions USD with the weighted average variable cost per case approximately 8 thousand USD. In face of a 125 thousand USD HD 3D camera system using standing laparoscopic instrument, it is a tough decision which would be a more economical option.

2 Conclusion

Technology advances exponentially every day. Over the past two decades, there are monumental leaps in the developments of 3D technology in the commercial and medical field. 3D laparoscopic surgeries are widely adopted in practice nowadays with the potential benefits on training and surgical outcomes. Furthermore, it is known that procedures involving intracorporeal suturing are most challenging and requires advanced laparoscopic skills. With the evidence supporting the preponderance of 3D laparoscopy in such situation, the stereoscopic surgical view plays a crucial role of accurate appreciation of depth during intracorporeal suturing.

Let us not get too carried away by technology; let us not get too caught up in the midst of acquiring certain approaches and techniques; most importantly, let us never stop the quest in dissecting and uncoding the biology of the diseases and utilizing these approaches to the benefit in prevailing its effect on the health of humankind. Further studies are mandated to evaluate the cost-benefit of such technology.

References

1. Basiri A, et al. Comparison of retropubic, laparoscopic and robotic radical prostatectomy: who is the winner? World J Urol. 2018;36:609–21.
2. Eskicorapci SY, et al. Laparoscopic radical nephrectomy: the new gold standard surgical treatment for localized renal cell carcinoma. ScientificWorldJournal. 2007;7:825–36.
3. Wenzl R, Pateisky N, Husslein P. First use of a 3D video-endoscope in gynecology. Geburtshilfe Frauenheilkd. 1993;53:776–8.

4. Buchs NC, Volonte F, Pugin F, Toso C, Morel P. Three-dimensional laparoscopy: a step toward advanced surgical navigation. Surg Endosc. 2013;27:692–3.
5. Uluc K, Kujoth GC, Baskaya MK. Operating microscopes: past, present, and future. Neurosurg Focus. 2009;27:E4.
6. Buess G, et al. Technique of transanal endoscopic microsurgery. Surg Endosc. 1988;2:71–5.
7. Becker H, Melzer A, Schurr MO, Buess G. 3-D video techniques in endoscopic surgery. Endosc Surg Allied Technol. 1993;1:40–6.
8. Smith R, et al. Advanced stereoscopic projection technology significantly improves novice performance of minimally invasive surgical skills. Surg Endosc. 2012;26:1522–7.
9. Maier-Hein L, et al. Optical techniques for 3D surface reconstruction in computer-assisted laparoscopic surgery. Med Image Anal. 2013;17:974–96.
10. Poudel S, et al. Impact of 3D in the training of basic laparoscopic skills and its transferability to 2D environment: a prospective randomized controlled trial. Surg Endosc. 2017;31:1111–8.
11. Patel HRH, Ribal M-J, Arya M, Nauth-Misir R, Joseph JV. Is it worth revisiting laparoscopic three-dimensional visualization? A validated assessment. Urology. 2007;70:47–9.
12. Arezzo A, et al. The use of 3D laparoscopic imaging systems in surgery: EAES consensus development conference 2018. Surg Endosc. 2019;33:3251–74.
13. Bertolo R, et al. Current status of three-dimensional laparoscopy in urology: an ESUT systematic review and cumulative analysis. J Endourol. 2018;32:1021–7.
14. Dirie NI, Wang Q, Wang S. Two-dimensional versus three-dimensional laparoscopic systems in urology: a systematic review and meta-analysis. J Endourol. 2018;32:781–90.
15. Komatsuda A, et al. Technical improvement using a three-dimensional video system for laparoscopic partial nephrectomy. Asian Pac J Cancer Prev. 2016;17:2475–8.
16. Ruan Y, et al. Clinical evaluation and technical features of three-dimensional laparoscopic partial nephrectomy with selective segmental artery clamping. World J Urol. 2016;34:679–85.
17. Abou-Haidar H, et al. Laparoscopic pyeloplasty: Initial experience with 3D vision laparoscopy and articulating shears. J Pediatr Urol. 2016;12:426.e1–5.
18. Xu W, et al. Comparison of three dimensional and two dimentional laparoscopic pyeloplasty for ureteropelvic junction obstruction. Zhonghua Wai Ke Za Zhi. 2014;52:771–4.
19. Aykan S, et al. Perioperative, pathologic, and early continence outcomes comparing three-dimensional and two-dimensional display systems for laparoscopic radical prostatectomy--a retrospective, single-surgeon study. J Endourol. 2014;28:539–43.
20. Bove P, et al. 3D vs 2D laparoscopic radical prostatectomy in organ-confined prostate cancer: comparison of operative data and pentafecta rates: a single cohort study. BMC Urol. 2015;15:12.
21. Zhou J, et al. A comparative study of distinct ocular symptoms after performing laparoscopic surgical tasks using a three-dimensional surgical imaging system and a conventional two-dimensional surgical imaging system. J Endourol. 2015;29:816–20.
22. Kinoshita H, et al. High-definition resolution three-dimensional imaging systems in laparoscopic radical prostatectomy: randomized comparative study with high-definition resolution two-dimensional systems. Surg Endosc. 2015;29:2203–9.

Kidney Transplantation

Angelo Territo, Iacopo Meneghetti, Julio Francisco Calderón Cortez,
Romain Boissier, and Alberto Breda

Abbreviations

BD	brain-dead
BMI	body mass index
CT	computed tomography
DCD	donation after cardiac death
ERUS	EAU Robotic Urology Section
ESRD	end-stage renal disease
GMV	grafts with multiple vessels
KT	kidney transplantation
OKT	open kidney transplantation
RAKT	robot-assisted kidney transplantation

1   Introduction and Kidney Procurement

Kidney transplantation (KT) confers a higher long-term survival rate and a better quality of life in comparison to dialysis [1] and is more cost-effective over the long term [2].

As a result of the growing discrepancy between the need for and the availability of donor kidneys, the concept of non-heart-beating donation, standard in the early days of transplantation when no living donor was available, has once again been taken up. Deceased donors can be divided into two groups: brain-dead (BD) (or heart-beating) donors and donation after cardiac death (DCD) donors. Although BD

A. Territo (✉) · I. Meneghetti · J. F. C. Cortez · A. Breda
Department of Urology, Fundació Puigvert, Autonomous University of Barcelona,
Barcelona, Spain

R. Boissier
Department of Urology, Aix-Marseille University, APHM, La Conception Academic Hospital,
Marseille, France
e-mail: romain.boissier@ap-hm.fr

© The Author(s), under exclusive license to Springer Nature
Switzerland AG 2021
D. Veneziano, E. Huri (eds.), *Urologic Surgery in the Digital Era*,
https://doi.org/10.1007/978-3-030-63948-8_5

79

donors are considered dead, the donor's heart continues to pump and maintain circulation, which permits surgeons to start operating while the organs are still perfused.

Kootstra et al. [3], along with other pioneers, proposed the use of non-heart-beating donors and identified different types of DCD donation (Maastricht categories of donation after circulatory death), leading to expansion of the pool of kidneys from deceased donors. Other authors [4] have since further expanded these criteria. The modified Maastricht classification (Table 1) distinguishes uncontrolled donors from controlled donors, the latter being the most suitable for initiation of a DCD program. The use of kidneys from DCD donors has led to an expansion in the pool of kidneys from deceased donors, but the use of DCD kidneys is not permitted all over the world.

The indications for and the technical description of the kidney withdrawal go beyond the scope of this chapter.

Compared with KT from deceased donors, KT from living donors has better results, such as improved long-term patient survival, better transplant survival, avoidance of a long waiting time for transplantation, less aggressive immunosuppressive regimens, and a global increase in the kidney transplant rate [5–7].

Right and left laparoscopic living donor nephrectomy are similar in terms of surgery and postoperative graft function, but the left kidney is preferred for donation as the left renal vein is longer than the right renal vein. When there is a difference in the function of the two kidneys, the lesser functioning kidney is used for donation in order to limit the risks for the donor [8–10].

Open nephrectomy for donation may offer an advantage in challenging cases, such as grafts with multiple vessels and/or vascular anomalies and cases with prior abdominal surgery. Furthermore, the open approach may be preferred in centers with little experience in laparoscopy and/or a low case volume of living donor nephrectomies [11].

The *laparoscopic approach* is the preferred technique for living donor nephrectomy in established KT programs [12]. At our institution, we perform living donor nephrectomies with the minimally invasive transperitoneal laparoscopic approach, using the linear port configuration as described by Harper et al. [13]. This trocar

Table 1 Modified Maastricht classification from cadaveric donor

Category	Description	Circumstances
I	Cardiocirculatory death outside hospital (with or without witnesses and rapid resuscitation attempt)	Uncontrolled
II	Unexpected cardiocirculatory death in hospital	Uncontrolled
III	Expected cardiocirculatory death in Intensive Care Unit or Operating Room	Controlled
IV	Expected or unexpected cardiocirculatory arrest in a brain-dead donor	Controlled
V	Medically assisted cardiocirculatory death in ward or Operating Room	Controlled

arrangement has the aim of offering an excellent ergonomic position for the surgeon and camera holder (Fig. 1).

Robot-assisted surgery offers clear advantages over conventional laparoscopy thanks to the use of EndoWrist instruments, the three-dimensional view, enhanced visualization of the operative field (×12), and, possibly, a shorter learning curve [14, 15].

2   Conventional Open KT Technique

Below we describe the open kidney transplantation (OKT) technique, which still represents the gold standard approach for KT [16].

Back Table Preparation of the Kidney Both the renal vein and the renal artery are carefully inspected, including with regard to any endothelial damage or atherosclerotic plaques (Fig. 2). All side branches are ligated and divided, and care must be taken to avoid extensive dissection of the vessels into the hilum or compromise of the vascularization of the proximal ureter or the renal pelvis. Any vascular reconstruction that might be necessary can be done at this point (Fig. 3). This can consist in shortening of a long aortic patch in the case of multiple renal arteries spread or repair of any damaged vessels. During the bench procedure, renal biopsy can also be performed if there is doubt about the quality of the parenchyma prior to transplantation.

Creation of the Operative Field and Graft Allocation A conventional OKT is performed in a heterotopic position in one of the lower quadrants via an extraperitoneal approach. An incision is usually made in the right (or left) lower abdominal quadrant (Gibson incision) for access to the retroperitoneal space. Generally, the kidney graft is placed in the right side because of greater accessibility to the iliac

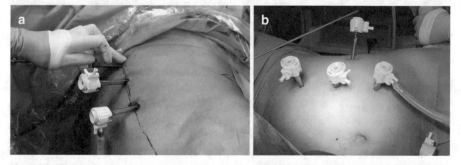

Fig. 1 (**a**) Linear port configuration along the left pararectal line, with the camera placed at the most cephalic position (at the 12th rib level). (**b**) An additional trocar is used to raise the kidney during the section of the vessels. A Pfannenstiel incision is made to introduce endovascular stapler and the 15-mm EndoCatch bag for organ extraction

Fig. 2 Kidney graft from cadaveric donor

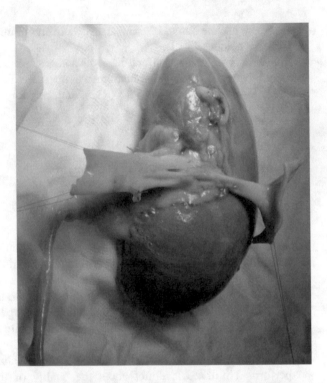

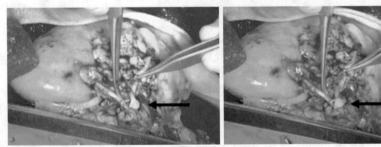

Fig. 3 Bench table preparation of the graft from living donation with double artery. In the picture above details of reconstruction of the arteries joined as a pantaloon

external vessels and the inferior vena cava. Currently, the tendency in nearly all conventional KTs is to place the anastomosis in the external iliac vessels, using an end-to-side suture. After the operative field has been created, the graft is placed in the retroperitoneal space to decide upon the best position to perform the anastomosis without moving the kidney. The position of the anastomosis is usually planned before surgery, according to the recipient preoperative computed tomography (CT) scan of the aorta and iliac vessels. Therefore, the iliac vessels are dissected but this should be limited to the area of the anastomosis. Limited dissection and correct ligation of the perivascular lymph vessels can reduce the incidence of lymphoceles.

Venous Anastomosis Usually, the vein is the first vessel to be anastomosed. The previously selected site for the anastomosis in the iliac vein is isolated using a Satinsky clamp and a venotomy is performed using a scalpel. It is convenient to have the vein full of blood to avoid any injury to the posterior aspect of the vein when performing the venotomy. The venotomy can be expanded by resecting a small strip of one of the edges. Diluted 4% heparin is instilled in the vein lumen to wash out traces of blood and avoid clot formation. The end-to-side anastomosis is performed using two running sutures of non-absorbable 5-0 or 6-0 monofilament thread. One suture is placed at each pole of the venotomy and two running sutures are carried out on both sides to complete the anastomosis (Fig. 4). Once the venous anastomosis has been completed, a Bulldog clamp is placed at the proximal end of the graft vein and the Satinsky clamp is released. If any bleeding of the suture or vein occurs, it must be repaired before proceeding to the arterial anastomosis. In the presence of multiple veins, only the biggest vein should be reimplanted, while smaller ones can be ligated.

Arterial Anastomosis An end-to-side anastomosis of the renal artery to the external iliac artery (or common iliac artery) is usually performed using an appropriately trimmed cuff of aorta attached to the renal artery (the Carrel patch—Fig. 5). Vascular clamps are applied to the external iliac artery proximally and distally if an end-to-side

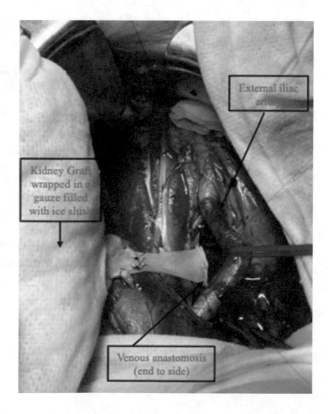

Fig. 4 The external iliac vessels are dissected in the right side (right iliac fossa). The venous end-to-side anastomosis is performed using two running sutures of non-absorbable 5-0 or 6-0 monofilament

Fig. 5 An end-to-side
anastomosis of the renal
artery to the external iliac
artery is performed using
the Carrel patch

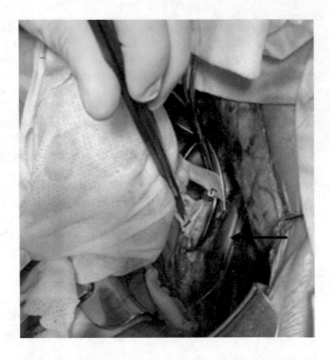

anastomosis is to be performed, with care being taken to avoid clamping diseased
segments of artery wherever possible. An arteriotomy, appropriately placed, is performed in the external iliac artery, and the lumen is flushed out again with heparin-
ized saline; when the donor artery has no Carrel aortic patch, a hole punch is used
to create a suitably sized hole for anastomosis. The anastomosis is done with a
continuous 5-0 or 6-0 monofilament vascular suture although an interrupted technique may be necessary where no Carrel patch exists. Particular care should be
taken to ensure that all the intima on the recipient artery is secured back in position
during the anastomosis to prevent a dissection propagating along the distal artery on
reperfusion. In very severe cases of calcification of the recipient artery, it may be
necessary to carry out a formal endarterectomy of the iliac artery, with the distal
intima stitched in place to prevent formation of a flap and subsequent dissection.
Figure 6 shows different techniques for arterial anastomosis. In the case of small
polar arteries, an evaluation of renal parenchyma perfusion can be done with intra-
arterial injection of indigo carmine (or methylene blue). The risk/benefit of reimplantation of polar arteries should be discussed based on the size of the perfused
zone and the diameter of the polar arteries as the arterial vascularization of the
kidney is terminal and non-reimplanted artery will lead to non-function of the perfused zone.

In the presence of multiple arteries, anastomosis can be done with a common
patch if the arterial ostia are closed to each other or with a dedicated patch if the
distance between the arterial ostia is too long.

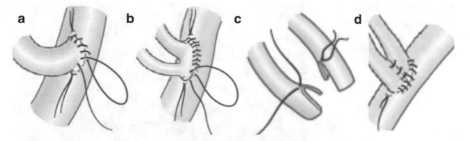

Fig. 6 Variations of renal artery anastomosis. (**a**) End-to-side anastomosis. (**b**) Two renal arteries on a patch. (**b**) Two arteries joined as a pantaloon

As an alternative to the classic end-to-side anastomosis of the graft artery on the external iliac artery, end-to-side anastomosis of the common iliac artery or end-to-end anastomosis with the internal iliac artery can be done.

Ureterovesical Anastomosis The Lich-Gregoir extravesical technique protected by a ureteral stent is preferred because it is fast to do, does not require a separate cystotomy, requires less ureteric length, and is associated with fewer urinary tract infections, fewer leaks, and less hematuria than intravesical techniques for minimization of urinary tract complications [16, 17]. Technically, a longitudinal oblique incision is made for approximately 2 cm until the bladder mucosa bulges into the incision. The bladder is partially drained via the urethral catheter, and the mucosa is dissected away from the muscularis on both sides to facilitate later creation of a submucosal tunnel for the ureter. The bladder mucosa is incised and 5-0 monofilament absorbable sutures are placed through both ends of the incision. The ureter is brought up to the wound, the mucosal sutures are passed through the toe and heel of the spatulated end, and the ureter is parachuted onto the bladder. The ureter is then anastomosed to the bladder mucosa with running sutures between the ureter and the mucosa of the bladder. Specifically, it is recommended to anchor the toe of the ureter with a horizontal or vertical mattress suture placed in the toe of the ureter and passed submucosally through the seromuscular layer of the bladder and tied about 5 mm distal to the cystotomy. Once the ureteric anastomosis has been completed, the seromuscular layer is closed over the ureter with interrupted absorbable sutures (Fig. 7).

Anastomosis of the native ureter in the pelvis of the graft is an alternative to ureterovesical anastomosis [18]. Absence of vesicoureteral reflux and/or reflux nephropathy is mandatory for performance of this technique and should be identified during the preoperative checkup. Ligation of the native ureter is well tolerated in the postoperative period, even in patients who still have residual diuresis and do not need excision of the native kidney.

Fig. 7 The ureter is fixed to the bladder mucosa with two running sutures and a double-J stent is placed into the urinary cavity

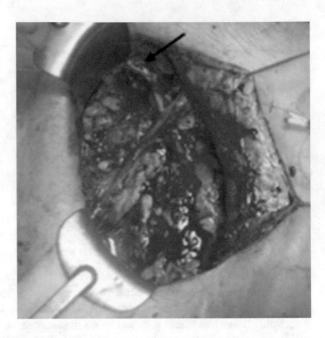

3 The Minimally Invasive Approach in Kidney Transplantation

A few attempts at *laparoscopic KT* have been reported [19–21], but the obvious limitations of laparoscopic suturing techniques have precluded widespread adoption of laparoscopy for renal transplantation.

In this scenario, robot-assisted kidney transplantation (RAKT) extends the options for recipients to minimally invasive techniques. RAKT is a safe technique with possible advantages such as low intra- and postoperative complication rates, better cosmetic results, and superlative vision that could result in better quality of the vascular and ureteral anastomoses [22–25].

4 Robot-Assisted Kidney Transplantation (RAKT)

In 2002 Hoznek et al. [26] described the possibility of performing a robotic anastomosis in KT, and in 2010 the first pure RAKT was performed by Giulianotti et al. [27] in the United States. In Europe, the first RAKT was performed in 2011 by Boggi et al. [28], who carried out the vascular anastomosis robotically and the ureteral reimplantation in open fashion. For this reason, the procedure may be considered as a "hybrid RAKT".

In 2014 Menon at al [29]. standardized the technique with use of the transperitoneal approach and regional hypothermia; this is known as the Vattikuti-Medanta technique as a result of the collaborative effort of Menon's team and the Medanta

Hospital team in India using the IDEAL (idea, development, exploration, assessment, and long-term monitoring) framework.

The initial European experience of pure RAKT was reported by Breda et al. [24] and Doumerc et al. [30], who, in 2015, performed the first two procedures in Spain and France respectively. In 2016 the ERUS RAKT working group was created by Dr. Alberto Breda with the aim of collecting and analyzing data from eight different European centers that perform RAKT. In 2017 the group was able to report the results in 120 patients, demonstrating that RAKT is associated with low complication rates, rapid recovery, and excellent graft function [31]. One year later, Territo et al. [32] addressed the functional results of RAKT from living donors at 1 year of follow-up. Until now, these are the largest series published on RAKT from living donations.

Furthermore, the ERUS group was able to analyze different scenarios for RAKT, such as RAKT using grafts with multiple vessels, described by Siena et al. [33]; the evaluation of RAKT in obese recipients, coordinated by colleagues from the University of Toulouse; and the RAKT program with grafts from deceased donors developed at the University of Florence (Italy) and reported by Vignolini et al. [34] Finally, the learning curve required in RAKT was studied by Gallioli et al. [35]

At our institution, we perform RAKT using a transperitoneal procedure which offers a greater field exposure while maintaining easier accessibility to iliac vessels for the anastomoses in comparison with an extraperitoneal approach.

However, the robotic extraperitoneal approach may potentially reduce gas filling-related consequences for the renal vasculature and the risk of bowel injuries. As regards graft introduction, it is usually carried out via a periumbilical incision, which is certainly the preferred option for obese patients. On the other hand, the Pfannenstiel incision may reduce the risk of incisional hernia and could be preferred in order to achieve better cosmetic results.

5   Key Steps in the RAKT Technique

When using the da Vinci Si® or X® system, the patient is positioned in the lithotomy position whereas if the da Vinci Xi® system is used, the patient is positioned in dorsal decubitus. A 20°–30° Trendelenburg position is recommended. A 12-mm camera port is inserted in the supraumbilical area and then the other three extra robotic 8-mm ports are placed under vision. Figure 8 shows the main steps of RAKT.

Accurate dissection of the external iliac vessels is performed and a retroperitoneal pouch is created to allocate the kidney and avoid pedicle torsion.

A GelPOINT® device replaces the camera trocar through a 6- to 8-cm periumbilical incision. This GelPOINT® device is used to introduce the graft and slushed ice in the abdominal cavity.

After clamping of the external iliac vein, a longitudinal venotomy using cold scissors is performed and an end-to-side anastomosis between the graft renal vein and the external iliac vein is created using a 6-0 continuous non-absorbable suture. Next, the graft vein is clamped and the bulldog clamps are removed from the

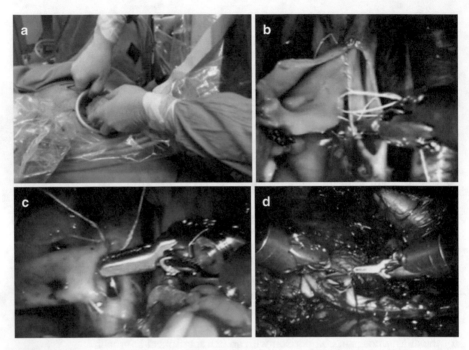

Fig. 8 Key steps in RAKT. (**a**) The graft is introduced into the abdominal cavity. (**b**) The graft renal vein is anastomosed in an end-to-side continuous fashion to the external iliac vein. (**c**) Arterial anastomosis. (**d**) Ureteroneocystostomy performed according to the Lich-Gregoir technique

external iliac vein and positioned on the external iliac artery, first proximally and then distally. The artery is incised with the cold scissors or a scalpel, and arterial anastomosis is then performed.

After completing the arterial anastomosis, a clamp is positioned on the graft artery while the external iliac artery is declamped. If no sign of bleeding is observed, the graft vein and artery are declamped.

After flipping the kidney on the psoas and retroperitonealization of the graft, the ureteroneocystostomy is performed according to the Lich-Gregoir technique using a Monocryl or PDS 5-0 continuous suture. A double J stent is inserted to protect the anastomosis and removed after 3 weeks.

6 Anatomic Variants and Challenges in Kidney Transplantation

6.1 Grafts with Multiple Vessels

Anatomic variations in the renal vasculature are common, being reported in 25–40% of kidneys. Supernumerary or accessory renal arteries and, to a lesser extent, renal veins, represent the most common variations [36]. Several retrospective studies, using different techniques for vascular reconstruction, have demonstrated the feasibility and safety of KT using grafts with multiple vessels (GMV) [37, 38].

GMV pose a technical challenge for KT. Previous studies have reported a potential increased rate of ureteral complications for grafts with accessory lower pole arteries, although this is still matter of controversy [39–41].

When using GMV, the following reconstruction techniques have been employed according to the case-specific vascular anatomy:

– Conjoined (side-to-side) arterial anastomosis (in a pantaloon fashion—Fig. 3), in cases with multiple renal arteries of almost equal caliber;
– Reimplantation (end-to-side) of a polar artery into the main renal artery;
– A combination of these techniques in the presence of more than two renal arteries and/or complex vascular anatomy;
– Ligation during bench surgery of small accessory renal arteries supplying the upper pole and with a diameter of less than 2–3 mm. Grafts with one artery and one vein after ligation of small accessory arteries are not considered grafts with multiple vessels.

The advantages of robotic technology for accurate vascular anastomoses are crucial also in cases of KT using GMV (Fig. 9). In these cases, the surgeon may decide to perform either extracorporeal reconstruction of graft vessels according to the specific graft and recipient anatomic characteristics. Moreover, robotic surgery may allow performance of precise vascular anastomoses even in the case of multiple vessels of very small caliber.

In experienced hands, RAKT using grafts with multiple vessels proved technically feasible and achieved optimal perioperative and early functional outcomes comparable to those of RAKT using grafts with conventional vascular anatomy [33]. Indeed, using appropriate vascular reconstruction techniques and a standardized operative protocol for RAKT [31], it was possible to perform single arterial and venous anastomoses in most cases, thereby reducing rewarming time and total ischemia time.

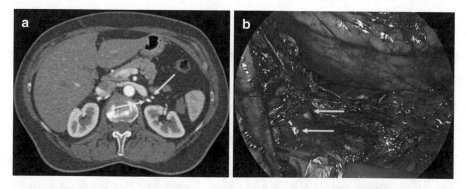

Fig. 9 (a) CT scan showing a double artery in the left kidney. (b) Laparoscopic dissection of the left renal arteries in preparation for the living donor nephrectomy

Despite longer cold and total ischemia times, probably reflecting the longer time required for extracorporeal bench vascular reconstruction, RAKT using GMV from living donors provided optimal early functional results that were comparable to those of RAKT using grafts with single vessels.

6.2   Obese Recipients

Many transplant centers tend to consider obese recipients unsuitable for KT because open surgery presents several challenges: access to the external iliac vessels, prolonged surgery and vascular anastomosis time, increased risk of surgical site complications (i.e., wound infection, lymphocele formation), and delayed graft function [42–45]. In view of these considerations, KT recipients and the obese population affected by ESRD are potentially the ideal candidates for a minimally invasive approach that avoids delay of transplant surgery due to the need to first perform bariatric surgery. In this context it is to be borne in mind that KT in obese recipients improves long-term survival and enhances quality of life, even though obesity is strongly associated with reduced long-term patient survival and graft failure, unlike non-obesity [46, 47].

Since the first case of RAKT in an obese recipient was reported in 2010 [27], more recent studies [48–50] have evaluated the feasibility and safety of RAKT in obese recipients in comparison with OKT. The ERUS RAKT working group analyzed data from 169 RAKT, dividing the population of recipients into three groups according to body mass index (BMI): obese recipients, BMI $\geq$ 30; overweight recipients, 25 < BMI < 30; non-overweight recipients, BMI < 25. They reported no statistically significant difference in console time or median times to complete arterial, venous, and ureterovesical anastomoses, and minor and major postoperative complication rates were similar between the groups. RAKT may, then, provide optimal graft function with a low complication rate and could represent a preferable surgical approach in patients with a high BMI. However, further studies and larger series are needed to confirm long-term functional outcomes.

6.3   Robotic Management of Atherosclerotic Plaques

The absence of touch or haptic feedback to the operating surgeon on the robotic console results in disadvantages with respect to the elimination of force and tactile cues [51]. The lack of tactile feedback in RAKT may be considered an important limitation of this emerging approach. The recipients, especially when in hemodialysis, have a high incidence of arterial atherosclerosis [52, 53], and since most of them have severe and multiple arterial calcified plaques, the absence of tactile feedback can potentially compromise arterial clamping and/or vascular anastomosis, with consequent further risk of distal embolism and/or thrombosis.

A CT scan is usually required to assess the presence of vascular calcifications and abnormalities but haptic aid always represents an additional diagnostic weapon that cannot be used with a robotic approach. In patients with severe calcification of the iliac and femoral artery, perfusion of the lower limb should be checked regularly to rule out plaque disruption and arterial embolism.

6.4 Maintenance of Cold Ischemia in KT

In both open and robotic KT, the most important aim is patient and graft survival. Graft function may be affected by ischemia/reperfusion injury and the ischemia time [54]. In order to protect the graft during vascular anastomosis in KT and avoid the risk of ischemia/reperfusion injury and, consequently, delayed graft function, ice slush is commonly used to maintain a low temperature. In order to keep the graft temperature below 20 °C before graft revascularization, some authors [29] have described the use of a gauze jacket filled with ice slush to cover the graft and modified Toomey syringes to introduce ice slush into the abdominal cavity on the kidney surface while performing vascular anastomosis. The limitation of this cooling approach is the gradual intra-abdominal melting of ice and the only partial control of the kidney temperature due to incomplete graft covering with ice, which might result in renal allograft impairment when there is an extended vascular anastomosis time. Another potential concern relates to potential injury generated by the ice slush as a result of development of local or systemic hypothermia. In particular, ileus has been reported to be a potential complication of local hypothermia, demonstrating that the ice slush could damage bowel function [55].

6.5 Grafts from Deceased Donors

RAKT from deceased donors faces primarily logistical challenges. Due to the time frame of organ preservation, it can be considered an unforeseeable "emergency" robotic procedure, which requires a structured multidisciplinary framework.

To fill this gap and move the field forward, the University of Florence group has recently developed a RAKT program from deceased donors that aims to safely and progressively increase the pool of patients who may benefit from minimally invasive KT[34].

The cornerstones of this program are:

– Extensive experience in OKT and robotic urologic surgery;
– A codified technique for RAKT [31];
– Structured modular training in RAKT, including e-learning, simulation, dry lab, wet lab, and training on animal models;

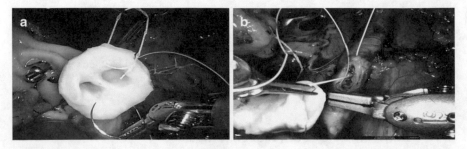

Fig. 10 RAKT from cadaveric donor. In (**a**) and (**b**) arterial anastomoses with and without Carrol's patch, respectively

- The availability of a multidisciplinary team (comprising urologists, anesthesiologists, nephrologists, and radiologists, as well as operating room support staff and nurses) with experience in KT and robotic surgery;
- The opportunity to perform RAKT at night and/or during the weekend in a dedicated operating room [34].

To date, exclusion criteria for RAKT from deceased donors include: age less than 18 years, severe comorbidities with contraindications to robotic surgery, significant atherosclerotic plaques at the level of the external iliac vessels, highly complex vascular graft anatomy (likely to require multiple anastomoses), multiple previous abdominal surgeries, and previous KT.

A specific challenge in the case of RAKT from deceased donors is management of the Carrel's patch for arterial anastomosis (Fig. 10). From a technical point of view, and thanks to the robotic platform, removing the Carrel's patch may provide the opportunity to perform a shorter arteriotomy, a more anatomic anastomosis thanks to the similar caliber of the graft renal artery and external iliac artery, with reduced risk of atherosclerotic plaques at the level of the graft renal artery (as compared with Carrel's aortic patch). The preliminary experience with robotic KT using grafts from deceased donors suggests that, mirroring the technique used in the setting of living donation, performance of arterial anastomosis without Carrol's patch is technically feasible and appears safer, especially in the presence of atherosclerotic plaques at the level of the renal artery's ostium [34].

References

1. Wolfe RA, Ashby VB, Milford EL, et al. Comparison of mortality in all patients on dialysis, patients on dialysis awaiting transplantation, and recipients of a first cadaveric transplant. N Engl J Med. 1999 Dec 2;341(23):1725–30.
2. Axelrod DA, Schnitzler MA, Xiao H, et al. An economic assessment of contemporary kidney transplant practice. Am J Transplant. 2018 May;18(5):1168–76.
3. Kootstra G, Daemen JH, Oomen AP. Categories of non-heart-beating donors. Transplant Proc. 1995 Oct;27(5):2893–4.

4. Detry O, Le Dinh H, Noterdaeme T, et al. Categories of donation after cardiocirculatory death. Transplant Proc. 2012 Jun;44(5):1189–95.
5. Liem YS, Weimar W. Early living-donor kidney transplantation: a review of the associated survival benefit. Transplantation. 2009 Feb 15;87(3):317–8.
6. Hariharan S, Johnson CP, Bresnahan BA, et al. Improved graft survival after renal transplantation in the United States, 1988 to 1996. N Engl J Med. 2000 Mar 2;342(9):605–12.
7. Banasik M. Living donor transplantation—the real gift of life. Procurement and the ethical assessment. Ann Transplant. 2006;11(1):4–6.
8. Wang K, Zhang P, Xu X, et al. Right Versus Left Laparoscopic Living-Donor Nephrectomy: A Meta-Analysis. Exp Clin Transplant. 2015 Jun;13(3):214–26.
9. Kumar A, Chaturvedi S, Gulia A, et al. Laparoscopic live donor nephrectomy: comparison of outcomes right versus left. Transplant Proc. 2018 Oct;50(8):2327–32.
10. Khalil A, Mujtaba MA, Taber TE, et al. Trends and outcomes in right vs. left living donor nephrectomy: an analysis of the OPTN/UNOS database of donor and recipient outcomes—should we be doing more right-sided nephrectomies? Clin Transpl. 2016 Feb;30(2):145–53.
11. Rampersad C, Patel P, Koulack J, et al. Back-to-back comparison of mini-open vs. laparoscopic technique for living kidney donation. Can Urol Assoc J. 2016 Aug;10(7-8):253–7.
12. Lennerling A, Lovén C, Dor FJ, et al. Living organ donation practices in Europe—results from an online survey. Transpl Int. 2013 Feb;26(2):145–53.
13. Harper JD, Leppert JT, Breda A, et al. Standardized linear port configuration to improve operative ergonomics in laparoscopic renal and adrenal surgery: experience with 1264 cases. J Endourol. 2011 Nov;25(11):1769–73.
14. Levi Sandri GB, de Werra E, Mascianà G, et al. The use of robotic surgery in abdominal organ transplantation: A literature review. Clin Transplant. 2017 Jan;31(1).
15. Giacomoni A, Di Sandro S, Lauterio A, et al. Robotic nephrectomy for living donation: surgical technique and literature systematic review. Am J Surg. 2016 Jun;211(6):1135–42.
16. Rodríguez Faba O, Boissier R, Budde K, et al. European association of urology guidelines on renal transplantation: update 2018. Eur Urol Focus. 2018 Mar;4(2):208–15.
17. Slagt IK, Dor FJ, Tran TC, et al. A randomized controlled trial comparing intravesical to extravesical ureteroneocystostomy in living donor kidney transplantation recipients. Kidney Int. 2014 Feb;85(2):471–7.
18. Timsit MO, Lalloué F, Bayramov A, et al. Should routine pyeloureterostomy be advocated in adult kidney transplantation? A prospective study of 283 recipients. J Urol. 2010 Nov;184(5):2043–8.
19. Bluebond-Langner R, Rha KH, Pinto PA, et al. Laparoscopic-assisted renal autotransplantation. Urology. 2004 May;63(5):853–6.
20. Rosales A, Salvador JT, Urdaneta G, et al. Laparoscopic kidney transplantation. Eur Urol. 2010 Jan;57(1):164–7.
21. Modi P, Pal B, Modi J, et al. Retroperitoneoscopic living-donor nephrectomy and laparoscopic kidney transplantation: experience of initial 72 cases. Transplantation. 2013 Jan 15;95(1):100–5.
22. Pein U, Girndt M, Markau S, et al. Minimally invasive robotic versus conventional open living donor kidney transplantation. World J Urol. 2020 Mar;38(3):795–802.
23. Territo A, Mottrie A, Abaza R, et al. Robotic kidney transplantation: current status and future perspectives. Minerva Urol Nefrol. 2017 Feb;69(1):5–13.
24. Breda A, Gausa L, Territo A, et al. Robotic-assisted kidney transplantation: our first case. World J Urol. 2016 Mar;34(3):443–7.
25. Breda A, Territo A, Gausa L, et al. Robotic kidney transplantation: one year after the beginning. World J Urol. 2017 Oct;35(10):1507–15.
26. Hoznek A, Zaki SK, Samadi DB, et al. Robotic assisted kidney transplantation: an initial experience. J Urol. 2002 Apr;167(4):1604–6.
27. Giulianotti P, Gorodner V, Sbrana F, et al. Robotic transabdominal kidney transplantation in a morbidly obese patient. Am J Transplant. 2010 Jun;10(6):1478–82.

28. Boggi U, Vistoli F, Signori S, et al. Robotic renal transplantation: first European case. Transpl Int. 2011 Feb;24(2):213–8.
29. Menon M, Sood A, Bhandari M, et al. Robotic kidney transplantation with regional hypothermia: a step-by-step description of the Vattikuti Urology Institute-Medanta technique (IDEAL phase 2a). Eur Urol. 2014 May;65(5):991–1000.
30. Doumerc N, Roumiguié M, Rischmann P, et al. Totally robotic approach with transvaginal insertion for kidney transplantation. Eur Urol. 2015 Dec;68(6):1103–4.
31. Breda A, Territo A, Gausa L, et al. Robot-assisted kidney transplantation: The European experience. Eur Urol. 2018 Feb;73(2):273–81.
32. Territo A, Gausa L, Alcaraz A, et al. European experience of robot-assisted kidney transplantation: minimum of 1-year follow-up. BJU Int. 2018 Aug;122(2):255–62.
33. Siena G, Campi R, Decaestecker K, et al. Robot-assisted kidney transplantation with regional hypothermia using grafts with multiple vessels after extracorporeal vascular reconstruction: results from the European association of urology robotic urology section working group. Eur Urol Focus. 2018 Mar;4(2):175–84.
34. Vignolini G, Campi R, Sessa F, et al. Development of a robot-assisted kidney transplantation programme from deceased donors in a referral academic centre: technical nuances and preliminary results. BJU Int. 2019 Mar;123(3):474–84.
35. Gallioli A, Territo A, Boissier R, et al. Learning curve in robot-assisted kidney transplantation: results from the European Robotic urological society working group. Eur Urol. 2020 Jan 9. pii: S0302-2838(19)30947-9.
36. Makiyama K, Tanabe K, Ishida H, et al. Successful renovascular reconstruction for renal allografts with multiple renal arteries. Transplantation. 2003 Mar 27;75(6):828–32.
37. Novick AC, Magnusson M, Braun WE. Multiple-artery renal transplantation: emphasis on extracorporeal methods of donor arterial reconstruction. J Urol. 1979 Dec;122(6):731–5.
38. Osman Y, Shokeir A, Ali-el-Dein B, et al. Vascular complications after live donor renal transplantation: study of risk factors and effects on graft and patient survival. J Urol. 2003 Mar;169(3):859–62.
39. Oh HK, Hawasli A, Cousins G. Management of renal allografts with multiple renal arteries resulting from laparoscopic living donor nephrectomy. Clin Transpl. 2003 Aug;17(4):353–7.
40. Kok NF, Dols LF, Hunink MG, et al. Complex vascular anatomy in live kidney donation: imaging and consequences for clinical outcome. Transplantation. 2008 Jun 27;85(12):1760–5.
41. Carter JT, Freise CE, McTaggart RA, et al. Laparoscopic procurement of kidneys with multiple renal arteries is associated with increased ureteral complications in the recipient. Am J Transplant. 2005 Jun;5(6):1312–8.
42. Lafranca JA, IJzermans JN, Betjes MG, et al. Body mass index and outcome in renal transplant recipients: a systematic review and meta-analysis. BMC Med. 2015 May 12;13:111.
43. Nicoletto BB, Fonseca NK, Manfro RC, et al. Effects of obesity on kidney transplantation outcomes: a systematic review and meta-analysis. Transplantation. 2014 Jul 27;98(2):167–76.
44. Furriel F, Parada B, Campos L, et al. Pretransplantation overweight and obesity: does it really affect kidney transplantation outcomes? Transplant Proc. 2011 Jan-Feb;43(1):95–9.
45. Tran MH, Foster CE, Kalantar-Zadeh K, et al. Kidney transplantation in obese patients. World J Transplant. 2016 Mar 24;6(1):135–43.
46. Gill JS, Lan J, Dong J, et al. The survival benefit of kidney transplantation in obese patients. Am J Transplant. 2013 Aug;13(8):2083–90.
47. Glanton CW, Kao TC, Cruess D, et al. Impact of renal transplantation on survival in end-stage renal disease patients with elevated body mass index. Kidney Int. 2003 Feb;63(2):647–53.
48. Spaggiari M, Lendacki FR, Di Bella C, et al. Minimally invasive, robot-assisted procedure for kidney transplantation among morbidly obese: Positive outcomes at 5 years post-transplant. Clin Transpl. 2018 Nov;32(11):e13404.
49. Garcia-Roca R, Garcia-Aroz S, Tzvetanov I, et al. Single center experience with robotic kidney transplantation for recipients with BMI of 40 kg/m^2 or greater: a comparison with the UNOS registry. Transplantation. 2017 Jan;101(1):191–6.

50. Oberholzer J, Giulianotti P, Danielson KK, et al. Minimally invasive robotic kidney transplantation for obese patients previously denied access to transplantation. Am J Transplant. 2013 Mar;13(3):721–8.
51. Amirabdollahian F, Livatino S, Vahedi B, et al. Prevalence of haptic feedback in robot-mediated surgery: a systematic review of literature. J Robot Surg. 2018 Mar;12(1):11–25.
52. Benz K, Hilgers KF, Daniel C, et al. Vascular calcification in chronic kidney disease: the role of inflammation. Int J Nephrol. 2018 Aug 13;2018:4310379.
53. Cianciolo G, Capelli I, Angelini ML, et al. Importance of vascular calcification in kidney transplant recipients. Am J Nephrol. 2014;39(5):418–26.
54. Hellegering J, Visser J, Kloke HJ, et al. Deleterious influence of prolonged warm ischemia in living donor kidney transplantation. Transplant Proc. 2012 Jun;44(5):1222–6.
55. Tuğcu V, Şener NC, Şahin S, et al. Robotic kidney transplantation: The Bakırköy experience. Turk J Urol. 2016 Dec;42(4):295–8.

Sacral Neuromodulation

Marco Torella, Antonio Schiattarella, Nicola Colacurci, and A. Di Gesu

Sacral nerve modulation (SNM) is a procedure used to treat patients with bladder and/or bowels conditions. Neuromodulation is based on the theory that a constant low amplitude stimulation directly or indirectly through the sacral nerve roots results in ascending signals to the micturition centers that modulate efferent signals to both the bladder and bowel. This treatment is usually offered as a third-line therapy after conservative treatments, lifestyle modification, and oral drugs have failed. The first neuromodulation procedure was performed in 1954 as deep brain stimulation (DBS) for the treatment of chronic pain. In 1988, Tanagho and Schmidt introduced SNM for lower urinary tract dysfunction (LUTD) therapy, including OAB treatment [1]. The Food and Drug Administration (FDA) approved SNM for the treatment of refractory OAB, frequency, and non-obstructive post-void residual urinary retention in 1997 and 1999. Recently, rechargeable and conditional magnetic resonance imaging (MRI)-safe devices (Axonics r-SNM SystemTM, Irvine, CA) have been introduced in both Europe and USA. The clinical effectiveness of this system appears to be similar to that of the current recharge-free InterStimTM II device (Medtronic, Minneapolis, MN). However, newer InterStim devices have been submitted for CE mark and FDA approval in order to improve patient preference and provide full-body MRI safety for both 1.5 and 3 Tesla with the latter field strength having become the clinical standard. Rechargeable batteries result in smaller volume implantable pulse generators (IPGs). These may result in more comfort for patients with low body mass index (BMI), and the much smaller size will be more attractive to the patient than the current InterStim II IPG.

M. Torella (✉) · A. Schiattarella · N. Colacurci
Department of Woman, Child and General and Specialized Surgery,
University of Campania "Luigi Vanvitelli", Naples, Italy

A. Di Gesu
St. Mary's Hospital. Imperial College, Paddington, London, UK

© The Author(s), under exclusive license to Springer Nature
Switzerland AG 2021
D. Veneziano, E. Huri (eds.), *Urologic Surgery in the Digital Era*,
https://doi.org/10.1007/978-3-030-63948-8_6

1   Mechanism of Action

The mechanism of action of SNM is still unclear. However, the electrical stimulation modulates nerves that supply the bladder, bowels, urinary and anal sphincters, and pelvic floor muscles. The intensity and frequency of the pulses can be modified by both the physician and the patient through an external programmer. The S3 nerve root is a primary target for SNM therapy in that it contains afferent sensory nerve fibers to the pelvic floor and parasympathetic fibers of the detrusor. The effect of SNM appears to be modulated by the activation of somatic afferents that in turn inhibit bladder sensory pathways and reflex bladder hyperactivity [2]. A possible mechanism of action on pain relies on the gate control theory. The stimulation of bigger Aβ fibers, such as with pressure or tactile stimuli, may activate inhibiting interneurons that in turn reduce the activity of smaller nociceptive Aδ and C fibers. A lower urinary tract neural control is showed in Fig. 1.

Cats models suggest that the inhibition of bladder activity occurs primarily in the central nervous system (CNS) by inhibition of the ascending or descending pathways of the spino-bulbo-spinal micturition reflex [3]. A recent work applying functional magnetic resonance on women treated with SNM for overactive bladder evidenced that SNM may directly influence brain activity [4]. The increasing of stimulation amplitude determined a progressive overall brain activation. A subsensory stimulation determined the deactivation of the pons and periaqueductal gray matter, with stable activation of the right inferior frontal gyrus. A sensory stimulation determined the activation of the insula and the deactivation of the medial and

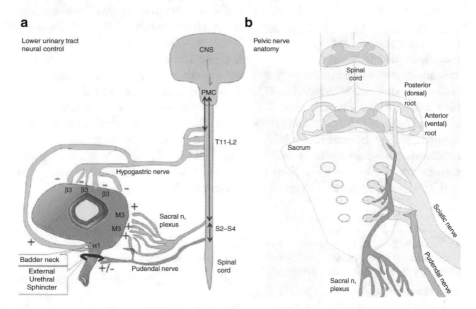

Fig. 1 Lower urinary tract neural control. *CNS* Central Nervous System, *PMC* Pontine micturition center

Fig. 2 Apposition of the sacral nerve stimulator

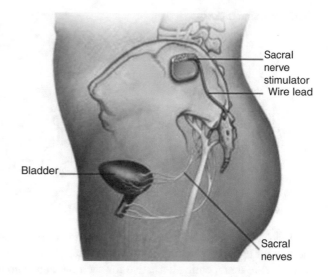

superior parietal lobes. A suprasensory stimulation determined the activation of multiple structures and the expected S3 somatosensory region. The device is inserted into the lower part of your back and is made up of a wire and a battery.

SNM comes in two stages: a basic evaluation (test phase) and a full system implant (permanent implant) (Fig. 2).

2 Indications

SNM is indicated for the treatment of urinary retention and symptoms of overactive bladder, including urinary incontinence and significant symptoms of urinary frequency, alone or in combination, in patients in whom more conservative therapies have failed or were not tolerated.

At the moment, the InterStim device (Medtronic, Fridley, MN) is the only FDA approved implantable SNM device for treatment of refractory urgency urinary incontinence, urgency-frequency, non-obstructive urinary retention and fecal incontinence (Fig. 3). It is also indicated for the treatment of chronic fecal incontinence (FI) in patients who have failed or are not candidates for more conservative treatments.

A Cochrane Review by Thaha et al. reported that SNM could improve continence in patients with fecal incontinence [5]. However, the study added that SNM did not improve symptoms in patients with constipation. SMN has also been evaluated as a fourth line treatment option for refractory interstitial cystitis/bladder pain syndrome (IC/BPS) [6]. Chronic pelvic pain and constipation is another area where off-label use of SNM has been trialed [7, 8]. Fowler's Syndrome or a primary disorder of external urethral sphinter relaxation, has been studied as a target for SNM [9].

Fig. 3 InterStim II Device

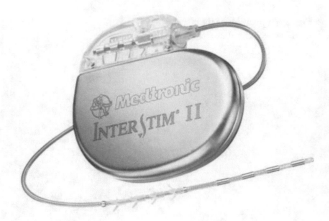

A study by Schober et al. proposed that sacral nerve stimulation is a valid adjunctive therapy for refractory pediatric lower urinary tract dysfunction [10]. SNM can constitute a safe therapeutic alternative for such patients who have undergone multiple failed treatments in their medical history. A meta-analysis performed by Kessler et al., which included patients with multiple sclerosis, Parkinson's disease, cerebrovascular accidents, spinal cord injuries, and other neurogenic LUTDs, revealed a success rate of 68% for the test phase and 92% for permanent neuromodulation [11].

3   Contraindications

SNM presents several contraindications such as:

- Mechanical outlet obstruction
- Diathermy use (shortwave, microwave, ultrasound)
- Inadequate response to test stimulation or inability to operate the device
- Magnetic resonance represents a relative contraindication for non-cranial indication.

However, safety and efficacy have not been determined for other conditions such as:

- Bilateral stimulation
- Pregnancy
- Unborn fetus and delivery
- Age younger than 16 years
- Patients with neurologic conditions such as multiple sclerosis

4 Precautions

The SNM system could adversely affect cardiac devices, electrocautery, defibrillators, ultrasonic equipment, radiation therapy, magnetic resonance imaging, theft detectors, and screening devices.

Individuals with very low perception thresholds may perceive fluctuations in the stimulation intensity as the battery nears depletion and may have to increase or decrease the amplitude to maintain symptom control. Patients should carry a control device at all times to be able to adjust and/or turn off the device.

The control device may affect other implanted devices and should not be placed over other implanted devices. The patient programmer should not be immersed in liquid or cleaned with bleach, nail polish remover, mineral oil, or other similar substances. When the programmer is in use, flammable or explosive atmospheres should be avoided.

5 Warnings

Sources of strong electromagnetic interference can result in dangerous injuries from heating of the implanted Interstim components and damage to surrounding tissue, damage to the Interstim requiring replacement, operational changes causing it to turn on or off or to reset to power-on-reset (POR) settings, and unexpected changes in stimulation causing an increase in stimulation or intermittent stimulation.

Damage to the case may result in leakage of battery chemicals, which can cause severe burns. The Interstim may affect the function of other implanted devices such as cardiac devices, other neurostimulators, and implantable drug pumps. To minimize interactions with cardiac devices, the Interstim should be programmed to bipolar configuration and a minimum rate of 60 Hertz and the cardiac device programmed to bipolar sensing. Defibrillators, when active, may damage the Interstim device. Activities that involve sudden, excessive, or repetitive bending, twisting, bouncing, or stretching (eg, gymnastics, mountain biking) can cause fracture or dislodgement.

Manipulation or rubbing of the system through the skin may result in damage to the system, lead dislodgement, skin erosion, or uncomfortable stimulation at the implant site.

Patients should not scuba dive below 10 meters (33 feet) or enter hyperbaric chambers of more than 2.0 atmospheres absolute (ATA). High altitudes do not affect the neurostimulator. However, skydiving or hiking may cause stress on the system, causing lead dislodgement or fractures.

6 Basic Evaluation Phase

Prior to the test phase, the patient is asked to complete a voiding diary, which will serve as a baseline. The initial test phase may be performed in the office or the operating room.

The test stimulator has 3 components.

- White verifier which is connected to the patient via a white cable and this delivers the stimulation.
- Handheld controller which is a touch screen and used to alter the intensity of the stimulation or to turn the device on/off.
- Thin wire which is inserted into the bottom of patient's back/spine in the sacrum.

The patient is placed in a prone position, and his or her lower back and gluteal region are prepared and draped. Socks are removed so that the physician can visualize the feet.

A portable c-arm and fluoroscopy are used to identify the midline of the spine and level of the S3 foramen. The skin is marked, and the area infiltrated with local anesthetic. A 20-gauge, 3.5-inch insulated foramen needle is then inserted into the S3 foramen on each side at a 60° angle relative to the skin under fluoroscopic guidance. A lateral image can be used to confirm the location and depth in the foramen.

The needles are then stimulated to confirm appropriate positioning. If the needles are in the correct position, there will be bellows contraction of the pelvic floor due to contraction of the levator muscles and plantar flexion of the great toe. The patient, if awake, will be able to confirm correct positioning with contraction or tingling of the pelvic floor muscles. If the needles are in the S2 foramen, plantar flexion of the whole foot with lateral rotation will occur with stimulation. If the needles are in the S4 foramen, there will be no lower extremity movement despite bellows response (Fig. 4).

Fig. 4 Needles apposition in sacral region

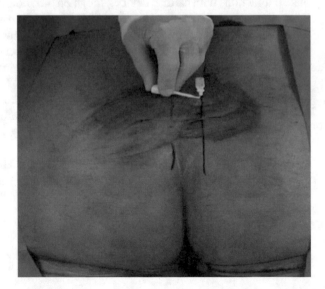

Once correct positioning of the needles has been confirmed, temporary lead wires are passed through the foramen needles, and the needles are removed carefully to prevent dislodgement of the leads. The temporary leads with unipolar electrodes are steri-stripped to the patient's back and a dressing placed.

The patient then goes home with an external stimulator after instruction regarding its use. Prophylactic antibiotics are often given while the temporary leads are in place. The temporary leads are typically left in place for 5–7 days while the patient completes treatment voiding diaries.

The patient should be instructed to avoid bending, stretching, or lifting heavy objects during the initial trial period to decrease the risk of wire dislodgment. The patient's response to treatment is compared to the baseline voiding diary. If the change in symptoms is 50% or greater, he or she is a candidate for placement of the permanent stimulator.

7 Advanced Evaluation (Tined Lead Test)

In some cases, with a not optimal test phase, maybe because the wire moved out of position early in the trial, an advanced evaluation with a tined lead could be performed. An advanced evaluation involves having the permanent tined lead/wire inserted in theatre with you asleep, but once again connected up to an external battery pack as described in the basic evaluation section. The benefit of this is that the permanent wire has small fixation points on it, called tines, which make it less likely to migrate out of position during the trial phase. The disadvantage of an advanced evaluation is that the wire needs to be put in in the operating room/theatre initially and you will then require a second surgical appointment 2–4 weeks after the insertion to either remove the wire if it has not worked, or attach the neurostimulator (battery) to the wire if you have had a significant improvement in symptoms. The process of lead insertion and subsequent neurostimulator attachment are outlined in the full system implant section below.

8 Permanent Implant Implant Phase

The second phase involves implantation of the permanent device. The InterStim device consists of:

- An implantable nerve stimulator (inside which is the battery) is inserted under the skin (just larger than a £2 coin). Usually in the buttock area.
- An electrode or thin wire with barbs/tines that carries the electrical pulses to the bladder nerves.
- A hand-held patient programmer that enables you to adjust the level of the stimulation and allows you to turn your implant on or off.

This is performed in the operating room under anesthesia. The patient is placed in a prone position and prepared and draped in a sterile fashion. Perioperative antibiotics are administered. The next step depends on whether a permanent quadripolar lead was placed during the first phase (often the case if the first phase is performed in the operating room) or temporary leads were placed (office based first phase). If the permanent quadripolar was placed during the first phase, the second phase is quick and does not require fluoroscopy. The incision where the temporary connector was placed in the buttock is opened and the permanent implantable pulse generator (IPG) is connected to the lead and buried in a deep subcutaneous pocket in the right buttock. It is important to ensure the IPG is functioning properly prior to closure of the incision. If the first phase was performed in the office and temporary leads are in place, fluoroscopy will be needed, and the quadripolar lead is placed on the side on which the patient had the best in-office test response. The lead is tunneled deeply through the subcutaneous fat to an incision in the buttock region, where the IPG will be placed. The lead is connected to the IPG and buried in the deep subcutaneous pocket.

9   Surgical Technique

The surgical technique involves placement of a quadripolar lead at the superior medial location of the S3 foramen with a standard transcutaneous image-guided approach, using a tined lead and a stylet. The curved stylet is an innovation from the straight stylet, allowing closer association with the S3 nerve and ultimately a higher percentage of therapeutic success. For lead placement, the goal is to achieve motor responses at low amplitudes (<2 mA) on all four electrodes. The optimal motor response needed for a successful lead placement continues to be an area of ongoing research. Gilleran et al. argued that obtaining motor responses in less than 4 electrodes does not negatively affect the rates of progressing to full implant or short-term revision rates [12].

Meanwhile, Pizarro et al. indicated that a higher number of electrodes that produced a toe motor response was associated with a lower likelihood of future lead revision while the higher number of bellows responses did not have the same association [13]. Thus, optimization of SNM lead placement is ongoing; however, the high rates of progression to full implant and efficacy for FDA-approved indications have been well established.

10   Monitoring & Follow-up

Once implanted, the neurostimulator is activated. The physician initially programs the device and adjusts the stimulator to optimize the therapy for each patient. The patient will also need instructions to adjust the intensity of the stimulation. Once an optimal strength and intensity of pulse stimulation has been determined, the patient can modulate the stimulator for maximal response. Periodic follow-up, usually every 6–12 months, is recommended to monitor the therapy's effectiveness.

11 Adverse Events

Several adverse events have been reported such as:

- Infections in lead site
- Migration of device
- Malfunctioning
- Pain at implantation site
- Spontaneous resolved seroma
- Surgical revision

Rare:

- urinary tract infections
- electrical shock sensation
- foreign-body sensation
- lower-limb numbness.

12 Outcomes

SNM has shown to achieve good long-term success in many patients, better than previous treatment methods. A review of neuromodulation devices showed at the long-term (>1 year) clinical response rates of SNM for urge incontinence and urgency frequency ranging around 50% or higher [14].

A study reported that 30% of patients had adverse effects with the most common being undesirable change in stimulation, 12% long-term complications of the SNM device showed that within the first 5 years about 30–40% of the devices had to be removed or replaced [15]. The main adverse events were pain at stimulator site, lead migration, infection or malfunctioning. However, if compared to drug therapies in OAB patients, SNS is considered more expensive, but more effective in a two-year period [16]. Carone et al. proved that SNM is effective and safe third-line treatments for OAB, non-obstructive urinary retention, and chronic pelvic pain/IC. The overall success rate of SNM ranges from 43% to 85%. The technique has demonstrated to be safe, with a low rate of complications and need of reintervention [17].

The InSite study trial showed a reduction of >50% of urinary leaks with a success rate of 76%, compared to standard medical therapy (SMT) that assessed at 49% (p = 0.002) [18]. A 3-years prospective evaluation of efficacy of the SNM arm was performed: the group of patients suffering of urgency incontinence, 43% returned to complete continence (p < 0.001), and there was a significant reduction of leaks episodes (from 3.1 ± 2.7 to 2.1 ± 2.3/24 h, p < 0.001). In the group of patients suffering of urgency without incontinence episodes, 66% of patients returned to a normal voiding frequency, with a significant reduction in number of voids/day (from 12.6 ± 4.5 to 4.8 ± 4.1) [19].

The ROSETTA trial (Refractory Overactive Bladder: Sacral Neuromodulation vs Botulinum Toxin Assessment), enrolled women suffering of OAB and randomized to two arms, SNM, and botulinum toxin injection. After a follow-up of 6 months, the results showed that both techniques lead to a significant decline in the main number of daily urgency incontinence events, which was greater for the botulinum toxin arm (−3.89 (−4.26/−3.52) vs −3.25 (−3.64/−2.87)). However, the Botulinum toxin arm was afflicted by a greater incidence of urinary tract infections (UTI), perhaps due to the higher need of self-intermittent catheterization [20]. Weil et al. in a smaller RCT, compared the results of SNM versus SMT with a follow-up of 18 months. It showed an increase in pad use in 85% of patients, with a significant reduction in leakage severity and mean number of leakage episodes [21]. Two smaller RCT by Hassouna et al. and Schmidt et al., compared the results of SNM to SMT with 6 months follow-up. The first study showed a significant reduction of daily number of voids in 56% of patients (vs 4% in the SMT group) and degree of urgency and a significant increase of voided volume per void (226 ± 124 vs 123 ± 75, p < 0.0001) [22]. The second study demonstrated a significant reduction in the daily number of urinary leakage (2.6 ± 5.1 vs 11.3 ± 5.9, p < 0.001) and leakage severity (0.03 ± 0.9 vs 3.9 ± 3.8, p < 0.0001) [23]. After the turn off of the stimulation, the results were comparable to baseline, pointing out that an active stimulation may be needed to achieve the curative effect of SNM.

Nobrega et al. demonstrated that a cohort of 99 consecutive patients with 47% response after first stage tined lead placement, that there was no significant difference in any urodynamic parameter between first stage success and failure groups. There was a tendency of having a lower compliance in the failure group, but it did not reach statistical significance [24]. Another study of Jadav et al., showed that female patients with pelvic floor dysfunction, demonstrated after a median 6.8 months follow-up a reduction on OAB symptoms from baseline with the use of ePAQ-PF score (20.9 ± 19.7 vs 28.5 ± 21.5, p < 0.05) with clinical benefit also in other domains such as bowel and sexual function [25]. Sutherland et al. in retrospective series of 83 patients treated with SNM with a mean follow-up of 22 months evidenced a decrease in daily mean number of voids (8.5 ± 5.0 vs 12.4 ± 5.1, p < 0.0001), mean night voids (1.6 ± 2.2 vs 2.3 ± 1.8, p = 0.0091), mean daily leakage episodes (1.0 ± 1.4 vs 5.0 ± 4.7, p < 0.0001), and number of daily pads (0.3 ± 0.7 vs 2.3 ± 2.6, p < 0.0001) [26]. In another retrospective study, Peeters et al. evidenced in a cohort of 104 patients, with a mean follow-up of 46.8 months, a significant decrease in urinary incontinence (70%) and urgency/frequency symptoms (68%). A smaller group of 94 patients suffered of idiopathic retention (32 patients with a diagnosis of Fowler's syndrome) and showed good results even in this peculiar subgroup with a success rate (symptom reduction >50%) of 73% in idiopathic retention and a cure rate of 62.5% in the Fowler's syndrome group and 53% in the remainder patients [27]. Another prospective study on 31 patients with non-obstructive urinary retention with a longer follow-up of 49.3 months showed a success rate of 58% with regard to the average number of daily catheters (1.9 ± 2.8 vs 5.3 ± 2.8, $p < 0.001$) and of 71% with regard to the average volume per catheter (109.2 ± 184.3 vs 379.9 ± 183.8, $p < 0.001$) [28]. There is a lower number of good quality studies on the treatment of IC/BPS with SNM. In a small retrospective study on 44 patients with IC/BPS with a long follow-up of 61.5 months, Gajewski and Al-Zahrani reported an 80% improvement of the global response assessment (GRA) and a 43% clinical success. They reported the need of surgical revision in 50% of patients, with an explant rate of 28%, in four cases due to painful stimulation [29]. A multicenter cross-sectional observational study evaluated the impact of pregnancy in SNM treatment. Roulette et al. enrolled a group of 21 women with SNM implant carrying 27 pregnancies. In all, 18.5% of women turned off the device while trying to conceive, all the remainder in the first trimester and during all pregnancy. Before pregnancy, SNM was effective in 76.19% of patients; during pregnancy, urinary symptoms were recurrent in all but one patient. In all, 74% of patients reactivated the SNM after pregnancy and 20% reported a reduction in efficacy, in two of four cases due to a displacement of the electrode. Three of four patients with chronic retention resumed self-catheterization and 25.9% of patients had complications, mainly UTI and one case of pelvic pain [30].

SNM is an effective therapy for CPP in both IC/BSP and non-IC/BSP patients, with better results in non-IC/BSP patients. Outcomes of the antegrade caudal approach were comparable with the standard retrograde approach [7]. SNM in women with pelvic floor disorders, especially bladder dysfunction, seems to have a positive effect on sexual function. Studies reported a positive effect of SNM on sexual function. Pooled analysis of data from 11 studies involving 573 patients before SNM and 438 patients after SNM showed significant improvement in sexual function [31]. SNM was superior to PTNS in Wexner score reduction and improvement in weekly FI episodes. SNM showed greater improvement in Fecal Incontinence Quality of Life (FIQL) domains of coping and depression as compared with PTNS [32].

References

1. Tanagho EA, Schmidt RA. Bladder pacemaker: scientific basis and clinical future. Urology. 1982;20:614–9. https://doi.org/10.1016/0090-4295(82)90312-0.
2. Abrams P, Blaivas JG, Fowler CJ, Fourcroy JL, Macdiarmid SA, Siegel SW, Van Kerrebroeck P. The role of neuromodulation in the management of urinary urge incontinence. BJU Int. 2003;91:355–9. https://doi.org/10.1046/j.1464-410x.2003.04105.x.
3. Yoshimura N, Chancellor MB. Neurophysiology of lower urinary tract function and dysfunction. Rev Urol. 2003;5(Suppl 8):S3–S10.
4. Dasgupta R, Critchley HD, Dolan RJ, Fowler CJ. Changes in brain activity following sacral neuromodulation for urinary retention. J Urol. 2005;174:2268–72. https://doi.org/10.1097/01.ju.0000181806.59363.d1.

5. Thaha MA, Abukar AA, Thin NN, Ramsanahie A, Knowles CH. Sacral nerve stimulation for faecal incontinence and constipation in adults. Cochrane database Syst Rev. 2015; CD004464, https://doi.org/10.1002/14651858.CD004464.pub3.
6. Han E, Nguyen L, Sirls L, Peters K. Current best practice management of interstitial cystitis/bladder pain syndrome. Ther Adv Urol. 2018;10:197–211. https://doi.org/10.1177/1756287218761574.
7. Mahran A, Baaklini G, Hassani D, Abolella HA, Safwat AS, Neudecker M, Hijaz AK, Mahajan ST, Siegel SW, El-Nashar SA. Sacral neuromodulation treating chronic pelvic pain: a meta-analysis and systematic review of the literature. Int Urogynecol J. 2019;30:1023–35. https://doi.org/10.1007/s00192-019-03898-w.
8. Maeda Y, Kamm MA, Vaizey CJ, Matzel KE, Johansson C, Rosen H, Baeten CG, Laurberg S. Long-term outcome of sacral neuromodulation for chronic refractory constipation. Tech Coloproctol. 2017;21:277–86. https://doi.org/10.1007/s10151-017-1613-0.
9. Swinn MJ, Kitchen ND, Goodwin RJ, Fowler CJ. Sacral neuromodulation for women with Fowler's syndrome. Eur Urol. 2000;38:439–43. https://doi.org/10.1159/000020321.
10. Schober MS, Sulkowski JP, Lu PL, Minneci PC, Deans KJ, Teich S, Alpert SA. Sacral nerve stimulation for pediatric lower urinary tract dysfunction: development of a standardized pathway with objective urodynamic outcomes. J Urol. 2015;194:1721–6. https://doi.org/10.1016/j.juro.2015.06.090.
11. Kessler TM, La Framboise D, Trelle S, Fowler CJ, Kiss G, Pannek J, Schurch B, Sievert K-D, Engeler DS. Sacral neuromodulation for neurogenic lower urinary tract dysfunction: systematic review and meta-analysis. Eur Urol. 2010;58:865–74. https://doi.org/10.1016/j.eururo.2010.09.024.
12. Gilleran JP, Killinger K, Boura J, Peters KM. Number of active electrodes at time of staged tined lead interstim implant does not impact clinical outcomes. Neurourol Urodyn. 2016;35:625–9. https://doi.org/10.1002/nau.22766.
13. Pizarro-Berdichevsky J, Gill BC, Clifton M, Okafor HT, Faris AE, Vasavada SP, Goldman HB. Motor response matters: optimizing lead placement improves sacral neuromodulation outcomes. J Urol. 2018;199:1032–6. https://doi.org/10.1016/j.juro.2017.11.066.
14. Yamashiro J, de Riese W, de Riese C. New Implantable tibial nerve stimulation devices: review of published clinical results in comparison to established neuromodulation devices. Res Reports Urol. 2019;11:351–7. https://doi.org/10.2147/RRU.S231954.
15. Janssen DA, Martens FM, de Wall LL, van Breda HM, Heesakkers JP. Clinical utility of neurostimulation devices in the treatment of overactive bladder: current perspectives. Med Devices (Auckl). 2017;10:109–22. https://doi.org/10.2147/MDER.S115678.
16. Sukhu T, Kennelly MJ, Kurpad R. Sacral neuromodulation in overactive bladder: a review and current perspectives. Res Reports Urol. 2016;8:193–9. https://doi.org/10.2147/RRU.S89544.
17. Ammirati E, Giammò A, Manassero A, Carone R. Neuromodulation in urology, state of the art. Urologia. 2019;86:177–82. https://doi.org/10.1177/0391560319866075.
18. Siegel S, Noblett K, Mangel J, Griebling TL, Sutherland SE, Bird ET, Comiter C, Culkin D, Bennett J, Zylstra S, et al. Results of a prospective, randomized, multicenter study evaluating sacral neuromodulation with InterStim therapy compared to standard medical therapy at 6-months in subjects with mild symptoms of overactive bladder. Neurourol Urodyn. 2015;34:224–30. https://doi.org/10.1002/nau.22544.
19. Siegel S, Noblett K, Mangel J, Griebling TL, Sutherland SE, Bird ET, Comiter C, Culkin D, Bennett J, Zylstra S, et al. Three-year follow-up results of a prospective, multicenter study in overactive bladder subjects treated with sacral neuromodulation. Urology. 2016;94:57–63. https://doi.org/10.1016/j.urology.2016.04.024.
20. Amundsen CL, Richter HE, Wallace D. Pelvic floor disorders network OnabotulinumtoxinA vs sacral neuromodulation for urgency incontinence-reply. JAMA. 2017;317:535–6. https://doi.org/10.1001/jama.2016.19566.
21. Weil EH, Ruiz-Cerdá JL, Eerdmans PH, Janknegt RA, Bemelmans BL, van Kerrebroeck PE. Sacral root neuromodulation in the treatment of refractory urinary urge inconti-

nence: a prospective randomized clinical trial. Eur Urol. 2000;37:161–71. https://doi.org/10.1159/000020134.

22. Hassouna MM, Siegel SW, Nÿeholt AA, Elhilali MM, van Kerrebroeck PE, Das AK, Gajewski JB, Janknegt RA, Rivas DA, Dijkema H, et al. Sacral neuromodulation in the treatment of urgency-frequency symptoms: a multicenter study on efficacy and safety. J Urol. 2000;163:1849–54.

23. Schmidt RA, Jonas U, Oleson KA, Janknegt RA, Hassouna MM, Siegel SW, van Kerrebroeck PE. Sacral nerve stimulation for treatment of refractory urinary urge incontinence. Sacral Nerve Stimulation Study Group. J Urol. 1999;162:352–7.

24. Nobrega RP, Solomon E, Jenks J, Greenwell T, Ockrim J. Predicting a successful outcome in sacral neuromodulation testing: are urodynamic parameters prognostic? Neurourol Urodyn. 2018;37:1007–10. https://doi.org/10.1002/nau.23383.

25. Jadav AM, Wadhawan H, Jones GL, Wheldon LW, Radley SC, Brown SR. Does sacral nerve stimulation improve global pelvic function in women? Color Dis. 2013;15:848–57. https://doi.org/10.1111/codi.12181.

26. Sutherland SE, Lavers A, Carlson A, Holtz C, Kesha J, Siegel SW. Sacral nerve stimulation for voiding dysfunction: one institution's 11-year experience. Neurourol Urodyn. 2007;26:19–28.; discussion 36. https://doi.org/10.1002/nau.20345.

27. Peeters K, Sahai A, De Ridder D, Van Der Aa F. Long-term follow-up of sacral neuromodulation for lower urinary tract dysfunction. BJU Int. 2014;113:789–94. https://doi.org/10.1111/bju.12571.

28. van Kerrebroeck PEV, van Voskuilen AC, Heesakkers JPFA, Lycklama á Nijholt AAB, Siegel S, Jonas U, Fowler CJ, Fall M, Gajewski JB, Hassouna MM, et al. Results of sacral neuromodulation therapy for urinary voiding dysfunction: outcomes of a prospective, worldwide clinical study. J Urol. 2007;178:2029–34. https://doi.org/10.1016/j.juro.2007.07.032.

29. Gajewski JB, Al-Zahrani AA. The long-term efficacy of sacral neuromodulation in the management of intractable cases of bladder pain syndrome: 14 years of experience in one centre. BJU Int. 2011;107:1258–64. https://doi.org/10.1111/j.1464-410X.2010.09697.x.

30. Roulette P, Castel-Lacanal E, Sanson S, Caremel R, Phé V, Bart S, Duchêne F, De Sèze M, Even A, Manunta A, et al. Sacral neuromodulation and pregnancy: results of a national survey carried out for the neuro-urology committee of the French Association of Urology (AFU). Neurourol Urodyn. 2018;37:792–8. https://doi.org/10.1002/nau.23349.

31. Khunda A, McCormick C, Ballard P. Sacral neuromodulation and sexual function: a systematic review and meta-analysis of the literature. Int Urogynecol J. 2019;30:339–52. https://doi.org/10.1007/s00192-018-3841-x.

32. Simillis C, Lal N, Qiu S, Kontovounisios C, Rasheed S, Tan E, Tekkis PP. Sacral nerve stimulation versus percutaneous tibial nerve stimulation for faecal incontinence: a systematic review and meta-analysis. Int J Color Dis. 2018;33:645–8. https://doi.org/10.1007/s00384-018-2976-z.

Injections and Biomaterials

Ömer Acar and Ervin Kocjancic

1 Introduction

Coincident with the "digital era", there has been a trend in performing minimally invasive procedures to treat urological disorders. This concept has been driven by the aim of causing less harm while providing at least noninferior benefit when compared with the conventional and usually more invasive treatment alternatives. The potential advantages of a truly minimally invasive procedure include the absence of the adverse events associated with medical treatment, the lack of compliance issues that occur with long-term oral medication, the lack of an urgent need for anesthesia and the minimal risk of technical adverse effects and complications. In times of dramatically rising health-care costs in an aging population, economic aspects are of critical importance and a cost-effective, easy-to-perform and efficient therapy performed in an office-based setting is desirable.

Injection of certain substances or chemicals and utilizing natural or synthetic biomaterials may serve well to meet the expectations of some patients by improving (if not curing) the symptoms related to their urological condition which may otherwise necessitate a treatment with questionable benefit and lead to morbid complications. The progress that has been achieved with drug development and delivery systems together with the growing interest in regenerative urology boosted the research efforts testing the safety and efficacy of treatment alternatives including the use of injectables and biomaterials which might have a therapeutic role in a wide spectrum of conditions including (but not limited to) stress urinary incontinence (SUI), benign prostatic obstruction, erectile dysfunction, Peyronie's disease, pelvic organ prolapse (POP), urethral strictures, and lower urinary tract dysfunction.

Ö. Acar (✉) · E. Kocjancic
Department of Urology, University of Illinois College of Medicine, Chicago, IL, USA
e-mail: oacar2@uic.edu

D. Veneziano, E. Huri (eds.), *Urologic Surgery in the Digital Era*,
https://doi.org/10.1007/978-3-030-63948-8_7

Herein, we'll review and discuss the relevant literature about the use of injections and biomaterials for the management of urological disorders. Our focus will be concentrated on the studies conducted in human subjects in an effort to provide insight about the potential application of these rather underutilized treatment modalities in the clinical setting.

2 Injections

2.1 Urethral Bulking Therapy for SUI

Midurethral sling (MUS) placement represents the gold standard surgical treatment option for female SUI [1]. However, there is a need for less invasive alternatives especially for patients who are unfit for and/or unwilling to undergo surgeries, for those who have recurrent SUI after failed anti-incontinence procedure(s) and for those in whom surgical options are limited (e.g., prior radical pelvic surgery or pelvic radiotherapy) [2–5]. Additionally, the use of MUS has been plagued due to the concerns about mesh-related complications including infection, chronic pain and erosion, which have led to their withdrawal from the market in several countries [6]. Endoscopic injection of urethral bulking agents (or urethral bulking therapy (UBT)) is a minimally invasive, well tolerated, outpatient procedure which is associated with acceptable success rates especially in the short-term. As a result, UBT can have a role in the management of these "non-index" clinical scenarios as well as some selected primary cases, especially when symptomatic palliation meets patient's goals.

The ideal bulking agent should be nonimmunogenic; permanent; nonmigratory; nonerosive; noninflammatory; easily stored, handled, and injected; painless; have no long-term side effects; be cost-effective; should provide durable clinical improvement; and possess a high safety profile. However, the currently available urethral bulking agents do not completely fulfill these criteria and the search for the ideal one is ongoing. Many different bulking agents have been investigated to be used for UBT (Table 1) and there is an unmet need for comparative outcome analysis between various bulking agents. Overall, the efficacy of UBT usually ranges from 50% to 70% in terms of early subjective improvement which is not sustainable and destined to diminish after longer follow-up [7].

2.2 Stem Cell Therapy for SUI

Functionality of the urethral rhabdosphincter relies on the integrity of anatomic constituents (such as a connective tissue layer encompassing rich vascular supply, striated and smooth muscle groups, somatic and autonomic nervous structures) and the synergic coordination among them. Age-related changes (such as apoptosis, fatty

Table 1 Past and current injectable bulking agents used for UBT

Injectable Bulking Agent		Constituents	Year of FDA approval	Time period when the agent was available on the market	Primary reason for withdrawal from the market
Biological	Nonautologous:				
	Collagen (Contigen™)	Bovine dermal collagen (95% type 1 and 5% type 3) cross-linked with glutaraldehyde	1993	1993–2011	Hyper-sensitivity reactions
	Porcine dermis (Permacol™)	Collagen and elastin harvested from porcine dermis	N/A	On the market, as of 2009 (used also for fecal incontinence, hernia repair, etc.)	N/A
	Autologous:				
	Autologous fat	Adipose tissue harvested from the abdominal wall	N/A	N/A (described for SUI in 1989)	N/A, Not being used for SUI due to the risk of pulmonary fat embolism

(continued)

Table 1 (continued)

Injectable Bulking Agent		Constituents	Year of FDA approval	Time period when the agent was available on the market	Primary reason for withdrawal from the market
Synthetic	Historical:				
	Sodium morrhuate, Dondren	Sclerosing agents	N/A	1930s–1960s	Particle migration
	Teflon	Polytetrafluoroethylene (PTFE)	N/A	Described for SUI in 1973	N/A, Not being used for SUI due to the risk of particle migration
	Ethylene vinyl alcohol copolymer (Tegress™, Uryx™)	Ethylene vinyl alcohol copolymer bound to dimethyl sulphoxide	2004	2004–2007	Urethral erosion
	Dextranomer/hyaluronic acid (Deflux™, Zuidex™)	Hydrophilic dextran polymer with a hyaluronic acid base	N/A	On the market but not used for female SUI (FDA approved for vesicoureteral reflux since 2001)	N/A, Not being used for SUI due to injection site collections (sterile abscess, etc.)
	Polydimethylsiloxane (Macroplastique™)	Polydimethylsiloxane macroparticles in a hydrogel of polyvinylpyrrolidone	2006	Still on the market (US and Europe)	N/A
	Carbon-coated zirconium (Durasphere™)	Carbon-coated zirconium beads in polysaccharide carrier gel	1999	Still on the market (US and Europe)	N/A
	Calcium hydroxyapatite (Coaptite™)	Calcium hydroxylapatite bioceramic microspheres in aqueous gel carrier	2005	Still on the market (US and Europe)	N/A
	Polyacrylamide hydrogel (Aquamid™, Bulkamid™)	Cross-linked polyacrylamide with non-pyrogenic water	N/A	On the market, as of 2006 (Europe)	N/A
	Vinyl dimethyl polydimethylsiloxane (Urolastic™)	Silicone elastomer cross-linked with dimethylpolydimethylsiloxane	N/A	On the market, as of 2009 (Europe)	N/A

Adapted from reference [7]

degeneration, fibrosis) or acquired insults (such as radical prostatectomy, pelvic radiotherapy) that disrupt the morphology and function of the sphincteric unit may lead to intrinsic sphincter deficiency (ISD) and consequent SUI [8]. Current treatment options that can be employed in the setting of SUI secondary to ISD include urethral bulking therapy (UBT), MUS, pubovaginal slings (PVS), and artificial urinary sphincter (AUS) implantation. However, none of these treatment options target the main etiology underlying SUI and aim to provide symptomatic improvement via varying degrees of extrinsic urethral support. Additionally, each has some drawbacks such as the modest clinical efficacy and limited durability of UBT, the possibility of de-novo voiding dysfunction following PVS, concerns and complications related to the use synthetic material in MUS surgery, and the greater likelihood of complications (such as infection, erosion, and malfunction) after AUS implantation.

Stem cell therapy holds promise as an alternative modality to treat sphincteric SUI. Owing to their regenerative potential, stem cells can differentiate into different functional cell types and secrete paracrine factors in order to salvage the exact deficiency that the individual sphincteric unit is facing. Embryonic and adult stem cells constitute the two main groups of stem cells that can be used for clinical purposes [9]. Due to ethical concerns and the possible teratogenicity, the use of embryonic stem cells has been limited in most of Western Europe and North America. The adult, somatic, stem cells can be obtained from any vascularized tissue as it is currently thought that they constitute the pericytes of the vessels within the tissue [10]. The common donor sites for adult stem cells are the bone marrow, the skeletal muscle, and the adipose tissue.

Atala et al. tested the utility of muscle precursor cells for the restoration of irreversibly damaged sphincter function in an animal model. Stem cell injection was done through the transurethral route with cystoscopic guidance and the clinical efficacy was tested using urethral pressure profilometry. They showed that static urethral pressure was significantly higher (at 1, 2, 3, and 6 months) in the stem cell group when compared with the measurements recorded in the control group. Parallel to this finding, leak point pressure (LPP) was higher in the stem cell group, with the difference being statistically significant only in the 1-month time point. Cystourethrographic images at 6 months demonstrated near-normal urethral caliber at the sphincteric level in the stem cell group, while that part of the urethra and bladder neck was significantly dilated in the control arm [11].

Shi et al. assessed a tissue-engineered bulking agent composed of adipose derived stem cells and silk fibroin microspheres for the treatment of ISD in an animal model. At 4, 8, and 12 weeks, LPP was significantly higher in the combined injection group compared to the animals who received either bulking agent or sham procedure. Accordingly, luminal cross-sectional area was significantly lower in the combined group throughout the study timeline [12].

Table 2 outlines the results reported in selected clinical studies that focused on the safety and efficacy of stem cell injections for SUI. To sum up, striated muscle- and adipose tissue-based stem cells were much more commonly tested than the other alternatives in human studies, suggesting the relative easiness and less complicated nature of their harvest. Majority of the relevant literature is composed of studies including females with SUI as a result of ISD. Very few studies have dealt

Table 2 Selected clinical studies about stem cell injection therapy for SUI

Study	N	Follow-up (year)	Change in LPP/ MUCP (cmH₂O)	Non-urodynamic assessment
Mitterberger et al. 2007–2008 STRIATED MUSCLE [13–15]	123 ♀	1	MUCP: 11.7 ± 28.1, %40.6	Cure: %79 Significant improvement: %13
	63 ♂	1	LPP: 21.9 ± 41.4, %47.3	Cure: %65 Significant improvement: %27
	20 ♀	2	MUCP: 66.4 ± 28.1, %45.9 (1 year) MUCP: 15.2 ± 25.4, %56.2 (2 year)	Cure: %80 Significant improvement: %20
Gerullis et al. 2012 STRIATED MUSCLE [16]	222 ♂	1	N/A	Cure: %12 Significant improvement: %42 Failure: %46
Stangel-Wojcikiewicz et al. 2014, STRIATED MUSCLE [17]	16 ♀	1	MUCP: 21.5 ± 46, %71.9	Cure: %50 Significant improvement: %25
Kuismanen et al. 2014, ADIPOSE TISSUE + COLLAGEN + SALINE [18]	5 ♀	1	MUCP: no significant change	Significant improvement: %60 Failure: %40

LPP leak point pressure, *MUCP* maximal urethral closing pressure

with post-prostatectomy incontinence. Mean follow-up duration is in the range of 6–12 months and almost half of the studies tested the clinical benefit of stem cell injection by non-urodynamic means. The studies, which included urodynamic assessment, resulted in a 40–50% increase in maximal urethral closing pressure (MUCP) or LPP. Almost ¼ of the patients achieved dryness with stem cell injection therapy, while more than 50% reported decreased severity of SUI. Some of the studies have reported a positive correlation between symptomatic improvement and concentration of injected stem cells. No clinically significant adverse events have been reported in human studies.

The lack of standardization in the technique, dosage and frequency of stem cell injections together with the absence of data with regard to the comparative efficacy of stem cell therapy vs. conventional treatment options and limited long-term follow-up in the available series precluded widespread adoption of its utility.

2.3   Stem Cell Therapy for ED

The recent increase in modifiable risk factors for ED, such as obesity and metabolic syndrome, has caused an increase in the prevalence of ED [19]. Restorative treatment options for ED target the main pathophysiological mechanism underlying ED and aim to lessen or cure symptomatology without causing adverse effects. Stem cell therapy (SCT) holds promise within this context as a regenerative therapy for ED.

Considering the clinical trials conducted in the last decade, which included patients aged between 50 to 70 years and had a sample size and follow-up ranging between 4 to 21 and 6 months to over 60 months, respectively, SCT was shown to improve erectile function as reflected by enhanced penile vascular flow, and the changes recorded in International Index of Erectile Function-15 item (IIEF-15), and Erectile Hardness Scale scores. No serious adverse effects have been reported in these trials and there were no tolerance issues with regards to the harvesting and injection of stem cells [20].

Some of these trials focused on "difficult-to-treat" ED subpopulations, such as those with concomitant diabetes mellitus (DM) and patients who underwent radical prostatectomy (RP). Haahr et al. tested the safety and efficacy of autologous adipose-derived regenerative cells in 21 patients with ED following RP. At 12 months follow-up, 8 of the 15 (53%) continent men reported erectile function sufficient enough for sexual intercourse. None of the patients who were incontinent or had preoperative ED were able to regain erections. Median IIEF-5 scores of the continent men increased significantly at 12 months (from 6.0 to 8.0) [21]. Bahk et al. assessed the efficacy of umbilical cord derived mesenchymal stem cells for the treatment of ED in 10 patients (7 patients in treatment arm vs. 3 patients in control arm who received saline injection) with type II DM. At 2 months follow-up, 6 of 7 patients experienced morning erections, which were maintained for at least 3 months. None of the patients in the control group reported such an improvement. However, the degree of erection was not sufficient for penetration and 2 of the 7 patients in the treatment arm eventually underwent implantation of penile prosthesis [22].

Currently, SCT is not listed as one of the recommended treatment options for ED. It has been regarded as an experimental treatment modality that warrants further research in large scale randomized clinical trials.

2.4 Injectables for BPO-LUTS

Minimally invasive treatments have been developed to offer rapid and effective relief of lower urinary tract symptoms (LUTS) with less perioperative and postoperative morbidity than is associated with conventional procedures such as transurethral resection of the prostate or open prostatectomy. Novel agents for intraprostatic treatment of LUTS associated with benign prostatic hyperplasia (BPH) include botulinum neurotoxin A (BoNT-A), NX-1207 and PRX302.

2.4.1 BoNT-A

BoNT-A inhibits the release of acetylcholine from the cholinergic neurons into the neuromuscular junction through interaction with synaptosomal protein 25. BoNT-A has become increasingly attractive in the urological field for the treatment of lower urinary tract dysfunction with excessive motor activity such as detrusor sphincter dyssynergia, detrusor overactivity and bladder pain syndrome/interstitial cystitis [23–25]. Owing to its neuromodulatory effect on sympathetic, parasymphathetic, and sensory nerve terminals in the prostate; BoNT-A has also emerged as a promising treatment option in LUTS caused by BPH. Experimental evidence has shown that BoNT-A addresses the static component of BPO-LUTS by causing atrophy by apoptosis and decreased cell proliferation. BoNT-A injection treats the dynamic component by causing downregulation of the α1A-adrenoceptor and reduction in prostatic smooth muscle contractility [26].

Despite promising preclinical data, there are few randomized, placebo-controlled clinical trials about the efficacy of BoNT-A for LUTS/BPH. The first study of this kind included 30 patients who were randomly assigned to receive 200 U BoNT-A (specifically Botox®) or saline solution via the transperineal route. When compared with baseline values, the reduction in prostate volume and postvoid residual (PVR) urine amount together with the increase in mean peak urinary flow rate and the improvement in symptom score were significantly in favor of the treatment arm. These outcomes were stable for 12 months. Notably, no significant adverse events were reported [27]. On the contrary, results of another randomized, double-blind, placebo-controlled study (n = 380), revealed insignificant differences between BoNT-A and placebo arms. This study tested different dosages of Botox® and the route of administration (from transperineal to transrectal) and injected volumes were modified throughout the course of study. Side-effect profile was favorable with no negative impact on sexual function [28]. To sum up, current data is insufficient to justify the use of BoNT-A for the management of LUTS/BPH.

2.4.2   NX-1207

NX-1207 is a novel cysteine-containing linear protein of proprietary composition with prostate-selective proapoptotic properties. It was designed for transrectal ultrasonography-guided intraprostatic injection which can be done as an outpatient procedure without local or general anesthesia and does not necessitate catheterization. Apoptosis-induced atrophy of the encroaching prostatic tissue is supposed to result in short-term and long-term symptomatic relief of LUTS [29]. However, the pivotal US-based phase III trials failed to meet the primary efficacy end points [26].

2.4.3   PRX302

PRX302 is a genetically engineered precursor toxin derived from the highly toxic bacterial pore-forming protein, aerolysin. It requires proteolytic processing by PSA for activation which means that its activity is confined to the prostate tissue and supports its potential safety. Elhilali et al. conducted a prospective, randomized, double-blind clinical trial which included 92 patients who were randomly assigned to receive PRX302 or the vehicle control. Mean decrease in IPSS and mean change in qmax were similar between study groups. Adverse events reported in the treatment arm were mild to moderate in severity and subsided with conservative measures after a mean duration of <2 days [30]. The US-based phase III trial of PRX302 failed to meet the primary endpoints on interim analysis [26].

2.5 Intralesional Therapy for Peyronie's Disease

Peyronie's disease (PD) is a progressive fibrotic disorder of the tunica albuginea that causes penile deformity and painful erection, making sexual intercourse difficult. Conservative treatment options for PD aim to treat patients in the early stages of the disease. Injection therapies have been utilized to reduce penile pain, plaque size, and/or penile curvature. Until now various injectables have been studied in the context of PD including calcium channel blockers, interferon α-2B (IFNα-2B) and hyaluronic acid (HA). In 2013, collagenase Clostridium histolyticum (CCH) was introduced as the only Food and Drug Administration- and European Medicines Agency-approved treatment option for PD.

2.5.1 Calcium Channel Blockers (Verapamil or Nicardipine)

The randomized placebo controlled trial which compared intralesional verapamil (10 mg) vs. saline injection demonstrated a significantly higher degree of reduction of curvature in the treatment arm (37.7° to 29.6° for verapamil vs. 33.6° to 31.4° for placebo). The reduction in plaque size and preservation of sexual function indices were similarly in favor of verapamil group [31].

Soh et al. performed a randomized placebo-controlled study to investigate the effects of 10 mg nicardipine injections versus placebo which failed to show any beneficial effect on the degree of curvature. However, those who received intralesional nicardipine injections reported less penile pain than those subjected to placebo [32].

Based on the results of a recently published systematic review, the evidence is not robust enough to support the use of intralesional injection therapy with calcium channel blockers and does not suggest a meaningful improvement in penile curvature compared with placebo [33].

2.5.2 IFNα-2B

Kendirci et al. demonstrated superiority of IFNα-2b in terms of the improvement recorded in penile curvature (36.8° vs 44.1°) in their randomized placebo controlled trial. A similarly meaningful benefit was not achieved for plaque size reduction [34]. Another randomized controlled trial showed the superiority of IFNα-2b in treating penile curvature and reducing plaque size over placebo. However, the difference was statistically insignificant with regards to erectile function and penile pain [35].

2.5.3 Hyaluronic Acid

A non-placebo-controlled study compared injection of 20 mg HA with a control group of patients who did not receive any treatment. At 12 months follow-up, penile curvature was stabilized in the HA group while a mean change of +15.4° was recorded in the control group. HA injections also reduced the size of the plaque and improved erectile function. Pain scores were similar between study groups [36].

2.5.4 Collagenase Clostridium Histolyticum

The results from the pivotal randomized controlled trials (IMPRESS I and II) demonstrated the superiority of CCH over placebo in terms of percentage improvement in penile curvature (34% and 18.2%, respectively), erectile function (mean change in IIEF-15 of +1.0 and +0.4, respectively), and penile length (0.4 and 0.2 cm, respectively), but not when considering penile pain. Of note, CCH injections were coupled with penile modelling in these trials which has a putative role of improving outcomes in men with PD and is potentially more efficacious than placebo as a monotherapy. Subjects who received CCH injections reported higher degree of improvement in patient-reported PD bother compared to the placebo arm [37].

2.6 Intrasphincteric Injection of BoNT-A

BoNT-A is currently licensed for use in treating urinary incontinence associated with idiopathic overactive bladder and neurogenic detrusor overactivity. However, its application has also involved injections into the external urethral sphincter (EUS) with the aim of reducing urethral resistance, by inducing a striated muscle paralysis to treat various aspects of voiding dysfunction including chronic urinary retention due to Fowler's syndrome, detrusor underactivity, after pelvic surgery, pelvic floor spasticity, and idiopathic voiding dysfunction.

Galien et al. conducted the largest randomized placebo-controlled trial which included 86 patients with multiple sclerosis (MS) and detrusor sphincter dyssnergia (DSD). Herein, two groups were constructed; BoNT-A 100 U vs 0.9% saline, with treatment administered through a single electromyography-guided transperineal injection. There was no significant difference between the BoNT-A and placebo arms with regard to PVR which was the primary endpoint. On the other hand, the difference in terms of voided volumes (+54%) and maximal detrusor pressures (−21%) were in favor of BoNT-A injection [38].

Kuo et al. conducted a non-placebo-controlled study without randomization in which BoNT-A was injected into the EUS in an effort to reduce resistance in patients with persistent voiding dysfunction after radical hysterectomy. Twenty patients received 100 U BoNT-A, while 10 received ongoing medical treatment as a control arm. The improvement in clinical and urodynamic parameters were significantly higher in the BoNT-A arm and this trend was evident for up to 9 months. Half of those (3 out of 6) who were in complete retention resumed spontaneous voiding, while 8 of 10 who performed CIC were able to either reduce their CIC frequency or eventually discontinue it [39].

2.7 Platelet-Rich Plasma Injection for ED

Platelet-rich plasma (PRP) is autologous blood plasma that is highly concentrated with platelets and growth factors such as vascular endothelial growth factor (VEGF), platelet-derived growth factor (PDGF), epidermal growth factor (EGF), insulin-like growth factor (IGF), and fibroblast growth factor (FGF) [40]. Preclinical evidence documented the potential positive impact of these growth factors (especially, VEGF which mediates its effect through endothelial nitric oxide synthase pathway) on erectile function [41].

Intracavernous injection of PRP was tested in a total of 5 patients with mild and/or moderate ED. There were no major adverse outcomes. However, the study lacked a placebo arm and the protocol for PRP injection was not consistent (median number of injections: 2, the amount of injectable PRP: 2–9 mL). Post-treatment IIEF improved 4 points on average [42].

Currently available data suggest that PRP treatment for ED carries a low risk of adverse events. However, it is not possible to draw conclusions on its efficacy regarding ED treatment since the relevant literature consists low patient numbers without controls, and reports questionable clinical efficacy.

3 Biomaterials

3.1 Biomaterials in POP/SUI Surgery

Weakened support from the connective tissues, ligaments, and muscles of the pelvic floor contributes to POP and SUI. Strategies to correct these disorders may include correcting for the tissue defects with cell-based treatments (as previously discussed in stem cell injection for SUI) or the use of biomaterials to augment the natural tissue support.

Biomaterials may be synthetic or natural. Natural biomaterials, which are typically decellularized, can be autologous (harvested from the patient), allograft (harvested from cadaveric tissue) or xenograft (harvested from animal tissue). Disadvantages of allografts and xenografts include increased cost of production, inconsistent mechanical strength, risk of disease transmission to the host and unpredictable host response. Whereas, limitations related to the availability of material, added OR time and increased morbidity related to graft harvest represent the main concerns surrounding autologous biomaterials. Lastly, any natural biomaterial may be susceptible to matrix degrading enzymes if the underlying host pathophysiology is not addressed properly [43].

Pore size, filament type, local tissue durability, and stiffness characterize synthetic biomaterials (Table 3). Multifilament materials may increase the risk of erosion and biomaterials with smaller pore size would allow integration of bacteria and not of host cells. Although there are lower erosion rates with absorbable meshes, long-term anatomical success rate of non-absorbable mesh-based POP repair is

Table 3 Amid classification of synthetic non-absorbable meshes used in pelvic floor reconstruction

Type	Pore size	Structure	Polymer	Examples of trade names
I	Macroporous (>75 μm)	Monofilament	Polypropylene	Uretex, Gynecare TVT, Bard Mesh, Sparc, In-Fast, Monarc, Lynx, Obtryx, Gynecare Prolift, Atrium, Marlex
		Multifilament	Copolymer of glycolide (90%) and lactide (10%)	Vicryl
			Polypropylene and polyglecaprone	Vypro, Ultrapro
			Polyglycolic acid	Dexon
II	Macroporous (<10 μm)	Multifilament	Expanded PTFF	GORE-TEX
			Polyethylene terephthalate	Mersuture
III	Macroporous with microporous components (>75 μm)	Multifilament	PTFE	Teflon
			Polyethylene terephthalate	Mersilene
			Polypropylene	IVS Tunneller
			Woven polyester	Protegen
IV	Nanoporous (<1 μm)	Multifilament	Silicon-coated polyester	Intermesh
			Dura mater substitute	PRECLUDE MVP Dura substitute
			Expanded PTFE, pericardial membrane substitute	PRECLUDE Pericardial Membrane

higher than that achieved with absorbable material. Finally, a stiff graft will have good mechanical strength, but will lack compliance. Conversely, a flaccid graft would better adapt to the patient's anatomy, but may lack the needed strength to correct SUI or POP [44].

Mesh-based POP repairs have been shown to yield superior anatomical outcomes when compared to native tissue-based corrections. Additionally, native-tissue based POP repairs have a higher recurrence rate in the long run [45]. The main disadvantages of synthetic meshes are the complications of erosion (graft material in the urethra or bladder) and extrusion (graft material in the vaginal lumen). Moreover, pelvic pain and dyspareunia which can be chronic in nature and bothersome in severity might complicate the postoperative course of mesh-based POP and SUI repairs. These complications, which are not product-specific, can be the result of host, operative and biomechanical factors [46]. Furthermore, mesh-related complications can be reduced by training and proper patient selection. Nevertheless, local authorities have banned the use of synthetic mesh in transvaginal POP repair in many countries across the globe. Considering the dramatic rise in legal claims and the heightened public sensitivity about mesh-related complications, surgeons have also become reluctant to do anti-incontinence procedures involving the use of synthetic material. Consequently, autologous fascial slings have started to regain their popularity.

To conclude, the "ideal" biomaterial for pelvic support should provide the following: biocompatibility, enhanced tissue repair, maintain mechanical strength over time, and easily customizable including biodegradability. However, none of the currently available biomaterials fulfill these criteria [47].

3.2 Biomaterials in Bladder Reconstruction

Many efforts have been made to replace or augment bladder without using intestinal segments in an effort to avoid the long-term complications associated with bowel interposition such as infection, mucous production, stone formation, metabolic disturbances, intestinal perforation, and tumorigenicity. Natural acellular biomaterials have been commonly evaluated for the purpose of bladder augmentation and reconstruction. They can be produced, stored, and used as "off-the-shelf" materials, thereby reducing the need for technically demanding and expensive cell-based and patient-specific procedures which are beyond the scope of this chapter.

Herein, an acellular biomaterial graft is used as a tissue implant, which becomes incorporated through the ingrowth of cells from the surrounding native host bladder. The most commonly investigated natural decellularized materials are xenogenic extracellular matrices (ECM) [46].

Constituents of xenogenic ECMs after the decellularization process include collagen, glycosaminoglycans, fibronectin, laminins and growth factors that facilitate host ingrowth through a regenerative tissue remodeling response. During the preparation process, ECM scaffolds can be manipulated by prefabrication with collagen bioactive recognition sites and growth factors for directed cell interaction on the scaffold prior to in-vivo implantation. Porcine small intestinal submucosa (SIS), porcine urinary bladder matrix (UBM)/bladder-derived acellular matrix (BAM) and BAM allograft represent favorable tissue substitutes that can be used for urinary tract reconstruction [48].

Unseeded (bare ECM scaffold to provide a framework for ingrowth and regeneration of native tissue) SIS and UBM were effective for regenerating small urinary tract defects in animal models through the release of stimulatory growth factors and absorbable bioactive factors [48]. BAM allograft was first used in rats for bladder augmentation was after partial cystectomy. Histological examination documented the presence of epithelialization, smooth muscle regeneration, neovascularization, and neural element formation after grafting remnant bladder tissue with BAM [49]. Subsequent studies have reported graft contraction in association with an extensive fibrosis and incomplete tissue layer formation [50].

As a hollow organ, the successful regeneration of bladder requires functional muscle layers, which may limit the application of decellularized BAMs. Jayo et al. used a synthetic polymer matrix seeded with autologous urothelial and smooth muscle cells in a subtotal cystectomy canine model. They reported formation of a three-layered detrusor muscle tissue within the follow-up of 2 years. Urodynamic studies demonstrated favorable viscoelastic characteristics and the dogs were able to void by increasing their abdominal tone [51].

Based on the promising preclinical data, further research tested the feasibility of using cell-seeded grafts in the clinical setting, whereby bladder-derived autologous

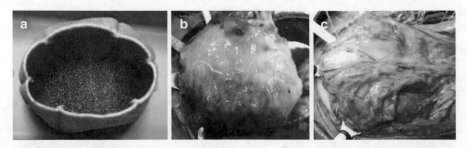

Fig. 1 Construction of engineered bladder: (**a**) scaffold seeded with cells; (**b**) engineered bladder anastomosed to native bladder with running 4–0 polyglycolic sutures; and (**c**) implant covered with fibrin glue and omentum [52]

cells were expanded in-vitro for 7 to 8 weeks and then seeded onto collagen or collagen-polyglycolic acid scaffolds to generate bioengineered tissue constructs. These "patches" were used for augmentation cystoplasty in 7 patients (aged 4 to 19 years) with neurogenic bladder (Fig. 1). After a follow-up period ranging from 22 to 61 months, the investigators were able to demonstrate increase in bladder capacity and decrease in filling pressures. None of the patients suffered from metabolic derangements or stone formation in the urinary tract. Moreover, the ultimate goal of renal functional preservation was achieved in all 7 patients [52].

A subsequent clinical trial, in which autologous cell seeded polyglycolide/polylactide composite scaffold was applied for augmentation cystoplasty in paediatric patients with spina bifida (n = 10), could not replicate these results. No improvement in bladder capacity was noted. Adverse events occurred in 4 patients with 5 patients requiring re-operation in the form of ileocystoplasty [53].

3.3 Biomaterials in Urethroplasty

The regeneration-based therapeutic potential of collagen-enriched BAM was tested in 28 patients with urethral strictures ranging from 1.5–16 cm in length. The bioengineered urethral tissue was created by anastomosing the matrix in an onlay fashion to the urethral plate. At 36–48 months follow-up, 86% of the patients had a successful outcome without the need for additional treatment [54]. Palminteri et al. achieved a similar success rate with the use of SIS in penile and bulbar urethroplasties [55].

Autologous cell-seeded matrices may be similar to native urethra and may be offered as an alternative for tubularized urethral repair. After proof of concept animal studies, Raya-Rivera et al. used polyglycolic acid: poly(lactide-co-glycolide acid) scaffolds seeded with autologous epithelial cells and muscle cells for urethral repair in 5 patients [56]. They were able to demonstrate promising results with this approach as reflected with stricture-free luminal patency and adequate urinary flow at median follow-up of 71 months (Fig. 2).

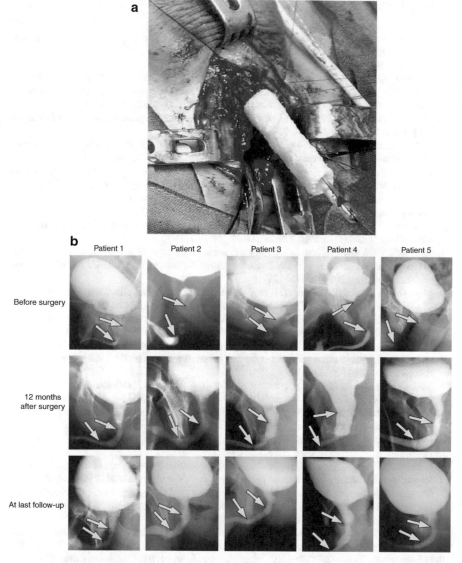

Fig. 2 (**a**) Tubularized urethral reconstruction with autologous cell-seeded matrix. (**b**) Voiding cystourethrograms of all 5 patients before surgery (arrows show the abnormal margins), 12 months after surgery (arrows show margins of tissue engineered urethras), and at last follow-up (arrows show margins of tissue engineered urethras) [56]

The existing data suggests a future role of biomaterials and tissue engineering approaches in the treatment of POP, SUI, urethral strictures, and LUTD and the field has seen significant progress in recent years. However, the translation of tissue-engineering into urological practice is still at an early stage and relatively few applications have yet reached a clinical standard in urology.

References

1. Serati M, Salvatore S, Uccella S, et al. Surgical treatment for female stress urinary incontinence: what is the gold-standard procedure? Int Urogynecol J Pelvic Floor Dysfunct. 2009;20:619–21.
2. Sassani P, Aboseif SR. Stress urinary incontinence in women. Curr Urol Rep. 2009;10:333–7.
3. Keegan PE, Atiemo K, Cody J, McClinton S, Pickard R. Periurethral injection therapy for urinary incontinence in women. Cochrane Database Syst Rev. 2007;3:CD003881.
4. Chapple CR, Wein AJ, Brubaker L, et al. Stress incontinence injection therapy: what is best for our patients? Eur Urol. 2005;48:552–65.
5. Plotti F, Zullo MA, Sansone M, et al. Post radical hysterectomy urinary incontinence: a prospective study of transurethral bulking agents injection. Gynecol Oncol. 2009;112:90–4.
6. Siddiqui ZA, Abboudi H, Crawford R, Shah S. Intraurethral bulking agents for the management of female stress urinary incontinence: a systematic review. Int Urogynecol J. 2017;28:1275–84.
7. Kocjancic E, Mourad S, Acar Ö. Complications of urethral bulking therapy for female stress urinary incontinence. Neurourol Urodyn. 2019;38(Suppl 4):12–20.
8. Herschorn S. Female pelvic floor anatomy: the pelvic floor, supporting structures, and pelvic organs. Rev Urol. 2004;6(Suppl 5):2–10.
9. Kocjancic E, Motiani K, Joneja J. Stem cells for the treatment of stress urinary incontinence. In Gopal Badlani editor. Minimally invasive therapy for urinary incontinence and pelvic organ prolapse, Springer; 2014, p. 115–121.
10. Meirelles L, Fontes AM, Covas DT, et al. Mechanisms involved in the therapeutic properties of mesenchymal stem cells. Cytokine Growth Factor Rev. 2009;20:419–27.
11. Eberli D, Aboushwareb T, Soker S, Yoo JJ, Atala A. Muscle precursor cells for the restoration of irreversibly damaged sphincter function. Cell Transplant. 2012;21:2089–98.
12. Shi LB, Cai HX, Chen LK, et al. Tissue engineered bulking agent with adipose-derived stem cells and silk fibroin microspheres for the treatment of intrinsic urethral sphincter deficiency. Biomaterials. 2014;35:1519–30.
13. Mitterberger M, Marksteiner R, Margreiter E, et al. Autologous myoblasts and fibroblasts for female stress incontinence: a 1-year follow-up in 123 patients. BJU Int. 2007;100:1081–5.
14. Mitterberger M, Marksteiner R, Margreiter E, et al. Myoblast and fibroblast therapy for postprostatectomy urinary incontinence: 1-year followup of 63 patients. J Urol. 2008;179:226–31.
15. Mitterberger M, Pinggera GM, Marksteiner R, et al. Adult stem cell therapy of female stress urinary incontinence. Eur Urol. 2008;53:169–75.
16. Gerullis H, Eimer C, Georgas E, et al. Muscle-derived cells for treatment of iatrogenic sphincter damage and urinary incontinence in men. ScientificWorldJournal. 2012;2012:898535.
17. Stangel-Wojcikiewicz K, Jarocha D, Piwowar M, et al. Autologous muscle-derived cells for the treatment of female stress urinary incontinence: a 2-year follow-up of a Polish investigation. Neurourol Urodyn. 2014;33:324–30.
18. Kuismanen K, Sartoneva R, Haimi S, et al. Autologous adipose stem cells in treatment of female stress urinary incontinence: results of a pilot study. Stem Cells Transl Med. 2014;3:936–41.
19. Schulster ML, Liang SE, Najari BB. Metabolic syndrome and sexual dysfunction. Curr Opin Urol. 2017;27:435–40.
20. Lokeshwar SD, Patel P, Shah SM, Ramasamy R. A systematic review of human trials using stem cell therapy for erectile dysfunction. Sex Med Rev. 2020;8:122–30.
21. Haahr MK, Harken Jensen C,Toyserkani NM, et al. A 12-month follow-up after a single intracavernous injection of autologous adipose-derived regenerative cells in patients with erectile dysfunction following radical prostatectomy: An open-label phase I clinical trial. Urology 2018;121. 203.e6203.e13. https://doi.org/10.1016/j.urology.2018.06.018.
22. Bahk JY, Jung JH, Han H, et al. Treatment of diabetic impotence with umbilical cord blood stem cell intracavernosal transplant: preliminary report of 7 cases. Exp Clin Transplant. 2010;8:150–60.

23. Dykstra DD, Sidi AA, Scott AB, Pagel JM, Goldish GD. Effects of botulinum A toxin on detrusor-sphincter dyssynergia in spinal cord injury patients. J Urol. 1988;139:919–22.
24. Karsenty G, et al. Botulinum toxin A (Botox) intradetrusor injections in adults with neurogenic detrusor overactivity/neurogenic overactive bladder: a systematic literature review. Eur Urol. 2008;53:275–87.
25. Smith CP, et al. Botulinum toxin a has antinociceptive effects in treating interstitial cystitis. Urology. 2004;64:871–5.
26. Magistro G, Stief CG, Gratzke C. New intraprostatic injectables and prostatic urethral lift for male LUTS. Nat Rev Urol. 2015;12:461–71.
27. Maria G, et al. Relief by botulinum toxin of voiding dysfunction due to benign prostatic hyperplasia: results of a randomized, placebo-controlled study. Urology. 2003;62:259–64.
28. Marberger M, et al. A randomized double-blind placebo-controlled phase 2 dose-ranging study of onabotulinumtoxinA in men with benign prostatic hyperplasia. Eur Urol. 2013;63:496–503.
29. Shore N, Cowan B. The potential for NX-1207 in benign prostatic hyperplasia: an update for clinicians. Ther Adv Chronic Dis. 2011;2:377–83.
30. Elhilali MM, et al. Prospective, randomized, double-blind, vehicle controlled, multicenter phase IIb clinical trial of the pore forming protein PRX302 for targeted treatment of symptomatic benign prostatic hyperplasia. J Urol. 2013;189:1421–6.
31. Rehman J, Benet A, Melman A. Use of intralesional verapamil to dissolve Peyronie's disease plaque: a long-term single-blind study. Urology. 1998;51:620–6.
32. Soh J, Kawauchi A, Kanemitsu N, et al. Nicardipine vs. saline injection as treatment for Peyronie's disease: a prospective, randomized, single-blind trial. J Sex Med. 2010;7:3743–9.
33. Russo GI, Milenkovic U, Hellstrom W, Levine LA, Ralph D, Albersen M. Clinical efficacy of injection and mechanical therapy for Peyronie's disease: a systematic review of the literature. Eur Urol. 2018;74:767–81.
34. Kendirci M, Usta MF, Matern RV, Nowfar S, Sikka SC, Hellstrom WJ. The impact of intralesional interferon alpha-2b injection therapy on penile hemodynamics in men with Peyronie's disease. J Sex Med. 2005;2:709–15.
35. Hellstrom WJG, Kendirci M, Matern R, et al. Single-blind, multicenter, placebo controlled, parallel study to assess the safety and efficacy of intralesional interferon a-2b for minimally invasive treatment for Peyronie's disease. J Urol. 2006;176:394–8.
36. Gennaro R, Barletta D, Paulis G. Intralesional hyaluronic acid: an innovative treatment for Peyronie's disease. Int Urol Nephrol. 2015;47:1595–602.
37. Lipshultz LI, Goldstein I, Seftel AD, et al. Clinical efficacy of collagenase Clostridium histolyticum in the treatment of Peyronie's disease by subgroup: results from two large, double-blind, randomized, placebo-controlled, phase III studies. BJU Int. 2015;116:650–6.
38. Gallien P, Reymann JM, Amarenco G, Nicolas B, de Seze M, Bellissant E. Placebo controlled, randomised, double blind study of the effects of botulinum A toxin on detrusor sphincter dyssynergia in multiple sclerosis patients. J Neurol Neurosurg Psychiatry. 2005;76:1670–6.
39. Kuo HC. Effectiveness of urethral injection of botulinum A toxin in the treatment of voiding dysfunction after radical hysterectomy. Urol Int. 2005;75:247–51.
40. Sampson S, Gerhardt M, Mandelbaum B. Platelet rich plasma injection grafts for musculoskeletal injuries: a review. Curr Rev Musculoskelet Med. 2008;1:165–74.
41. Epifanova MV, Gvasalia BR, Durashov MA, et al. Platelet-rich plasma therapy for male sexual dysfunction: myth or reality? Sex Med Rev. 2020;8:106–13.
42. Matz EL, Pearlman AM, Terlecki RP. Safety and feasibility of platelet rich fibrin matrix injections for treatment of common urologic conditions. Invest Clin Urol. 2018;59:61–5.
43. Rizk DE, El-Safty MM. Female pelvic floor dysfunction in the Middle East: a tale of three factors—Culture, religion and socialization of health role stereotypes. Int Urogynecol J Pelvic Floor Dysfunct. 2006;17:436–8.
44. Maher C, Baessler K, Glazener CM, et al. Surgical management of pelvic organ prolapse in women: a short version Cochrane review. Neurourol Urodyn. 2008;27:3–12.

45. Mettu JR, Colaco M, Badlani GH. Evidence-based outcomes for mesh-based surgery for pelvic organ prolapse. Curr Opin Urol. 2014;24:370–4.
46. Zhang C, Murphy SV, Atala A. Regenerative medicine in urology. Semin Pediatr Surg. 2014;23:106–11.
47. Aboushwareb T, McKenzie P, Wezel F, Southgate J, Badlani G. Is tissue engineering and biomaterials the future for lower urinary tract dysfunction (LUTD)/pelvic organ prolapse (POP)? Neurourol Urodyn. 2011;30:775–82.
48. Davis NF, et al. Biomaterials and regenerative medicine in urology. Adv Exp Med Biol Cell Biol Transl Med. 2018;3:189–98.
49. Sutherland RS, Baskin LS, Hayward SW, Cunha GR. Regeneration of bladder urothelium, smooth muscle, blood vessels and nerves into an acellular tissue matrix. J Urol. 1996;156:571–7.
50. Probst M, Piechota HJ, Dahiya R, et al. Homologous bladder augmentation in dog with the bladder acellularmatrix graft. BJU Int. 2000;85:362–71.
51. Jayo MJ, Jain D, Ludlow JW, et al. Long-term durability, tissue regeneration and neo-organ growth during skeletal maturation with a neo-bladder augmentation construct. Regen Med. 2008;3:671–82.
52. Atala A, Bauer SB, Soker S, Yoo JJ, Retik AB. Tissue-engineered autologous bladders for patients needing cystoplasty. Lancet. 2006;367:1241–6.
53. Joseph DB, Borer JG, De Filippo RE, Hodges SJ, McLorie GA. Autologous cell seeded biodegradable scaffold for augmentation cystoplasty: phase II study in children and adolescents with spina bifida. J Urol. 2014;191:1389–95.
54. El-Kassaby AW, Retik AB, Yoo JJ, Atala A. Urethral stricture repair with an off-the-shelf collagen matrix. J Urol. 2003;169:170–3.
55. Palminteri E, Berdondini E, Colombo F, Austoni E. Small intestinal submucosa (SIS) graft urethroplasty: short-term results. Eur Urol. 2007;51:1695–701.
56. Raya-Rivera A, Esquiliano DR, Yoo JJ, Lopez-Bayghen E, Soker S, Atala A. Tissue- engineered autologous urethras for patients who need reconstruction: an observational study. Lancet. 2011;377:1175–82.

Robot-Assisted Surgery

P. Umari, E. Mazzone, R. De Groote, K. Maes, and A. Mottrie

1 Introduction: Robotic Surgery

The introduction of novel technologies substantially changed our approach to patients with surgical indications over the last decade. The number of robotic procedures performed per year is rapidly increasing all over the world and more and more centers are equipping with this technology [1]. Data suggest an overall trend for conversion from open surgery to robotic-assisted surgery in many surgical specialities [2]. The da Vinci Surgical System has dramatically changed the landscape of minimally invasive surgery providing the surgeon with substantial advantages in dexterity of the instruments, tremor filtration and a better visualization of the surgical field with primary surgeon camera control compared to laparoscopy [3]. The

P. Umari (✉)
Department of Urology, Onze-Lieve-Vrouw (OLV) Hospital, Aalst, Belgium

Department of Translational Medicine, University of Eastern Piedmont, Novara, Italy

Ospedale maggiore della Carità di Novara, University of Eastern Piedmont,
Novata (NO), Italy

E. Mazzone
Department of Urology, Onze-Lieve-Vrouw (OLV) Hospital, Aalst, Belgium

Division of Oncology/Unit of Urology, URI, IRCCS Ospedale San Raffaele, Milan, Italy

ORSI Academy, Melle, Belgium

R. De Groote · A. Mottrie
Department of Urology, Onze-Lieve-Vrouw (OLV) Hospital, Aalst, Belgium

ORSI Academy, Melle, Belgium

K. Maes
Center for Robotic and Minimally Invasive Surgery, Hospital Da Luz, Luz Sáude, Portugal

© The Author(s), under exclusive license to Springer Nature
Switzerland AG 2021
D. Veneziano, E. Huri (eds.), *Urologic Surgery in the Digital Era*,
https://doi.org/10.1007/978-3-030-63948-8_8

129

main advantages are observed when operating in a deep and narrow field and when intracorporeal suturing and fine tissue dissection are required [4].

The increasing implementation of robotic systems determined profound changes in the surgical practice in particular in Urology, Genecology, Cardiac, General and Thoracic surgery. There was a profound change in the management of patients with prostate, bladder and kidney disease. For example, when considering the case of prostate cancer, robot-assisted radical prostatectomy (RARP) has now become the gold standard surgical treatment modality in many centers [5]. A robot-assisted approach for partial nephrectomy (RAPN) has shown benefits over the open approach including a reduced blood loss, postoperative pain and length of stay [6]. Finally, a recent systematic review comparing robot-assisted radical cystectomy (RARC) with open cystectomy showed that RARC benefited from fewer periopera-tive complications, greater lymph node yield, lower blood loss and a shorter length of stay [7].

The aim of this chapter is to review the evolution of robotic surgery and focus on the technical innovations that has been developed since the first robotic system obtained the approval from the FDA for laparoscopic surgery in 2000.A special emphasis was placed on the development of novel devices and their potential future clinical applicability.

2   Evolution: History of Robotic Surgery

The term "robot" derives from "*robota*" which is a Check term to describes a forced labour or *activity* [8]. The use of robots is commonplace in industry, where the machines can undertake ultra-precise and pre-programmed tasks many times, while in medicine they have only been recently adopted to enhance the delivery of care.

The definition of robot suggests a machine capable of performing repetitive tasks autonomously with, if any, different amount of artificial intelligence. There are many types of robotic systems currently available in the healthcare sector. *Active* systems essentially work autonomously and undertake pre-programmed tasks. *Semi-active* systems allow for a surgeon-driven element to complement the pre-programmed element of these robot systems. Lastly the *master–slave* systems lack any of the pre-programmed or autonomous elements of the previous systems. They are entirely dependent on the activity of the surgeon, in fact they just replicate the hand movements of the surgeon and transmit them to laparoscopic surgical instru-ments. Most of the robots adopted in the healthcare are not true robots because they lack independent motions or pre-programmed actions. They are rather master-slave machines that assist the surgeon in various procedures, rather than independently perform tasks [9].

The first robotic system adopted in medicine was the PUMA 560. Kwoh et al. used this robotic system to undertake neurosurgical biopsies with greater accuracy

[10]. The same system was later used by Davies et al. to undertake a transurethral resection of the prostate (TURP) [11]. Later the Integrated Surgical Supplies Ltd developed the PROBOT which was specifically designed to undertake a TURP. In essence, it was a robot with a rotating blade able to complete the process of prostatic resection [12]. In the non-urological field, the ROBODOC system was developed to improve the precision of hip replacement surgery and was the first to achieve a formal Food and Drug Administration (FDA) approval [13].

The United States (US) military were first to recognise the potential significance of linking doctors (distant from the battlefield) to soldiers, in order to reduce the mortality and morbidity during the fields of conflict. A similar concept was used to develop innovation in medical field in particular in minimally invasive surgery. The idea was to connect surgeons to the surgical field with technology [14].

The ZEUS platform developed by Computer Motion and the DaVinci platform by Intuitive Surgical were the pioneers that have dominated the field of robotic surgery for a decade pushing back the frontiers of minimally invasive surgery. After that the Intuitive Surgical acquired Computer Motion in 2004 [15] and after a successful US FDA regulatory approvals, for almost 2 decades [1].

The Computer Motion was founded by Dr. Yulun Wand in 1990 and the goal was initially to build an endoscopic holder. Computer Motion developed the first automated endoscopic system for optimal positioning (AESOP). It essentially enabled surgeons to voice control the positioning of a laparoscopic camera system. It was the first surgical robot to receive FDA clearance [16].

The ZEUS system was a three arms system where one arm held the camera and a further two arms were used to hold surgical instruments. When launched, the ZEUS system was using the AESOP camera system [17]. The surgical console included a high-backed chair with armrests, controlling the instruments with dedicated chopstick like handles. The surgical field was visualized on a two (2D) or three-dimensional (3D) video system and the instruments provided only 4 degrees of freedom. The Conformite Europeenne (CE) and the FDA approvals were obtained in 1999 for cardiovascular surgery. The most impressive demonstration of this system was performed by Marescaux et al. Surgeons in New York City successfully removed a gallbladder from a 68-year-old woman in Strasbourg, France [18]. In the Urological field there were only few human urological applications of the ZEUS system, such as pelvic lymph node dissection and pyeloplasty [19].

3   Current Robots Available

Four generations of the da Vinci system have been introduced over the last 20 years. Technological refinements has been continuously implemented and at currently, the American company Intuitive Surgical owns >1500 patents.

3.1   DaVinci Family

Intuitive Surgical was founded by Dr. Fred Moll, his assistant Dr. John Freund and the Engineer Robert Younge [16]. The system takes its name from the artist Leonardo da Vinci and it is inspired by his study of human anatomy and his development of automatons and robots. The da Vinci platform developed by Intuitive Surgical is a three-to-four-armed system with the central arm holding a binocular lens. Besides the superior 3D vision a unique selling point were advanced instruments with artic- ulated wrist to seven degrees of freedom (Endowrist technology). The da Vinci sys- tem had the CE mark in 1999 and full FDA approval since 2001.

The da Vinci platform was designed for robot-assisted coronary artery surgery, and the first cases were performed at the Heart Centre of Leipzig [20]. The first Robot-assisted laparoscopic radical prostatectomy was pioneered in 2001 in the Henry Ford Hospital [21].

3.1.1   Da Vinci Standardand S-HD

Intuitive Surgical, Inc. was founded in 1995 and the first (standard) da Vinci robotic surgical system was introduced to the market in 1999. The da Vinci robot technol- ogy including three-dimensional vision, EndoWrist instrumentation, Intuitive motion, ergonomic superiority and surgical precision, and has surmounted the dif- ficulties preventing the widespread adoption of laparoscopic RP (LRP). The first up grade occurred in 2003, with the addition of a fourth robotic arm, allowing the console surgeon greater control of retraction. In 2006, the da VinciS system was released, offering high definition vision and TilePro, a multi-image display feature. The latest model, da Vinci ® Si (2009), has dual console capability, allowing for collaborative surgical opportunities.

The first da Vinci surgical system (Standard) was launched to the market in 1999. It was a closed console robot with three robotic arms mounted on a chart offering a 3D vision, EndoWrist instrumentation, superior ergonomic and surgical precision (Fig. 1). The first upgrade occurs in 2003 with the addition of a fourth robotic arm, allowing the surgeon a better control during retraction. In 2006 the da Vinci S sys- tem was released, offering a better range of motion, longer instruments, implemen- tation of bipolar energy, and an optional high definition video system and the possibility to install the fourth arm (Fig. 2).

The unique features of the da Vinci systems were its Endowrist technology with 7 degrees of freedom and loop-like handles enabling ergonomic working, including a clutch mechanism. The operative surgeon sits at the surgeon console, views the surgical site in a three-dimensional binocular viewer, and controls movements of the surgical instruments using two master controllers and dedicated foot switches. The technical support of the da Vinci Standard and S ended in 2015 and 2018 respectively.

Fig. 1 da Vinci Standard
robotic system

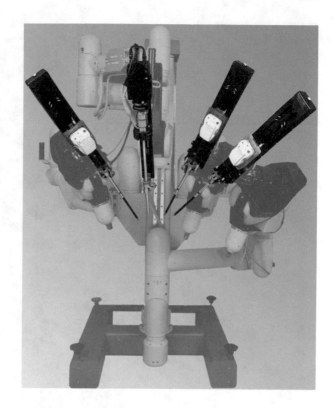

3.1.2   Da Vinci Si

The da Vinci Si system was launched in 2009 with full CE mark and FDA approval.
Its unique features were high definition (HD) video technology, finger-based clutch
mechanism and the possibility to use the intraoperative fluorescence (Fire-Fly technology) with an optional camera (Fig. 3). The surgeon console has been equipped
with a touch screen display for setting up preferences and operating parameters, and
a newly designed foot switch that allows the surgeon to toggle between operating
modes and activation of electrosurgical energy to instruments. The da Vinci Si dual
console allows two surgeons to collaborate during surgery, representing an ideal
training platform (Fig. 4). The da Vinci Si system also allows use of the Intuitive
Surgical single-site platform, providing flexible instruments with only 4 degrees of
freedom (VesPa system) [22, 23].

3.1.3   Da Vinci Fourth Generation (Xi, X)

The da Vinci Xi robot has been completely redesigned compared to the previous
generations (Fig. 5). Has been launched in 2014 with CE mark and FDA approval.
It consists of four arms mounted on a rotating boom that allows the docking of the

Fig. 2 da Vinci S-HD
robotic system

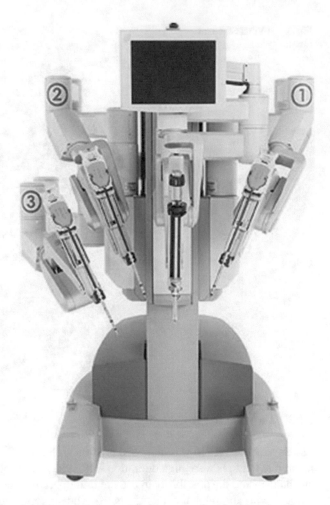

robot from any side (Fig. 6a). A new laser guided system for docking has been
implemented. A green target is projected from the cart's overhead boom, which is
aligned to camera port. When the camera is inserted and the "targeting button"
pressed, the remaining robotic arms automatically optimise their positions in order
to minimize clacking (Fig. 6b). The arms architecture has been completely redesigned in order to minimize the instrument clashing and to allow the positioning of
trocar ports closer than the previous version and in in line fashion (Fig. 6c). A
unique feature is the new 8-mm 3D high definition (HD) camera that can be liber-
ally placed in any of the four ports ('camera hopping') (Fig. 6d). This feature can be
important for specific multi-quadrant procedures, such as colorectal surgery.
Moreover the 30° up and down function allows to change the vision directly from
the console. The Fire fly technology is incorporated in the camera and it should not
be acquired as an optional. An advanced and specifically designed operating table is
available as optional. It can be connected to the system and moved while the robotic

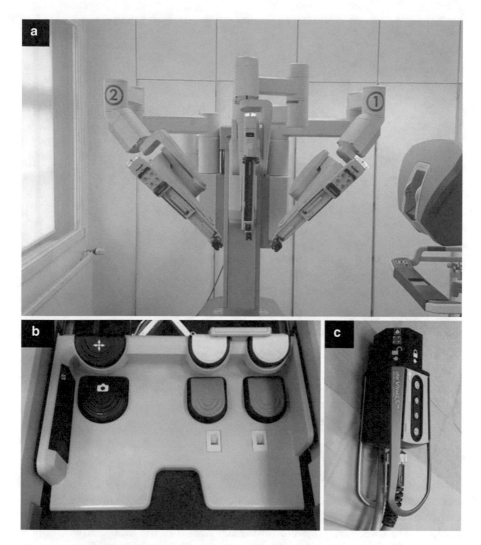

Fig. 3 (**a**) da Vinci Si robotic system, (**b**) da Vinci Si pedals, (**c**) da Vinci Si camera

arms are connected ('table motion' technology) (Fig. 7). Many technological advancements are available for the new Xi robotic platform, including new stapling devices and 7 degrees of freedom flexible instruments for single-site surgery. Finally this system is compatible with the new robotic SP platform designed for robotic single-port surgery (SP999).

In 2018, Intuitive Surgical introduced the da Vinci X system with the intent to offer a more affordable version of the Xi platform (Fig. 8). The X system is equipped with all the most advanced technologies present of the Xi model mounted on a Si system-like chart. It uses the same instruments and the same camera as the Xi

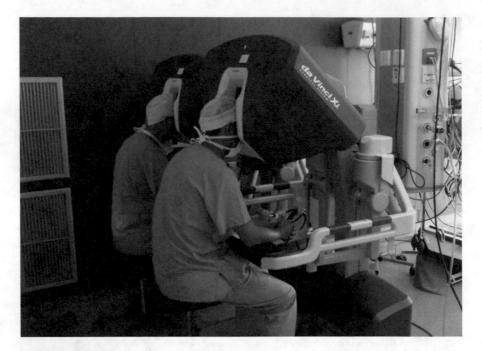

Fig. 4 da Vinci dual console

model, however it doesn't offer the docking flexibility and the compatibility for SP platform as the big brother.

3.1.4 DaVinci SP

To date, the experience of robotic laparo-endoscopic single site (R-LESS) surgery has involved modification of existing robotic systems using single-access ports, specialised semi-rigid curved instruments, and software modifications (VesPa system) [22, 23]. The disadvantages were principally related to the availability of only 4 degrees of freedom instruments and the extremely difficult bed-side assistance due to limited range of motion and impossible simultaneous use of multiple instruments [24].

The da Vinci SP (single port) robotic platform has been specifically created for single site surgery in order to overcome many limitations of up to date R-LESS surgery (Fig. 9). Moreover it has been designed to offer advantages over the standard multi-arm systems, when operating in spaces with difficult access. Indeed all the instruments are included in a single port, which is introduced trough a single abdominal wall incision. Once introduced, the flexible instruments, including the optic, can separate and achieve triangulation thanks to a snake-style wrist [25].

The da Vinci SP platform has several unique and novel features compared to the multiport systems [25]. This platform is equipped with a single robotic arm docked

Fig. 5 da Vinci Xi robotic
system

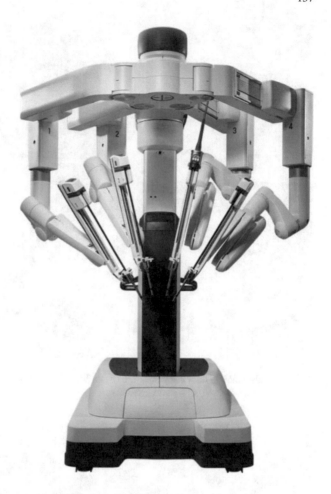

to a 25 mm multichannel port (Fig. 10a). It has a fully articulating 12 × 10-mm oval
camera and three 6 mm instruments able of 7 degrees of freedom (Fig. 10b). All
instruments and the camera have a double articulating design (i.e., wrist and elbow)
(Fig. 10c). A virtual guidance system allows the surgeon to visualize the spatial
relations of each arm and the camera during surgery. An extra-clutch has been
designed, by which the surgeon can move the camera and working arms independently or as a single unit during surgery. The surgeon console design on the da Vinci
SP Surgical System is identical to the standard da Vinci system except for an the
already mentioned extra foot switch [26] (Fig. 10d).

The first generation SP platform (SP999) was designed to use the same base and
column of the da Vinci XI patient side cart, but with a different configuration of the
surgical arms and manipulators in order to drive the unique SP instruments and
camera through a single port. The Intuitive Surgical da Vinci SP999 platform gained
FDA approval for single-port surgery in urology in 2014 [27]. However Intuitive
decided not to market and instead focus on developing the purpose-built platform,

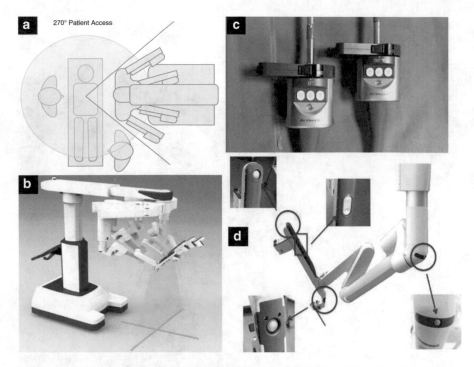

Fig. 6 (**a**) da Vinci Xi docking flexibility, (**b**) da Vinci Xi docking laser, (**c**) da Vinci Xi 0 and 30° digital camera, (**d**) da Vinci Xi arm architecture

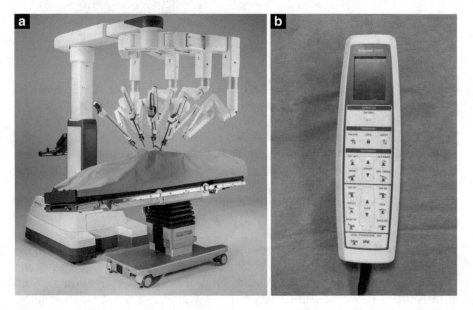

Fig. 7 (**a**) da Vinci table with table motion technology, (**b**) da Vinci table remote controller

Fig. 8 da Vinci X robotic system

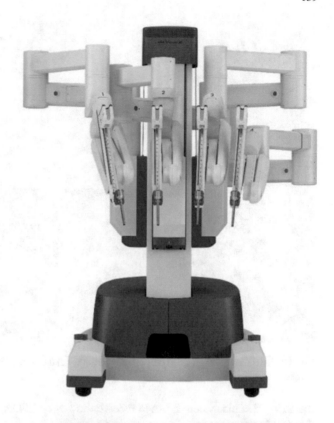

Fig. 9 da Vinci SP robotic system

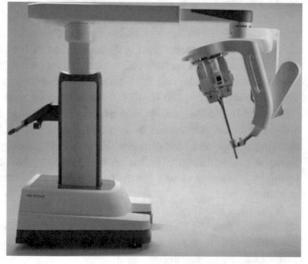

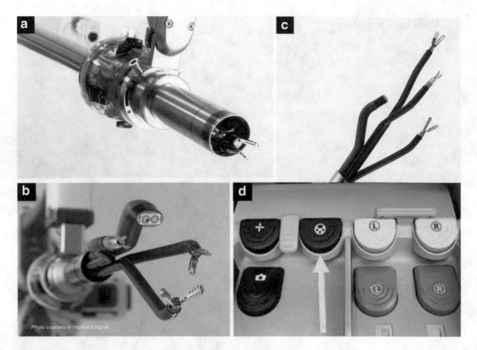

Fig. 10 (**a**) da Vinci SP port, (**b**) da Vinci SP camera, (**c**) da Vinci SP instruments, (**d**) da Vinci SP extra clutch pedal

the SP1098. This system is yet to receive the CE and FDA approval and remains in the development stage.

The second generation SP surgical system (SP1089) is equivalent to the predicate device SP999 in terms of technological characteristics, and has identical indications for use. It basically an updated version of the first generation SP999. The surgeon console, vision and patient cart were modified to incorporate the latest mechanical, electrical, and user interface technology of the cleared multi-port da Vinci Xi Surgical System (IS4000). An integrated monopolar energy monitor was also added to the Vision Cart. Modifications were also made to the EndoWrist SP instruments and accessories to improve manufacturability, robustness, reliability, cleaning ability, and ease of use while enhancing safety and maintaining the same ability to perform surgical tasks. In order to accommodate the modified instruments and to improve ease of use, the instrument arm and instrument drives were updated as well.

It has been investigated in pre-clinical trials involving a small number of patients and showed that R-LESS with the second generation SP1098 platform is feasible, however it will require further investigation to compare with conventional multi-port robotic surgery [28–30].

3.2 CMR Versius

The Versius Surgical System is the new tele-operated robotic surgical system designed to assist surgeons in performing minimally-invasive surgery designed by CMR Surgical (Cambridge, UK).

The design of the Versius differs significantly from that of the Da Vinci Surgical System. The robotic arms are modular providing an increased arm positioning and flexibility. Each instrument and visualisation arm is attached to its own wheeled cart to form a compact and mobile bedside unit (Fig. 11). Each bedside unit is connected with cables to the console representing the world's smallest clinical robot on the market. It is a reconfigurable system, the number of bed side units that can be used per surgery varies between 3 and 5. The bed side units or robotic arms are mobile and can be interchanged. The robotic instruments mimics the articulation of the human arm and the wristed instrument tip provides seven degrees of freedom allowing greater surgical access than standard laparoscopic surgery (Fig. 12). The Versius surgeon console is open, and can be operated at either a standing or a seated position, and all the robotic device control has been placed on-board handheld control units, removing the need for foot pedal controls (Fig. 13). The console has a 2D/3D screen and the surgeon sits straight with 3D glasses, while others can sit and watch the surgery behind the surgeon [31].

In 2019 the safety and effectiveness of the system has been demonstrated for urological [32] and general surgery [33] procedures in the preclinical setting. The assessment was performed on cadaveric and porcine models. Several types of

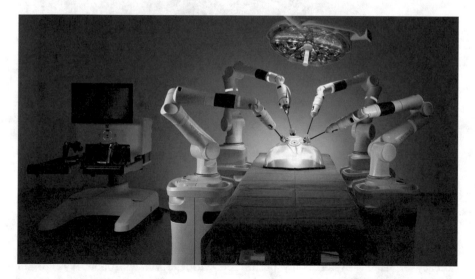

Fig. 11 Versius robotic system

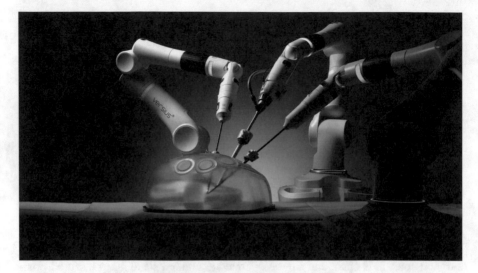

Fig. 12 Versius robotic arms during pelvic box training

Fig. 13 Versius handheld
control units

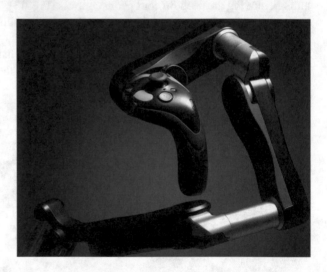

abdominal surgeries were tested in cadavers, with the lead surgeons evaluating a range of port and bedside units positions. All surgeries were completed successfully. A radical nephrectomy, a cholecystectomy and a small bowel enterotomy were also performed safely and effectively in a live animal model.

Finally, Puntambekar et al. has recently demonstrated the feasibility, safety and efficacy of radical hysterectomy performed with the Versius robotic systems in clinical setting on 30 patients [34].

3.3 Telelap ALF-X

Telelap ALF-X is a robotic platform designed by the Italian healthcare company Sofar Surgical Robotics (Milan, Italy). An initial patent was registered in 2007. In 2015 Sofar Surgical Robotics has been acquired by TransEnterix (Morrisville, NC, USA). Telelap ALF-X obtained the CE clearance for indications in general surgery, gynaecology, urology and thoracic surgery in 2016. The first devices has been sold in Italy and early clinical reports of robot-assisted hysterectomies were published by an Italian group in Rome (Italy) [35].

It uses an open console, laparoscopy-like handles and arms mounted on separate carts. The TELELAP Alf-X system offers a novel approach to remotely operated 3-dimension endoscopy by adding haptic sensation, an eye-tracking system, and a high degree of configuration versatility. The ALF-X system instruments are reusable with lower disposable costs compared to the present robots [36].

3.4 Senhance Robot

TransEnterix, a US medical device company is focused on the commercialization of a the Senhance robotic system. The platform received the FDA approval for laparoscopic surgical procedures in general, cardiac, colorectal, gynaecologic, head and neck, thoracic and urologic surgical procedures.

The robot system comprises three arms, each individually mounted on its own cart. Recently a fourth robotic arm has been approved by the company. Senhance instruments are similar to traditional laparoscopic instrumentation, however they provide haptic feedback from the cable-actuated arms, and 7 degrees of freedom. Additionally, the Senhance incorporates a novel eye-tracking technology, which centers the camera image at the point the surgeon is looking at. Finally the Senhance system is compatible with many of the currently available visualizations systems including fluorescence technology [2].

From November 2018 to March 2019 a total of 100 procedures using the Senhance robotic platform were performed in general and colorectal surgery, gynaecology, and urology at the in Klaipeda University Hospital (Klaipeda, Lithuania) with excellent outcomes [37].

4 Upcoming Robots

Nowadays the Da Vinci intuitive system is the only leader on the marked. New companies are engaged in designing new robotic systems in order to propose an alternative to the well-established DaVinci platform [35–40]. However, mainly because of issues related to patenting, their clinical applications remain limited. Nevertheless, the landscape of robotic surgery is expected to witness significant changes as new technologies might soon become available.

4.1 Avatera (The German Robot)

Since 2012, Avateramedical (Jena, Germany) have been developing the Avatera surgical platform in cooperation with Force Dimension (Nyon, Switzerland) and with Tubingen Scientific (Tubingen, Germany) (Fig. 14). The Avatera robot features a closed console with an integrated seat using a microscope-like technology for in-line 3D image with full HD resolution. Four robotic arms are mounted on a single cart and 5 mm instruments with 6 degrees of freedom are applied. Patents were registered in 2012 and 2013. The system has only been used in experimental animal trials. The validation process for CE certification was initiated in 2017 [38].

Fig. 14 Avatera robotic system ("the German robot")

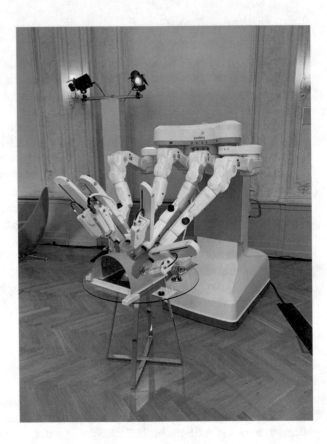

4.2   MicroSurge (Medtronic)

Medtronic is developing a new robotic platform together with German Aerospace Center (DRL). In 2010 the first experimental results of MiroSurge were published. The main strength of the system is its versatility, indeed the system has been designed to be expandable and useful in multiple surgical applications [41]. In 2015 Medtronic completed the acquisition of Covidien and the company became able to develop all necessary instruments and it is currently working on the tenth prototype of this system. MiroSurge consisted of three lightweight arms mounted on the operating table, and an open console with the surgeon sitting in front of an autofocusing monitor. The robotic arms are designed to have seven joints with serial kinematics, comparable to human arms. Instruments are driven by micro-motors providing tactile feedback via potentiometers. Patents were registered in 2012 and 2013. Medtronic plan has been to launch the device in the USA in 2018, however this is still not happening [42].

4.3   REVO-I (The Korean Robot)

In Korea, a new robotic platform has been developed, called REVO-I by the Yonsei University and other Korean academic and industry groups, Meerecompany (Hwasong, Korea). It consists of an open console and a four-arm system mounted on a single cart. The system uses 8 mm instruments with 6 degrees of freedom that are reusable for 20 surgical procedures. A tactile feedback system is an important feature in robotic surgery as it has been shown to decreased grasping forces and it may improve surgical outcomes [43]. The patent was registered in 2014 and the first experiments with this system were published in 2016. A RPN was successfully performed using the REVO-I robot platform on a porcine model. The only limitation was a lack of range of motion in the needle driver if compared to the Da Vinci surgical platform [39, 40]. The approval for human trials was received in South Korea.

5   Technology in Robotic Surgery

Technology is constantly affecting the field of minimally invasive surgery. Many innovations have been integrated within recent robotic surgical systems leading to numerous benefit for the surgeon and patients. New generation robotic systems are equipped with the newest technological refinements in order to improve vision, dexterity and assist the surgeon during the operation (image-guided surgery). Fluorescence imaging, Tactile feedback, Single site surgery, Virtual reality and Image-guided surgery and are all hot topics for the next generation robotic surgeons.

5.1 Fluorescence Imaging

Since 2011 the potential uses of near-infrared fluorescence imaging (NIRF) in surgery has been investigated. The technology of fluorescence imaging can be applied in several fields of minimally invasive surgery. It is able to provide an enhanced anatomical view of the surgical field with visual assessment of vessels, blood flow and tissue perfusion. It is capable to improve the identification of key anatomical landmarks and pathological structures for oncological and non-oncological procedures [39].

The indocyanine green (ICG) is a water-soluble molecule which binds albumin and immediately allows visualization of both the vasculature and contours of anatomic structures (Fig. 15). It has been approved for intravenous administration by FDA since 1959 [44]. It has been also proven to potentially improve the perioperative surgical outcomes during some procedures without compromising the oncological adequacy [45].

The last (fourth) generation of DaVinci platforms has been equipped with this technology by default, while on the previous (third) generation models it was available as an optional. Indeed a specific camera equipped with a near-infrared laser, easily recognizable by the green graphics is needed to use this technology. The system is called "Firefly System" and is capable to provide real-time endoscopic visible near-infrared fluorescence directly on the console and it is activable by the surgeon in any moment [46].

The applications of NIRF/ICG are multiple, as for example it permits to identify diseased parenchyma or assess the lymphatic pathways. This has made a significant impact on facilitating challenging reconstructive and oncologic robotic procedures. It has been proven to be effective for selective/super-selective clamping of arteries during robot-assisted partial nephrectomy and in differential perfusion assessment during renal mass resection [47, 48]. It allows to differentiate various types of adrenal pathologies (pheochromocytoma, metastatic RCC, lymphangioma,

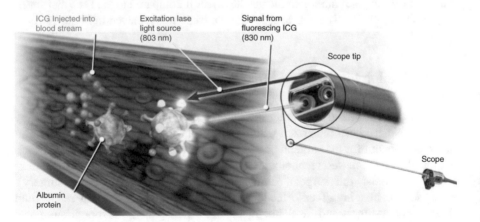

Fig. 15 Intuitive Firefly technology

adrenocortical adenoma, adrenal haemorrhagic cyst, adrenal simple cyst, cystic lymphangioma) and to perform a safe adrenal-sparing surgery [49, 50]. It has been found to achieve a more scrupulous diagnostic approach during extended pelvic lymph node dissection (ePLND) and sentinel node biopsy in patient with prostatic cancer [51, 52]. Recent studies have shown to reduce morbidity during superficial and deep inguinal nodes in patient with penile cancer [53]. Despite may applications the level of evidence is low, indeed further investigation is needed to improve the understanding of this technology (Fig. 16).

Moreover the near-infrared fluorescence imaging could be used also without ICG dye. In fact the white light of the endoscope illuminates green during Firefly mode allowing simultaneous vision of the surrounding tissues. In literature there is only a publication report three different procedures performed using Firefly mode without ICG [54].

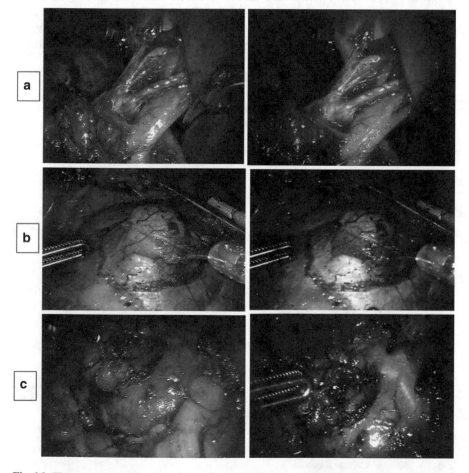

Fig. 16 Fluorescence applications: (**a**) renal pedicle dissection, (**b**) renal tumor excision, (**c**) renal hilum selective clamping

5.2 Tactile Feedback

A widely criticized disadvantage associated with robotic systems is the absence of tactile feedback. The physical connection between the surgeon's hands and the robotic instruments is removed when operating with robotic assistance and the haptic sensation such as the tension of a suture, texture of tissue, and even collisions between robotic arms is physically imperceptible. In addition, the robot system is capable of creating varying forces that far exceed tissue tolerances resulting in tissue tearing and the risk of suture ruptures [55] (Fig. 17).

The current most widely used robotic surgical system Da Vinci is limited by the lack of tactile or haptic feedback that may be useful when performing complex and delicate surgical tasks. At the same its clinical relevance in the performance of robot-assisted surgery is still controversial. Many expert robotic surgeons suggest that the lack of a tactile feedback can be adequately compensated using visual cues such as tissue deformation and retraction during tension. Moreover there are several technical and practical challenges that need to be overcome to implement direct haptic capabilities top the hands of the surgeon in complex surgical systems.

Reiley at al investigated the use of a visual force feedback during surgical knot tying with the da Vinci robotic system equipped with force-sensing instruments tips and real-time graphic overlays. The study showed a lower suture breakage rate and

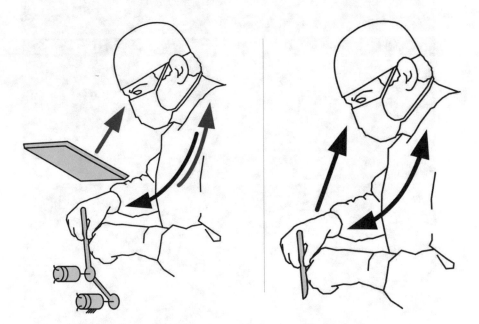

Fig. 17 Tactile and Visual feedback

peak applied forces when using the visual force feedback. Measurable benefits, however, were lacking among experienced users [56].

Another preliminary study investigated the feasibility and potential benefits of sensory substitution in providing haptic feedback in the context of robotic-assisted knot tying [57]. In conjunction with the Johns Hopkins University Department of Mechanical Engineering, a tension measuring device (TMD) was constructed, allowing the measurements of the tension (in newtons) on both the left and right hand during robotic assisted knot tying. A visual colour bar scale was developed to render applied suture tensions to the operating surgeon. The results demonstrated a significantly greater and more consistent tensions applied to suture materials, without breakage, during robotic knot tying with haptic feedback compared to knots tied without feedback.

An interesting research investigate the grasping forces with the application of a tactile feedback system in vivo and the incidence of tissue damage incurred during robotic tissue manipulation [43]. A waterproof sensor was mounted on da Vinci robotic instrument and was capable to evaluate the force output and data acquisition. A control system was designed to convert forces detected at the grasper tips to pressures at the surgeon's fingertips. Pneumatic actuators provided pressure stimuli to fingertips using hemispherical silicone balloons, targeting the slow-adapting mechanoreceptors through constant deformation of the finger pad. The in vivo application of integrated tactile feedback in the robotic system demonstrates significantly reduced grasping forces, resulting in significantly less tissue damage. This tactile feedback system may improve surgical outcomes and broaden the use of robotic-assisted minimally invasive surgery in a wider spectrum of clinical care [58].

Finally another study investigated the capability of the surgeon's experience to compensate for the lack of haptic feedback of the robotic system da Vinci Si HD [59]. 25 surgeons divided in two groups (experts vs non-experts) underwent a specific test to assess their ability to recognize the thickness of custom made membranes, without the availability of haptic feedback. The expert surgeons scored significantly better than the non-expert showing that the personal expertise seems to overcome the lack of a feedback haptic sensor. Moreover the high-definition images combined with 3D binocular vision cues of the da Vinci robotic surgical system compensates for the lack of tactile information.

5.3 Single Site Surgery

The concept of laparo-endoscopic single site (LESS) surgery has been proposed to minimise the surgical morbidity during minimally invasive procedures. The aim was further improve the benefits of conventional multiport surgery by decreasing the number of surgical incisions leading to improved cosmesis, postoperative pain, recovery time as well as postoperative incisional hernias [60]. At the same time a number of obstacles such as poor ergonomics, loss of triangulation, instrument clashing, limited tissue retraction and lack of space for surgical assistant ergonomic challenges and other technical difficulties precluded its widespread application [61].

Before the presentation of the new da Vinci SP platform, the Intuitive Surgical single-site platform was available for robotic laparo-edoscopic single site (R-LESS) surgery [62]. It represented a definitive step forward compared to standard LESS surgery. The main features were the 5 mm semi-rigid instruments allowing only 4 degrees of freedom, which were inserted through a couple of curved cannulas. The cannulas were placed in a crossing over fashion through a multi-trocar port which allowed the triangulation of the instruments. When the single-site instruments were docked into the da Vinci Si System, they were automatically reassigned so the right hand of the Surgeon's Control will control the left instrument and vice versa.

However the technical approach of R-LESS using the Intuitive Surgical single-site platform was limited by many drawbacks. The main were the non-availability of 7 degrees of freedom Endowrist technology for the instruments and the extremely difficult bed-side assistance due to limited range of motion and impossible simultaneous use of multiple instruments [28].

5.4 Virtual Reality

Originally developed for gaming, virtual reality is now spreading in many fields. The healthcare sector is one of the biggest adopters of virtual reality, in particular as a means of training the next generation of medical professionals. Virtual reality (VR) has played an important role in training robotic surgeons to gain valuable experience but in a safe environment. VR is a useful tool to improve familiarity with the robotic console, three-dimensional vision and wristed instruments [63, 64].

There are many VR simulator on the market. Thanks to the huge technological improvements of the last years, a wide array of VR simulator are available on the market. Many of them are designed for basic skill acquisition, while others are designed for the acquisition of entire procedures. The newest simulators are able to recreate an entire surgical procedure as for example a RARP. VR simulation has been demonstrated to improve surgical performances in a risk-free environment [65, 66].

5.5 Image-Guided Surgery

Image-guided surgery (IGS) is the use of a real-time correlation of the operative field to a preoperative imaging data set that reflects the precise location of a selected surgical instrument to the surrounding anatomic structures [67]. In many procedures, the surgeon has a limited view of the operating field and cannot visualize structures beyond the exposed surfaces. In minimally invasive surgeries, particularly during endoscopic procedures, the surgeon is also confronted with difficult hand-eye coordination problems. Better use of the three-dimensional imaging can improve surgical visualization and help the surgeons overcome these limitations. In particular, enhanced reality visualization, in which the surgeon's field of view is augmented with additional structural information, can provide useful guidance in planning and executing the surgery. Robotic surgery offers the unique opportunity to integrate 3D virtual renderings and real-time images from the endoscopic camera in the robotic console (Fig. 18).

Porpiglia et al. described the first clinical experience with a novel software for augmented-reality robot-assisted radical prostatectomy. Preoperatively, the MRI images were segmented in order to obtain a 3D reconstruction of the prostate and the surrounding structures. In order to allow a better visualization of the images during the operation an elastic 3D model was. Using the TilePro facility of the da Vinci surgical system the virtual image of the prostate was superimposed onto the endoscopic view of the surgical field. The surgeon was able to perform less invasive procedures when using IGS with potential better funcional outcomes for the patient [68].

ICG can be used also during robot-assisted partial nephrectomy in order to better visualize renal masses and perform a more effective selective clamping during the enucleation of the tumor [69].

There is an increasing interest in this technology among the new-generation robotic surgeons. It is gaining interest because of its potential to improve patient

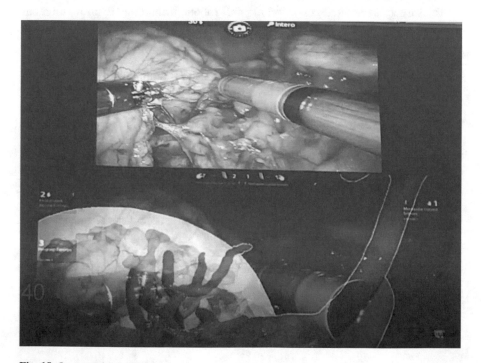

Fig. 18 Image guided surgery

outcome following oncologic surgery. At the same time, IGS is still in an embryonal phase of its development. Further investigation is needed to improve and make this technology usable and profitable [70].

6 The Future of Robotic Surgery

In the operating room of the future, robots will be an integral part of the surgical team, working alongside human surgeons to make surgeries safer, faster, more precise and more automated. In the meantime Telementoring and Telesurgery are progressing quickly as a subset of Telemedicine. With the amalgamation of technological communication and surgery, Telesurgery and Telementoring are having a tremendous impact on next generation surgeons.

6.1 Telementoring and Telesurgery

Telemedicine is an expanding field that can help clinicians connect with patients when in-person medical visits are not possible. During COVID pandemic for example it has been used as rescue management for chronic pain patients [71].

Telesurgery uses wireless networking and robotic technology to allow surgeons to operate on patients who are distantly located, while telementoring can be used as a guidance to by another expert surgeon who is in a different geographic location (Fig. 19). With the advancement of technology, both telementoring and telesurgery are becoming more practical and cost-effective also for minimally invasive urological surgery [72]. Indeed minimally invasive surgery lends itself well to telesurgery and telementoring techniques mainly because the images of the surgical field are projected via cable to the surgical console and to additional screens. As such, the exact same images as the primary surgeons can be seen on another screen. An impressive demonstration of Telesurgery was performed by Marescaux et al. when they performed a successful transatlantic gallbladder removal from a 68-year woman in Strasbourg [18].

Telementoring and Telesurgery can take various forms, based on the increasing level of interaction between proctor and trainee. Instruction from the mentor could be as simple as verbal guidance while the mentor is watching a real-time video of the operation. In its more advanced iterations, telementoring can progressively involve indicating target areas on the local monitor screen (telestration), taking over as the assistant by controlling the operative camera or an instrument via robotic arms (tele-assisted surgery), or actually performing the surgery remotely (telesurgery) [72].

Fig. 19 Telementoring

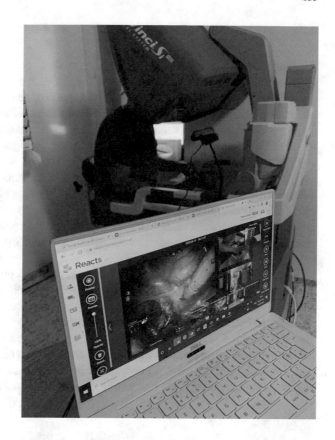

Telesugery and Telementoring can provide high-quality surgery where limited human and economic resources exists as for example in underserved locations, such as rural areas, battlefields, and spacecraft. They virtually eliminate the need for long-distance travels, allowing surgical collaboration amongst surgeons at different medical centers in real-time [73].

5th-Generation Mobile Communication (5G) offers a high potential for the further development of telemedicine. The high data transmission volume, low latency and a high quality of service are important requirements for real-time Telesurgery and Telementoring applications [74].

Advanced technology has opened new avenues for long-distance observation and interaction through telesurgery and telementoring. Although the medicolegal implications of an active surgical intervention by a proctor are not clearly defined, the role as an observer should grant immunity from malpractice liability. Legal and ethical implications linked to the use of telemedicine, telesurgery should be clarified [75].

6.2 Engineering of Robotics (Aerospace and Automation)

A robotics engineer is a designer, who is responsible for creating robots and robotic systems that are able to perform duties in Industries like manufacturing, aerospace and medicine. Through their creations, a robotics engineer helps to make jobs safer, easier, and more efficient, with many benefits even in healthcare.

Robot engineering is a wide field where professionals are working on and developing different type of projects. They are building, configuring, and testing, as well as designing software systems to control their robots. At the same time they are analysing and evaluating the prototypes they have created. Monitoring is generally a never-ending task, since technology is constantly changing and advancing. The cost calculation and technical support including the maintenance are essential to make the project beneficial, both for the producer and the costumer. Finally teaching plans and structured training curricula allow to make the best use of the robotic systems.

The goal of robotic technology in medicine is not to replace human surgeons, but to augment their capabilities and better assist during difficult operations. Indeed, human surgeons are essential during decision making process that can't be left to a robot (ex.to indicate a specific treatment or to develop a new surgical technique). On the other hand, a robot with high-power computing and sub-millimeter precision will be able to control complex instruments and navigate through spaces in the body that a human surgeon can't access. For this reason a close cooperation between engineers and surgeons is the best recipe to obtain the success.

References

1. Leal Ghezzi T, Campos CO. 30 years of robotic surgery. World J Surg. 2016;40(10):2550–7.
2. Peters BS, Armijo PR, Krause C, Choudhury SA, Oleynikov D. Review of emerging surgical robotic technology. Surg Endosc. 2018;32(4):1636–55.
3. Mazzone E, Mistretta FA, Knipper S, Tian Z, Larcher A, Widmer H, et al. Contemporary national assessment of robot-assisted surgery rates and total hospital charges for major surgical uro-oncological procedures in the United States. J Endourol. 2019;33(6):438–47.
4. Honda M, Morizane S, Hikita K, Takenaka A. Current status of robotic surgery in urology. Asian J Endosc Surg. 2017;10(4):372–81.
5. Lowrance WT, Eastham JA, Savage C, Maschino AC, Laudone VP, Dechet CB, et al. Contemporary open and robotic radical prostatectomy practice patterns among urologists in the United States. J Urol. 2012;187(6):2087–92.
6. Ghani KR, Sukumar S, Sammon JD, Rogers CG, Trinh QD, Menon M. Practice patterns and outcomes of open and minimally invasive partial nephrectomy since the introduction of robotic partial nephrectomy: results from the nationwide inpatient sample. J Urol. 2014;191(4):907–12.
7. Li K, Lin T, Fan X, Xu K, Bi L, Duan Y, et al. Systematic review and meta-analysis of comparative studies reporting early outcomes after robot-assisted radical cystectomy versus open radical cystectomy. Cancer Treat Rev. 2013;39(6):551–60.
8. Palep JH. Robotic assisted minimally invasive surgery. J Minim Access Surg. 2009;5(1):1–7.
9. Lane T. A short history of robotic surgery. Ann R Coll Surg Engl. 2018;100(6_sup):5–7.

10. Kwoh YS, Hou J, Jonckheere EA, Hayati S. A robot with improved absolute positioning accuracy for CT guided stereotactic brain surgery. IEEE Trans Biomed Eng. 1988;35(2):153–60.
11. Davies BL, Hibberd RD, Ng WS, Timoney AG, Wickham JE. The development of a surgeon robot for prostatectomies. Proc Inst Mech Eng H J Eng Med. 1991;205(1):35–8.
12. Harris SJ, Arambula-Cosio F, Mei Q, Hibberd RD, Davies BL, Wickham JE, et al. The Probot- -an active robot for prostate resection. Proc Inst Mech Eng H J Eng Med. 1997;211(4):317–25.
13. Subramanian P, Wainwright TW, Bahadori S, Middleton RG. A review of the evolution of robotic-assisted total hip arthroplasty. Hip Int. 2019;29(3):232–8.
14. Satava RM. Surgical robotics: the early chronicles: a personal historical perspective. Surg Laparosc Endosc Percutan Tech. 2002;12(1):6–16.
15. Binder J, Kramer W. Robotically-assisted laparoscopic radical prostatectomy. BJU Int. 2001;87(4):408–10.
16. George EI, Brand TC, LaPorta A, Marescaux J, Satava RM. Origins of robotic surgery: from skepticism to standard of care. J Soc Laparoendosc Surg. 2018;22(4):e2018.00039.
17. Reichenspurner H, Damiano RJ, Mack M, Boehm DH, Gulbins H, Detter C, et al. Use of the voice-controlled and computer-assisted surgical system ZEUS for endoscopic coronary artery bypass grafting. J Thorac Cardiovasc Surg. 1999;118(1):11–6.
18. Larkin M. Transatlantic, robot-assisted telesurgery deemed a success. Lancet (London, England). 2001;358(9287):1074.
19. Luke PP, Girvan AR, Al Omar M, Beasley KA, Carson M. Laparoscopic robotic pyeloplasty using the Zeus Telesurgical System. Can J Urol. 2004;11(5):2396–400.
20. Mohr FW, Falk V, Diegeler A, Autschback R. Computer-enhanced coronary artery bypass surgery. J Thorac Cardiovasc Surg. 1999;117(6):1212–4.
21. Pasticier G, Rietbergen JB, Guillonneau B, Fromont G, Menon M, Vallancien G. Robotically assisted laparoscopic radical prostatectomy: feasibility study in men. Eur Urol. 2001;40(1):70–4.
22. Cestari A, Buffi NM, Lista G, Lughezzani G, Larcher A, Lazzeri M, et al. Feasibility and preliminary clinical outcomes of robotic laparoendoscopic single-site (R-LESS) pyeloplasty using a new single-port platform. Eur Urol. 2012;62(1):175–9.
23. Mattevi D, Luciani LG, Vattovani V, Chiodini S, Puglisi M, Malossini G. First case of robotic laparoendoscopic single-site radical prostatectomy with single-site VesPa platform. J Robot Surg. 2018;12(2):381–5.
24. Gaboardi F, Pini G, Suardi N, Montorsi F, Passaretti G, Smelzo S. Robotic laparoendoscopic single-site radical prostatectomy (R-LESS-RP) with daVinci Single-Site® platform. Concept and evolution of the technique following an IDEAL phase 1. J Robot Surg. 2019;13(2):215–26.
25. Bertolo R, Garisto J, Gettman M, Kaouk J. Novel system for robotic single-port surgery: feasibility and state of the art in urology. Eur Urol Focus. 2018;4(5):669–73.
26. Aminsharifi A, Sawczyn G, Wilson CA, Garisto J, Kaouk J. Technical advancements in robotic prostatectomy: single-port extraperitoneal robotic-assisted radical prostatectomy and single-port transperineal robotic-assisted radical prostatectomy. Transl Androl Urol. 2020;9(2):848–55.
27. Kaouk JH, Haber GP, Autorino R, Crouzet S, Ouzzane A, Flamand V, et al. A novel robotic system for single-port urologic surgery: first clinical investigation. Eur Urol. 2014;66(6):1033–43.
28. Maurice MJ, Ramirez D, Kaouk JH. Robotic laparoendoscopic single-site retroperitioneal renal surgery: initial investigation of a purpose-built single-port surgical system. Eur Urol. 2017;71(4):643–7.
29. Ramirez D, Maurice MJ, Kaouk JH. Robotic perineal radical prostatectomy and pelvic lymph node dissection using a purpose-built single-port robotic platform. BJU Int. 2016;118(5):829–33.
30. Maurice MJ, Kaouk JH. Robotic radical perineal cystectomy and extended pelvic lymphadenectomy: initial investigation using a purpose-built single-port robotic system. BJU Int. 2017;120(6):881–4.

31. Atallah S, Parra-Davila E, Melani AGF. Assessment of the Versius surgical robotic system for dual-field synchronous transanal total mesorectal excision (taTME) in a preclinical model: will tomorrow's surgical robots promise newfound options? Tech Coloproctol. 2019;23(5):471–7.
32. Thomas BC, Slack M, Hussain M, Barber N, Pradhan A, Dinneen E, et al. Preclinical evaluation of the versius surgical system, a new robot-assisted surgical device for use in minimal access renal and prostate surgery. Eur Urol Focus. 2021;7(2):444–52.
33. Morton J, Hardwick RH, Tilney HS, Gudgeon AM, Jah A, Stevens L, et al. Preclinical evaluation of the versius surgical system, a new robot-assisted surgical device for use in minimal access general and colorectal procedures. Surg Endosc. 2021;35(5):2169–77.
34. Puntambekar SP, Goel A, Chandak S, Chitale M, Hivre M, Chahal H, et al. Feasibility of robotic radical hysterectomy (RRH) with a new robotic system. Experience at Galaxy Care Laparoscopy Institute. J Robot Surg. 2020; https://doi.org/10.1007/s11701-020-01127-x.
35. Rossitto C, Gueli Alletti S, Romano F, Fiore A, Coretti S, Oradei M, et al. Use of robot-specific resources and operating room times: The case of Telelap Alf-X robotic hysterectomy. Int J Med Robot. 2016;12(4):613–9.
36. Gidaro S, Buscarini M, Ruiz E, Stark M, Labruzzo A. Telelap Alf-X: a novel telesurgical system for the 21st century. Surg Technol Int. 2012;22:20–5.
37. Samalavicius NE, Janusonis V, Siaulys R, Jasėnas M, Deduchovas O, Venckus R, et al. Robotic surgery using Senhance® robotic platform: single center experience with first 100 cases. J Robot Surg. 2020;14(2):371–6.
38. Rassweiler JJ, Autorino R, Klein J, Mottrie A, Goezen AS, Stolzenburg JU, et al. Future of robotic surgery in urology. BJU Int. 2017;120(6):822–41.
39. Abdel Raheem A, Troya IS, Kim DK, Kim SH, Won PD, Joon PS, et al. Robot-assisted Fallopian tube transection and anastomosis using the new REVO-I robotic surgical system: feasibility in a chronic porcine model. BJU Int. 2016;118(4):604–9.
40. Kim DK, Park DW, Rha KH. Robot-assisted Partial Nephrectomy with the REVO-I Robot Platform in Porcine Models. Eur Urol. 2016;69(3):541–2.
41. Hagn U, Konietschke R, Tobergte A, Nickl M, Jörg S, Kübler B, et al. DLR MiroSurge: a versatile system for research in endoscopic telesurgery. Int J Comput Assist Radiol Surg. 2010;5(2):183–93.
42. meerecompany. Available from: http://www.meerecompany.com/en/product/surgical_01.asp
43. Wottawa CR, Genovese B, Nowroozi BN, Hart SD, Bisley JW, Grundfest WS, et al. Evaluating tactile feedback in robotic surgery for potential clinical application using an animal model. Surg Endosc. 2016;30(8):3198–209.
44. Nair R, Aggarwal R, Khanna D. Methods of formal consensus in classification/diagnostic criteria and guideline development. Semin Arthritis Rheum. 2011;41(2):95–105.
45. Tobis S, Knopf J, Silvers C, Yao J, Rashid H, Wu G, et al. Near infrared fluorescence imaging with robotic assisted laparoscopic partial nephrectomy: initial clinical experience for renal cortical tumors. J Urol. 2011;186(1):47–52.
46. Autorino R, Zargar H, White WM, Novara G, Annino F, Perdonà S, et al. Current applications of near-infrared fluorescence imaging in robotic urologic surgery: a systematic review and critical analysis of the literature. Urology. 2014;84(4):751–9.
47. Borofsky MS, Gill IS, Hemal AK, Marien TP, Jayaratna I, Krane LS, et al. Near-infrared fluorescence imaging to facilitate super-selective arterial clamping during zero-ischaemia robotic partial nephrectomy. BJU Int. 2013;111(4):604–10.
48. Angell JE, Khemees TA, Abaza R. Optimization of near infrared fluorescence tumor localization during robotic partial nephrectomy. J Urol. 2013;190(5):1668–73.
49. Kahramangil B, Kose E, Berber E. Characterization of fluorescence patterns exhibited by different adrenal tumors: determining the indications for indocyanine green use in adrenalectomy. Surgery. 2018;164(5):972–7.
50. Colvin J, Zaidi N, Berber E. The utility of indocyanine green fluorescence imaging during robotic adrenalectomy. J Surg Oncol. 2016;114(2):153–6.

51. Harke NN, Godes M, Wagner C, Addali M, Fangmeyer B, Urbanova K, et al. Fluorescence-supported lymphography and extended pelvic lymph node dissection in robot-assisted radical prostatectomy: a prospective, randomized trial. World J Urol. 2018;36(11):1817–23.
52. Mangano MS, De Gobbi A, Beniamin F, Lamon C, Ciaccia M, Maccatrozzo L. Robot-assisted nerve-sparing radical prostatectomy using near-infrared fluorescence technology and indocyanine green: initial experience. Urologia. 2018;85(1):29–31.
53. Sávio LF, Panizzutti Barboza M, Alameddine M, Ahdoot M, Alonzo D, Ritch CR. Combined partial penectomy with bilateral robotic inguinal lymphadenectomy using near-infrared fluorescence guidance. Urology. 2018;113:251.
54. Hockenberry MS, Smith ZL, Mucksavage P. A novel use of near-infrared fluorescence imaging during robotic surgery without contrast agents. J Endourol. 2014;28(5):509–12.
55. Mucksavage P, Kerbl DC, Pick DL, Lee JY, McDougall EM, Louie MK. Differences in grip forces among various robotic instruments and da Vinci surgical platforms. J Endourol. 2011;25(3):523–8.
56. Reiley CE, Akinbiyi T, Burschka D, Chang DC, Okamura AM, Yuh DD. Effects of visual force feedback on robot-assisted surgical task performance. J Thorac Cardiovasc Surg. 2008;135(1):196–202.
57. Bethea BT, Okamura AM, Kitagawa M, Fitton TP, Cattaneo SM, Gott VL, et al. Application of haptic feedback to robotic surgery. J Laparoendosc Adv Surg Tech A. 2004;14(3):191–5.
58. Toledo L, Gossot D, Fritsch S, Revillon Y, Reboulet C. Study of sustained forces and the working space of endoscopic surgery instruments. Ann Chir. 1999;53(7):587–97.
59. Meccariello G, Faedi F, AlGhamdi S, Montevecchi F, Firinu E, Zanotti C, et al. An experimental study about haptic feedback in robotic surgery: may visual feedback substitute tactile feedback? J Robot Surg. 2016;10(1):57–61.
60. Tugcu V, Ilbey YO, Mutlu B, Tasci AI. Laparoendoscopic single-site surgery versus standard laparoscopic simple nephrectomy: a prospective randomized study. J Endourol. 2010;24(8):1315–20.
61. McCrory B, Lowndes BR, Wirth LM, de Laveaga AE, LaGrange CA, Hallbeck MS. Ergonomic evaluation of laparoendoscopic single-site surgery ports in a validated laparoscopic training model. Work (Reading, Mass). 2012;41(Suppl 1):1884–90.
62. Escobar PF, Haber GP, Kaouk J, Kroh M, Chalikonda S, Falcone T. Single-port surgery: laboratory experience with the daVinci single-site platform. J Soc Laparoendosc Surg. 2011;15(2):136–41.
63. Fisher RA, Dasgupta P, Mottrie A, Volpe A, Khan MS, Challacombe B, et al. An over-view of robot assisted surgery curricula and the status of their validation. Int J Surg (London, England). 2015;13:115–23.
64. Beulens AJW, Vaartjes L, Tilli S, Brinkman WM, Umari P, Puliatti S, et al. Structured robot-assisted surgery training curriculum for residents in Urology and impact on future surgical activity. J Robot Surg. 2020; https://doi.org/10.1007/s11701-020-01134-y.
65. Wiener S, Haddock P, Shichman S, Dorin R. Construction of a urologic robotic surgery training curriculum: how many simulator sessions are required for residents to achieve proficiency? J Endourol. 2015;29(11):1289–93.
66. Menhadji A, Abdelshehid C, Osann K, Alipanah R, Lusch A, Graversen J, et al. Tracking and assessment of technical skills acquisition among urology residents for open, laparoscopic, and robotic skills over 4 years: is there a trend? J Endourol. 2013;27(6):783–9.
67. Teber D, Baumhauer M, Guven EO, Rassweiler J. Robotic and imaging in urological surgery. Curr Opin Urol. 2009;19(1):108–13.
68. Porpiglia F, Checcucci E, Amparore D, Autorino R, Piana A, Bellin A, et al. Augmented-reality robot-assisted radical prostatectomy using hyper-accuracy three-dimensional reconstruction (HA3D™) technology: a radiological and pathological study. BJU Int. 2019;123(5):834–45.
69. Shirk JD, Thiel DD, Wallen EM, Linehan JM, White WM, Badani KK, et al. Effect of 3-dimensional virtual reality models for surgical planning of robotic-assisted partial nephrectomy on surgical outcomes: a randomized clinical trial. JAMA Netw Open. 2019;2(9):e1911598.

70. Porpiglia F, Bertolo R, Amparore D, Checcucci E, Artibani W, Dasgupta P, et al. Augmented reality during robot-assisted radical prostatectomy: expert robotic surgeons' on-the-spot insights after live surgery. Minerva Urol Nefrol. 2018;70(2):226–9.
71. Ghai B, Malhotra N, Bajwa SJS. Telemedicine for chronic pain management during COVID-19 pandemic. Indian J Anaesth. 2020;64(6):456–62.
72. Hung AJ, Chen J, Shah A, Gill IS. Telementoring and telesurgery for minimally invasive procedures. J Urol. 2018;199(2):355–69.
73. Choi PJ, Oskouian RJ, Tubbs RS. Telesurgery: past, present, and future. Cureus. 2018;10(5):e2716.
74. Jell A, Vogel T, Ostler D, Marahrens N, Wilhelm D, Samm N, et al. 5th-generation mobile communication: data highway for surgery 4.0. Surg Technol Inte. 2019;35:36–42.
75. Saceanu SM, Angelescu C, Valeriu S, Patrascu A. Telesurgery and robotic surgery: ethical and legal aspect. J Commun Med Health Educ. 2015;5:355.

Robot-Assisted Upper Tract Surgery

Jens Rassweiler, Marcel Fiedler, Remzi Saglam, and Jan-Thorsten Klein

1 Introduction

Since the beginning of this century, robot-assisted surgery has gained significant importance in the field of laparoscopy ([1, 2]; Table 1). Recently, also in the management of urolithiasis, master-slave-systems have been tested [3–6]. Interestingly, the devices for extracorporeal shock wave lithotripsy have been already equipped with a lot of technology, such as navigation tools or video-systems for control of coupling quality [7]. However, in the meantime particularly flexible ureterorenoscopy (FURS) respectively retrograde intra-renal surgery (RIRS) has gained significant importance, which was enabled by the continuous improvement of the endourological armamentarium with miniaturization of the instruments and introduction of novel laser technologies [8–11].

However, FURS and RIRS are limited by ergonomic deficiencies during endoscopic manipulation, application of the laser, which may become cumbersome mainly when treating multiple stones or larger renal calculi and may even lead to orthopaedic problems among urologists [12, 13]. Based on the positive experience with master-slave-systems in laparoscopic surgery, cardiology and interventional radiology, several groups focused on the usefulness of such robotic devices for RIRS/FURS to overcome most of such methodological obstacles (Table 2).

J. Rassweiler (✉) · M. Fiedler
Department of Urology, SLK Kliniken Heilbronn, University of Heidelberg,
Heilbronn, Germany
e-mail: jens.rassweiler@slk-kliniken.de

R. Saglam
Department of Urology, Medicana International Hospital, Ankara, Turkey

J.-T. Klein
Department of Urology, Medical School Ulm, University of Ulm, Ulm, Germany

D. Veneziano, E. Huri (eds.), *Urologic Surgery in the Digital Era*,
https://doi.org/10.1007/978-3-030-63948-8_9

Table 1 Historical overview on most important robotic devices in surgery

Device	Description	Comment
Robodoc	Automated drilling of the shaft for hip-prothesis based on CT	Clinical problems (pain)
Caspar	Automated drilling for hip-prothesis based on CT	No more in clinical use
Probot	Automated resection of the prostate based on TRUS	No more in clinical use (only prototype)
Neuro-arm	Master-slave system with open console for neurosurgery	Developing company does not exist anymore
AESOP	Voice-controlled camera-arm for laparoscopy	Developing company does not exist anymore
ARTEMIS	Master-slave system with open console for laparoscopy	Only experimental Never produced
ZEUS	Master-slave system with open console for laparoscopy	Developing company does not exist anymore
Da Vinci	Master-slave system with closed console for laparoscopy	Still used in the fourth generation of device
Senhance	Master-slave system with open console for laparoscopy	First clinical experiences CE-mark
Sensei-Magellan	Master-slave system for angiography and cardiology	Not suitable for endourology (ie. FURS)
Avicenna Roboflex	Master-slave system with open console for flexible ureteroscopy	Still used in the third improved version CE-Mark
Monarch	Master-slave system with game-pad for bronchoscopy	First clinical cases
Focal One	Automated system to perform transrectal HIFU	Still used in the third improved version
Aquabeam	Automated system to perform TURP (Aquablation) based on TRUS	First clinical trials RCT-trials CE-mark

In this chapter, we want to focus on actual developments of robot-assisted upper tract surgery including recent evolutions in video-endoscopy, endoscopic armamentarium, and intraoperative navigation [3–6, 14–16].

2 The Ergonomic Deficiencies of Flexible Ureteroscopy

In classic FURS/RIRS the surgeon usually stands controlling the fluoroscopic system and the laser device each by a foot-pedal, while fixing the position of the endoscope with one hand and deflecting/rotating it with the other hand (Table 2). Additionally, the assistant needs to insert the laser fibre or any accessory instrument (basket, N-gage) and activate it according to the surgeon's demand. During this process surgeon and assistant have a very limited working space.

Table 2 Ergonomic requirements for classical flexible ureterorenoscopy (FURS/RIRS) during upper tract endoscopic surgery

Operative manoeuvre	Extremity used	Action by
Insertion of endoscope	Fingers of both hands (at meatus and instrument)	Surgeon
Deflection of endoscope	Hand holding hand piece Thumb at handle Fingers at meatus	Surgeon
Rotation of endoscope	Hand holding hand piece Fingers of the other hand At meatus	Surgeon
Fluoroscopic control	Right foot (foot-switch)	Surgeon (Radiotechnician)
Movement of XR-table/C-arm	Right Foot (foot-switch) Hand (manually)	Radiotechnician (Surgeon, Assistant)
Irrigation		
• By syringe	Hand	Nurse/Assistant
• By mechanic device	Foot	Nurse/Assistant (Surgeon)
• By pump	Finger activation (button)	Nurse/Technician
Laser		
• Insertion of fibre	Fingers at ureteroscope	Nurse/Assistant
• Laser settings	Finger (button)	Nurse/Technician
• Activation	Right foot (foot-switch)	Surgeon
Use of Basket/Grasper		
• Insertion	Fingers at ureteroscope	Nurse/Assistant
• Manipulation	Hand and thumb	Surgeon
• Closure	Fingers at handle	Nurse/Assistant

Thus the aim of a robotic device should mainly act also as a master-slave system trying to help the surgeon by offering an ergonomic working position and alleviating the manipulation of the endoscope without increasing the risk of damaging the urogenital system.

3 Historical Update of Development of Robotic Surgical Devices

3.1 Master-Slaves Systems for Laparoscopy

Already in 1996, Buess and Schurr et al. [17] developed the ARTEMIS-System and presented first experimental results, when successfully performing a telesurgical laparoscopic cholecystectomy in an experimental model (Fig. 1). Despite various promising experimental trials in abdominal and cardiac surgery, the device never made it beyond the experimental state (Table 1).

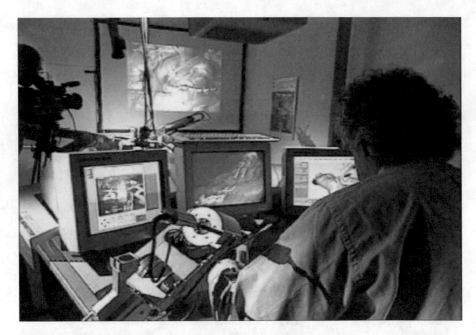

Fig. 1 ARTEMIS: First master-slave system used experimentally (G. Buess, German Nuclear Research Centre, Karlsuhe, Germany). Open console, 3D-videotechnology with polarizing glasses for the surgeon

Based on the voiced controlled camera-arm AESOP, the ZEUS-system (Computer motion Inc., Goleta, CA, USA) has been developed and used for cardiac surgery and gynecological procedures [18]. The ZEUS-System (Fig. 2) was based on the combination of a control unit and three tele-manipulators: All arms were mounted by hand on the rails of the operating table. The surgeon was seated on an open console with a high-backed chair with armrests, handling the instrument controllers. The most impressive demonstration with ZEUS represented the transatlantic laparoscopic cholecystectomy by Marescaux [19].

Parallel to ZEUS, the da Vinci Surgical system (Intuitive Surgical, Sunnyvale, United States) was introduced initially also designed for robot-assisted coronary artery surgery [20]. In 2000, Binder pioneered the first robot-assisted radical prostatectomy in Frankfurt followed by other European groups [21–23]. In 2001, FDA approved the use of the system for prostatic surgery [24]. Da Vinci 2000 by introducing the Endo-wrist™-technology addressed most ergonomic problems of classical laparoscopy sufficiently, such as limited depth perception, eye-hand coordination, and range of motion. A closed console offered a 3D-CCD-video-system with in-line view (Fig. 3). The cable-driven instruments with up to seven DOF and loop-like handles enabled an ergonomic working position due to the clutch-mechanism [16]. In the last decade, the company introduced further elaborated systems, such as Da Vinci SI, X, and XI (Fig. 4) which nowadays represent a very high standard [16, 25].

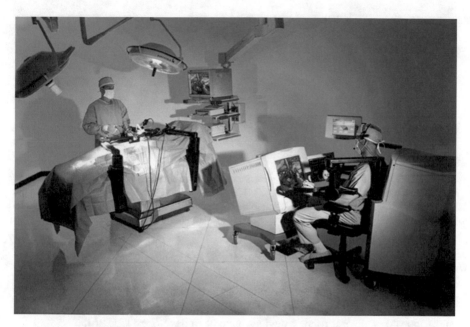

Fig. 2 ZEUS:First clinically used robotic-system for laparoscopic coronary artery revascularization. Open console, instruments with only 5 degrees of freedom (DOF). 3D-Video-technology using a helmet with two screens or only 2D-videotechnology

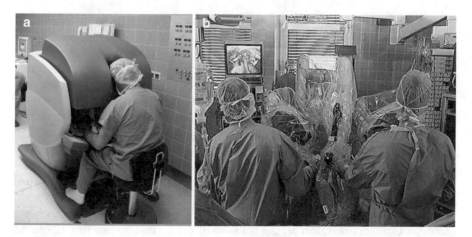

Fig. 3 DA VIN0CI 2000: First version of the Intuitive system, at that time without bipolar technology, but proving a closed console (**a**) with 7 degrees of freedom (Endowrist™) and three robotic arms (**b**)

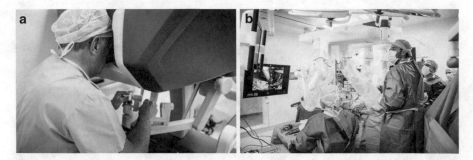

Fig. 4 DA VINCI XI: Console of last generation of robotic system for interdisciplinary use (**a**) In-line view with 3D-HD-videotechnology, 7 DOF for all instruments. Four-arm-system, telescope can be inserted via every port access. OR-table (Trumpf-Medical) can be moved without undocking of the robot

3.2 Master-Slaves Systems for Upper Tract Endourology

The development of robotic master-slave systems was not only limited to laparoscopy (Table 1). Also for neurosurgery, NOTES, interventional radiology, cardiology and endorology several robotic devices have been developed [25, 26].

3.2.1 Sensei-Magellan-System

In 2008, Desai described a robotic flexible ureteroscopy using the Sensei-Magellan-system (Hansen Medical, Mountain View, USA), which was designed for cardiology and angiography [3]. It provides an open console with a chair, armrests and a joystick to control the movement of the inserted catheter. The surgeon controls two screens for fluoroscopic and endoscopic images (Fig. 5a). The electronic rack contains computer hardware, power supplies and video distribution units.

The robotic flexible catheter system (manipulator) consists of an outer sheath (14/12F) and inner catheter guide (12/10F) (Fig. 5b). For robotic FURS, a 7.5F fibre-optic flexible ureteroscope was inserted and fixed in the inner catheter guide. Thus, remote manipulation of the catheter system manoeuvres the tip of the ureteroscope. The outer sheath was positioned at the ureteropelvic junction to stabilize navigation of the inner guide inside the collecting system (Fig. 5c). In this system, the ureteroscope was manipulated only passively, which proved to be a problem (Table 3). Consecutively, this project has been discontinued after the first 18 treated patients [4].

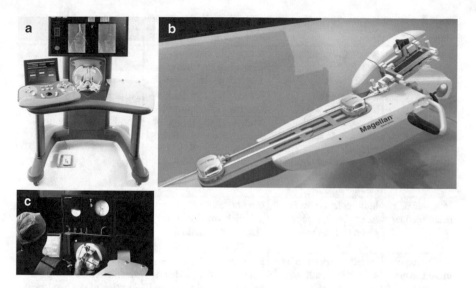

Fig. 5 Sensei-Magellan System (Hansen Medical, Mountain View, United States): (**a**) Master-slave system designed for angiography and transvascular cardiologic interventions, (**b**) Robotic arm mounted to the operating table, (**c**) Open console with the joy-stick analog endoscopic and fluoroscopic image during robotic flexible ureteroscopy. Joy-stick at the console controls the deflection and rotation of the inner sheath

3.2.2 Monarch

In March 2018, Monarch Platform was used in a clinical case of robotic bronchoscopy [29]. The system utilizes the common endoscopy procedure to insert a flexible robot into hard to reach places in the lung (Tables 1 and 3). A doctor trained on the system uses a video game-style controller to navigate inside, with help from 3D models (Fig. 6a). Like in the Sensei-Magellan-System, the technology is based on the robotic control of an external tube using two robotic arms (one for the outer and one for the endoscope) also to advance and retract the endoscope. However, the Monarch Platform also enables the additional movement of the flexible scope to reach small distal branches oft he bronchial system (Fig. 6b). An irrigation system is integrated. Another main feature of the device represents the integration of CT-imaging to guide the biopsy. The device is FDA-approved for bronchoscopy. In 2019, the manufacturer Auris has been acquired by Johnson & Johnson [30].

In the same year, Desai presented first videos of the clinical use of the Monarch System for robotic ureteroscopy using a single-use ureteroscope especially designed for the Monarch System [29] (Fig. 6c).

Table 3 Comparison of ergonomic features of Sensei™, Roboflex™, and Monarch™

Functions	Sensei	Roboflex	Monarch
Seat	Adjustable saddle-type seat No arm rest	Adjustable seat with integrated arm rest and foot pedal	No special seat provided
Imaging	Console with integrated Fluoroscopy and Endoscopic image screens Animation of position of catheter-tip (3D-navigation)	Console with integrated Endoscopic image screen Animation of position of ureteroscope in collecting system	No console only hand-held controller 2 Video-screen swith endoscopic image and fluoroscopy
Insertion of ureteroscope	Indirect insertion of inner sheath (scope glued to the sheath)	Fine-tunable by left joy-stick with numeric display of horizontal movement	Indirect insertion of the single-use scope in the steerable tube
Deflection of ureteroscope	Indirect deflection by the inner sheath based on single joy-stick	Fine-tunable deflection via wheel for right hand with display of grade and direction of deflection	Indirect deflection via the steerable tube using the joystick of the hand-held controller
Rotation of ureteroscope	Indirect rotation by the inner sheath (scope glued to the sheath)	Fine-tunable by sophisticated left joy-stick	Rotation of single-use ureteroscope inside the tube
Irrigation	No irrigation system included	Integrated irrigation pump activated by touch-screen	Integrated irrigation via the single-use ureteroscope
Laser	No function for laser fibre integrated	Integrated control of laser-fibre by touch-screen Activation by foot-pedal	Laser application via the working channel of the single-use ureteroscope with controlled advancement
Use of basket/ Grasper	No function for basket or grapser integrated	Activation of basket by the assistant at bed-side	Activation of basket by assistant at bed-side

3.2.3   Avicenna Roboflex

ELMED (Ankara, Turkey) is working on of a robot specifically designed for FURS since 2010 [5]. Roboflex Avicenna was continuously developed for flexible ureteroscopy providing all necessary functions [6]. The prototype consisted of a small console with an integrated flat-screen and two joysticks to move the endoscope (Fig. 7a), which is held by the hand-piece of the robotic arm (manipulator). This basic designed has not changed, however, several significant improvements have been accomplished during further development including size and design of the function screen, design of the joy-sticks to control rotation and deflection of endoscope, fine-adjustment of deflection of endoscope, and range of rotation of the manipulator (Table 3). Actually, Roboflex Avicenna represents the only robot, especially developed for FURS/RIRS [15]. The device has CE-mark since 2013, and FDA-approval is pending.

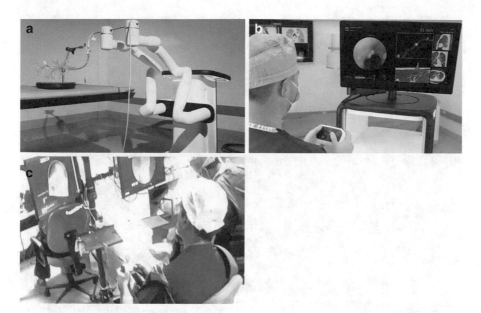

Fig. 6 Monarch (Auris Health, Redwood City, CA, United States): (**a**) Robot for flexible endoscopy designed for bronchoscopy. Two-arm-system for control of inner and outer sheath. Optional third arm for percutaneous access, (**b**) Movement of the robot is controlled by a handhold keypad like for computer games, (**c**) Experimental use of the device with a single-use robotic ureteroscope

4 Clinical Setting and Experience with Avicenna Roboflex

4.1 Design of the Device

The robot provides an open console and the manipulator of the flexible ureterorenoscope. The *manipulator* drives the flexible ureteroscope using its own mechanics (Fig. 7b). For this purpose the hand-piece of scope has to be attached directly to an especially designed master plate of the manipulator (Fig. 7c). Micromotors move the steering lever of the hand-piece for deflection with several ranges of motion. The robotic arm enables bilateral rotation, advancement and retraction of the ureteroscope. Additionally the height of the robotic arm can be adjusted according to the patient's size. Actually, there are five exchangeable master plates (Fig. 7d) available for three flexible digital ureteroscopes (Karl Storz Flex X2; Olympus URF-V2; Wolf Cobra/Viper digital) and two single-use devices (LithoVue, Boston Scientific, Pusen, Pusen Medical).

All functions of the robotic arm are controlled at the console providing an integrated adjustable seat with two armrests and two integrated foot-pedals for activation of fluoroscopy and the laser-lithotripter enabled via a pneumatic pedal-controller (Fig. 7e). The control panel at the console is used by touch-screen functions. The integrated HD-monitor displays the endoscopic image and all information about the

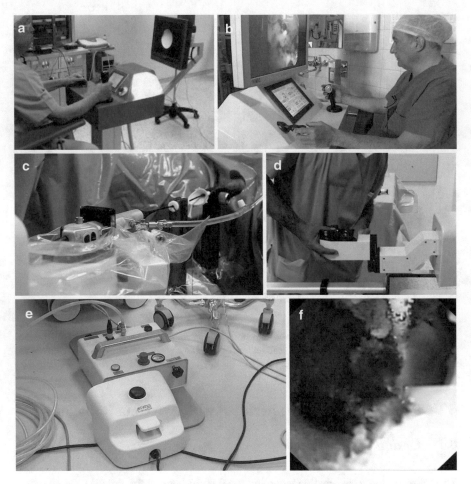

Fig. 7 Avicenna Roboflex System (ELMED, Ankara, Turkey): (**a**) Prototype with non-ergonomic handles and small screen, (**b**) Open console with sophisticated left-hand joystick for rotation and insertion/retraction and fine-tuned right-hand wheel for deflection. Touchscreen functions for laser activation, irrigation, and fine-tuning of movements, (**c**) Robotic arm with the hand-piece of a digital flexible ureteroscope (Flex XC, Karl Storz, Tuttlingen, Germany) fixed in the master plate and the flexible part supported by one or two stabilizers before entering the access sheath, (**d**) Exchange of the master-plate (i.e. when using a disposable device), (**e**) Pneumatic driven device for activation of the laser foot-pedal, (**f**) Endoscopic image of robot-assisted Thulium-laser ablation of upper tract urothelial carcinoma (single-kidney)

position of ureteroscope in the collecting system. All main manoeuvres to navigate the flexible endoscope can be fine-tuned at the control panel, such as horizontal movement (= insertion/retraction of the endoscope) with a range of 150 mm, bilateral rotation (220° to each side) and deflection of the scope (262° to each side). For this purpose the left hand controls a specifically developed joystick, whereas the right hand uses a wheel for deflection. All parameters of endoscope navigation are displayed on the control panel and the HD-screen. The deflection can be adjusted to

European respectively US-settings. Additionally, the infusion speed of the irrigation fluid can be adjusted together with a motorized insertion and retraction of the laser fibre.

4.2 Operative Technique

During the procedure the robotic arm is covered by a sterile plastic drape which is accomplished parallel to the anaesthesia of the patient. We have standardized our technique using routinely a 12/14F access sheath with hydrophilic coating (35–45–55 cm; Flexor parallel, Cook-Medical, Daniels Way, USA) enabling placement a safety guide-wire (Expert Nitinol wire 0.35i × 150 cm, IMP, Karlsruhe, Germany) parallel to the sheath. Position of the access sheath should be 1 cm below the UPJ, to allow enough flexibility of the ureteroscope. After arranging the position of seat and armrest by activating the memorized setting of each surgeon, the ureteroscope is inserted manually into the access sheath and fixed by one or two stabilizers (Fig. 7c). The definitive placement of the manipulator depends on the side of the stone and the size of the patient. Then the brakes of the manipulator are locked.

The endoscope is placed at the distal end of the access sheath with a horizontal value of 50 mm. Short-term digital fluoroscopy is used to determine the actual localization of stone and instrument. Once the endoscope has reached the renal pelvis, the scope needs to be rotated according to the axis of the kidney. Then, a systematic inspection of the entire collecting system is carried out. When the stone is visualized, the endoscope needs to be retracted and straightened slightly (<70°) to guarantee safe insertion of the laser fibre. Optionally Roboflex™ provides a memory function to guide the scope to its previous place once the laser fibre is inserted and the tip visualized endoscopically. However, with increasing experience there was no need to use this function.

Basically, any Holmium-YAG-laser can be used, but we strongly recommend a laser, which allows application of higher frequencies on low energy level such as Lumenis Pulse 120 (Lumenis, Yokneam, Israel) or Sphinx Jr. (LISA laser products, Katlenburg, Germany) with adequate small-calibre laser fibres (200-270 µ-fibre; Slimline™, Rigifib™). Laser-induced lithotripsy is initiated preferably aiming at pulverization respectively "dusting" of the stone (0.5 J, 15 Hz) by meander-like movement of the tip of the laser-fibre in the range of millimetres. The smaller fibre size allows sufficient bending of scope without deteriorating the efficacy of stone dusting respectively fragmentation (1.2 J, 10 Hz). Once fragmentation is progressing, increase of energy might be helpful to apply the "pop-corn-effect" or better "Jacuzzi-effect" for fine disintegration of the fragments similar to intracorporeal shock wave lithotripsy with a stable position of the laser fibre at the neck of the calyx.

If necessary, introduction of tip-less baskets or other forceps-like devices (i.e. Ngage™, Cook) for retrieval of fragments is performed. Here, the separation of the surgeon at the console from the assistant at the bedside is very helpful. Once the fragment is entrapped, the endoscope is driven back. Herein, the numeric demonstration of position of the tip of the endoscope along the horizontal axis is very helpful to anticipate, when the fragment will reach the distal end of the access sheath. When the fragment is pulled into the sheath, the assistant disconnects the ureteroscope from the distal stabilizer and extracts the stone. The endpoint of the treatment represents a stone-free status based on endoscopic inspection respectively remaining stone dust or fragments less than 2 mm. Then, the access sheath is retrieved under endoscopic inspection and a double J-stent placed. We usually introduce the stent with a string taped to the Foley catheter to be extracted the following morning.

We also have preliminary experience with intraluminal Thulium-laser ablation of low risk upper tract urothelial cancer (Fig. 7f). This can be accomplished primarily via the transureteral route or using a percutaneous access.

4.3   Clinical Studies

The clinical introduction of the device was accomplished according the IDEAL-system (idea, development, evaluation, assessment, long-term study) for the stages in surgical innovation [6]. First studies with the prototypes in Ankara were able to proof safety of the device [5]. Next step represented a proctored multi-centric study, where seven experienced surgeons treated 81 patients (mean age 42, range 6–68) with renal calculi (mean volume 1296 +/− 544, range 432–3100 mm^3) in an observational study (IDEAL stage 2) proctored by the urologist (R.S.) being involved in development and clinical introduction of the device. In this study the positive impact of Roboflex™ on ergonomics could be verified by use of a validated questionnaire [6].

The efficacy of the device in a real-life scenario was evaluated in a multi-centric phase II-study at two European centres (Ankara, Heilbronn) collecting data from 266 patients (Table 4). We could again proof safety and efficacy of the system, but of course comparing our results with the initial study docking time of the robot was longer (4 vs. 1 min), whereas time to visualize the stone was similar (4 vs. 3.7 min). According to the larger stone volume (1620 vs. 1300 mm^3) the console time was longer (96 vs. 53 min). Moreover, we were able to demonstrate that we could safely and successfully apply all modern techniques and protocols of flexible URS, such as laser dusting, using pop-corn/Jacuzzi-effect, and extraction of larger fragments [15]. In this setting, Avicenna Roboflex™ proved to be robust with only two cases of technical failure requiring conversion to classical FURS. The radiation exposure for the surgeon can be significantly reduced. In conclusion, we were able to integrate the device easily in our daily routine with now more than 500 successful cases performed by five surgeons.

Recently, Geavlete et al. [32] present a phase-3-study comparing robot-assisted versus classical FURS in 132 patients. Treatment time (51 vs 50 min.) and fragmentation time (37 vs 39 min.) were similar, but stone-free rate (92.4 vs 89.4%) favoured the robotic approach (Table 4).

Table 4 Comparison of clinical studies of robotic flexible ureteroscopy

Parameters	Desai et al. 2011	Saglam et al. 2014	Geavlete et al. 2016	Rassweiler et al. 2018
Robotic device	Sensei (Hansen-Medical)	Roboflex—prototype 2 (ELMED)	Roboflex—prototype 2 (ELMED)	Roboflex—final design (ELMED)
No. of patients	18 (12 males)	81 (56 males)	67 (27 males)	266 (176 males)
Stone size	10 (5–15) mm	13 (5–30) mm	21 (11–36) mm	14 (5–30) mm
Multiple stones	3 (16.7%)	52 (64.2%)	23 (34.3%)	192 (72.2%)
Total operating time	91 (60–130) min	74 (40–182) min	51 (38–103) min	96 (59–193) min
Robot docking	7 (4–18) min	1 (0.5–2) min	n.a.	4 (1–29) min
Console time	41 (21–70) min	53 (23–153) min	37 (27–86) min	65 (16–174) min
Stone localisation	9 (1–36) min	4 (2–8) min	n.a.	4 (1–12) min
Intraoperative complications	0	1 (1.2%) failure of device	0%	2 (0.7%) failures of device
Complete stone disintegration	17 (94.4%)	79 (96.2%)	65 (98.5%)	258 (96.9%)

n.a. not available

5 Discussion

5.1 Robotic Assistance for Upper Tract Endoscopic Surgery

During the last 30 years robot-assisted surgery has gained an established and irreversible role in urologic laparoscopic surgery [25]. The use of robotic master-slave-systems has not been limited to laparoscopic surgery. There are examples from gastroenterology, cardiology, interventional radiology, neurosurgery, and endourology ([26–28], Table 1).

In endourology first clinical applications tried to modify the Sensei-Magellan-system (Hansen, USA) designed for cardio-vascular intervention to perform robot-assisted flexible ureterorenoscopy [3, 4]. In this system, the surgeon sits in front of an open console manipulating a steerable flexible tube usually used for transvascular intra-cardiac interventions by use of a joystick (Fig. 2a). The remote manipulation system (Omega X, Force Dimension, Nyon, Switzerland) manoeuvres the outer and inner sheath of the device. To manipulate a flexible ureteroscope, the instrument tip had to be glued to the inner guide. This means that the ureteroscope could be manipulated only passively and its own deflection mechanics were not used. Such a system might be very useful for transvascular robotic atrial fibrillation ablation or any catheter-based angiographic procedure, but it proved to be insufficient for FURS [3, 4, 27].

The new Monarch™ system (Auris, USA) has been pushed significantly recently. It was developed for bronchoscopy, but the company sees also applications for other flexible endoscopes (ie FURS/RIRS) in the near future [31]. Interestingly, the device seems to work based on the some principles like the Sensei-Magellan™ without using the mechanics of the bronchoscope. The only difference is that the surgeon does not use a joystick, but controls the device via a hand-held keyboard similar to computer games. The two arms have an integrated cable driven system with small wheels similar to the da Vinci device This enables flexible movement of the tips of either the inner or outer sheath. Approximation of the arms results in advancement of the inner sheath. There are no specific functions (i.e. movement and activation of the laser fibre) integrated. Therefore the manufacturer developed a special single-use ureteroscope for robot-assisted flexible ureteroscopy (Table 4).

5.2   Important Features for Robotic FURS

Avicenna Roboflex has been developed specifically for FURS/RIRS. For robot-assisted flexible ureteroscopy specific technological features are of importance, such as chip-at-the-tip video-technology of the digital endoscope, easy manipulation of the endoscope, and activation of the laser and fluoroscopy. Roboflex uses the mechanical functions of the endoscope by digital control of the movement of the hand-piece. Such a system needs to be versatile. The exchangeable master plates enable the use of different kind of digital ureteroscopes including disposable devices (Fig. 3b). Also any holmium-YAG-laser lithotripter can be used and the laser-control device takes any laser-fibre. The main advantage of this concept represents the fact that all new developments of flexible ureteroscopes including video-technology, mechanics or the working channel can be immediately implemented.

Particularly, the two joysticks for navigation of the ureteroscope have been significantly improved during the developmental phase. Any necessary movement (insertion, retraction, rotation, deflection) can be fine-tuned according to the clinical situation. The range of rotation (210° in each direction = 420°) is beyond the human manual capabilities during classical FURS (max. 120°). During robot-assisted deflection 10° of movement with the wheel results in 3° deflection of the tip compared to 60° by manual use with thumb of the same endoscope.

5.3   Learning Curve of Robotic FURS

Surgical robots are mainly introduced to improve ergonomics of minimally invasive surgery. This can results in a shorter learning curve of the procedure, but also improve the quality and outcome of the procedure. One third of urologists have reported on hand-wrist and other ergonomic problems during classical FURS [12, 13], which was reflected by the recently published validated questionnaire comparing classical versus robot-assisted FURS [6]. Avicenna Roboflex™ provided a suitable platform improving ergonomics significantly (Table 4).

After only short introduction at the training model, all seven surgeons were able to perform robotic-assisted FURS safely and in a reasonable time frame compared to there own published series of classical FURS [33, 34]. Also in the second study involving more surgeons, the learning curve was short (maximal five cases). Of course, retrograde intra-renal surgery is less complicated compared to laparoscopic radical prostatectomy, particularly in case of small stones, which can be extracted by use of a Nitinol-basket. On the other side, the introduction of the device provides a safe and non-exhausting environment for the surgeon. Based on this we were able to extent the indication of FURS/RIRS to larger intra-renal calculi resulting to decrease of extracorporeal shock wave lithotripsy and percutaneous nephrolithotomy [15]. This means also a significant reduction of radiation exposure to patients and surgeons [35, 36].

5.4 Impact on the Lifetime of the Endoscope

Suboptimal ergonomics may be one of the reasons for imperfect performance of FURS mainly in complicated cases resulting in the need of second sessions and frequent repair of the endoscopes. Carey et al. [37] reported an 8.1% damage rate at a single tertiary centre with a 40–48 uses before the initial repair of new flexible ureteroscopes. Main reason for repair was errant laser firing (36%) and excessive torque (28%). Theoretically, the functions included in Roboflex™ such as insertion of laser fibre only in straight position of scope using a memory function, step-wise motorized advancement of laser fibre and force-controlled (maximal 1 N/mm^2) deflection of scope should contribute to a longer lifetime of ureterorenoscopes. However, the use of the device in a real-life scenario demonstrated various factors of breakage of an endoscope, such as inadequate handling during sterilization and cleaning of the instrument or technical failure of the chip. Not all of them can be avoided by use of the robot. Moreover the hygienic safety criteria have become much more stringent. The use of Cidex-sterilization is no more allowed. Thus, minimal leakage of the working channel may require complete repair exchange of the scope. On the other side, Roboflex™ proved to be very robust in clinical routing requiring only one exchange of the master plate after more than 500 cases.

5.5 Limitations of the Device: Cost Discussion

Obviously, there has been always criticism against the use of a robot for FURS. This concerns the issue of unnecessary costs, a robotic hype, and the final efficacy of the device [38]. It is evident, that main strength of the robot is to facilitate stone disintegration and extraction, where during classical FURS most ergonomic limitations are present (Table 2). Therefore, it is not surprising, that a recent in-vitro study using a simple model for endoscopic navigation no significant differences between both techniques could be demonstrated [39]. A possible limitation of the device may be the lack of tactile feedback. Similar to our experiences with Da Vinci-robot, lack of tactile feedback did not prove to be problematic during performance of robotic FURS mainly based on superior image quality of the used digital endoscope.

However, similar to classical FURS one has to follow certain guide-lines: (1) we recommend to place a guide-wire parallel to the sheath, (2) the ureteroscope should not be preloaded with a laser fibre when entering the collecting system, and (3) the access sheath should be placed 1 cm below the UPJ. The surgeon can always observe on the screen or console in which direction and how many degrees the endoscope is deflected. This has to be in accordance to the endoscopic image to minimize the risk of damage to the mucosa and/or instrument.

Like with all surgical robots, there is the discussion about costs. Possible financial revenues for robotic systems include longer durability of the endoscope, shorter operating times, less secondary procedures. Actually there is no demand from patients like with the Da Vinci system for radical prostatectomy. The ergonomic advantages and reduced radiation exposure for the surgeon should be considered, but similar to the other robotic systems have no financial benefit. On the other side, unlike Da Vinci, the Avicenna Roboflex represents a single investment without resulting to further costs (i.e. for instruments). Also adequate reimbursement of FURS/RIRS in relationship to PCNL may help the distribution of the device. Future studies have to focus more on these issues.

6 Conclusions

Despite its increased application, FURS may represent a challenging technique particularly in complicated cases. Robotic systems have been developed and tested. Avicenna Roboflex™ provides a suitable, safe, and robust platform for robotic FURS with significant improvement of ergonomics. However, future studies are necessary to evaluate the final role of robotics in upper tract endoscopic surgery.

References

1. Rassweiler JJ, Teber D. Advances in laparoscopic surgery in urology Nat. Rev Urol. 2016;13:387–99.
2. Rassweiler J, Binder J, Frede T. Robotic and telesurgery: will they change our future. Curr Opin Urol. 2001;11:309–20.
3. Desai MM, Aron M, Inderbir SG, Pascal-Haber Ukimura O, Kaouk JH, Stahler G, Barbagli O, Carlson C. Flexible robotic retrograde renoscopy: description of novel robotic device and preliminary laboratory experience. Urology. 2008;72:42–6.
4. Desai MM, Grover R, Aron M, Ganpule A, Joshi SS, Desai MR, Gill IS. Robotic flexible ureteroscopy for renal calculi: initial clinical experience. J Urol. 2011;186:563–8.

5. Saglam R, Kabakci AS, Koruk E, Tokatli Z. How did we designed and improved a new Turkish robot for flexible ureterorenoscopy. J Endourol. 2012;(26 suppl.1):A275 (MP44–12).
6. Saglam R, Muslumanoglu AY, Tokatlı Z, et al. A new robot for flexible ureteroscopy: development and early clinical results (IDEAL Stage 1-2b). Eur Urol. 2014;66:1092–100.
7. Rassweiler JJ, Knoll T, Köhrmann KU, McAteer JA, Lingeman JE, Cleveland RO, Bailey MR, Chaussy C. Shock wave technology and application: an update. Eur Urol. 2011;59:784–96.
8. Beiko DT, Denstedt JD. Advances in ureterorenoscopy. Urol Clin North Am. 2007;34:397–408.
9. Preminger GM, Tiselius HG, Assimos DG, Alken P, Buck AC, Gallucci M, Knoll T, Lingeman JE, Nakada SY, Pearle MS, Sarica K, Türk C, Wolf JS Jr; American Urological Association Education and Research, Inc; European Association of Urology. 2007 Guideline for the management of ureteral calculi. Eur Urol. 2007;52:1610–31.
10. Wright AE, Rukin NJ, Somani BK. Ureteroscopy and stones: current status and future expectations. World J Nephrol. 2014;3:243–8.
11. Rassweiler J, Rassweiler MC, Klein J. New technology in ureteroscopy and percutaneous nephrolithotomy. Curr Opin Urol. 2016;26:95–106.
12. Elkoushy MA, Andonian S. Prevalence of orthopedic complaints among endourologists are commen and their compliance with radiation safety measures very important. Endourol. 2011;25(10):1609–13.
13. Healy KA, Pak RW, Cleary RC, Colo-Herdman A, Bagley D. Hand and wrist problems among endourologists are very common. Endourology. 2011;25(12):1905–20.
14. Aron M, Haber GP, Desai MM, Gill IS. Flexible robotics: a new paradigm. Curr Opin Urol. 2007;17(3):151–5.
15. Rassweiler J, Fiedler M, Charalampogiannis N, Kabakci AS, Saglam R, Klein JT. Robot-assisted flexible ureteroscopy: an update. Urolithiasis. 2018;46:69–77.
16. Rassweiler JJ, Autorino R, Klein J, Mottrie A, Goezen AS, Stolzenburg JU, Rha KH, Schurr M, Kaouk J, Patel V, Dasgupta P, Liatsikos E. Future of robotic surgery in urology. BJU Int. 2017;120:822–41.
17. Schurr MO, Buess G, Neisius B, Voges U. Robotics and telemanipulation technologies for endoscopic surgery. A review of the ARTEMIS project. Surg Endosc. 2000;14:375–81.
18. Reichenspurner H, Damiano R, Mack M, et al. Use of the voice-controlled surgical system ZEUS for endoscopic coronary bypass grafting. J Thorac Cardiovasc Surg. 1999;118:11–6.
19. Marescaux J, Leroy J, Gagner M, et al. Transatlantic robot-assisted telesurgery. Nature. 2001;413:379–80.
20. Mohr FW, Falk V, Diegeler A, Autschbach R. Computer-enhanced coronary artery surgery. J Thorac Cardiovasc Surg. 1999;117:1212–5.
21. Binder J, Kramer W. Robotically assisted laparoscopic radical prostatectomy. BJU Int. 2001;87:408–10.
22. Abbou CC, Hoznek A, Salomon L, Olsson LE, Lobontiu A, Saint F, Cicco A, Antiphon P, Chopin D. Laparoscopic radical prostatectomy with a remote controlled robot. J Urol. 2001;165:1964–6.
23. Rassweiler J, Frede T, Seemann O, Stock C, Sentker L. Telesurgical laparoscopic radical prostatectomy. Eur Urol. 2001;40:75–83.
24. Menon M, Shrivastava A, Tewari A, et al. Laparoscopic and robot assisted radical prostatectomy: establishment of a structured program and preliminary analysis of outcomes. J Urol. 2002;168:945–9.
25. Leal Ghezzi T, Campos Corleta O. 30 years of robotic surgery. World J Surg. 2016;40:2550–7.
26. Sutherland GR, Maddahi Y, Gan LS, Lama S, Zareinia K. Robotics in the neurosurgical treatment of glioma. Surg Neurol Int. 2015;6(Suppl 1):S1–8.
27. Antoniou GA, Riga CV, Mayer EK, Cheshire NJ, Bicknell CD. Clinical applications of robotic technology in vacular and endovascular surgery. J Vasc Surg. 2011;53:463–99.
28. Gilling P, Reuther R, Kahokehr A, Fraundorfer M. Aquablation – image-guided robot-assisted water-jet ablation. BJU Int. 2016;117:923–9.

29. https://www.geekfence.com/2018/03/24/monarch-is-a-new-platform-from-surgical-robot-pioneer-frederic-moll/
30. https://www.medtechdive.com/news/jjs-auris-unveils-early-results-on-monarch-robot-for-lung-procedures/555223/
31. Desai M. Robotic URS. World Congress on Endourology 2019, Abu Dhabi, 29th October – 2nd November 2019.
32. Geavlete P, Saglam R, Georgescu D, Multescu R, Iordache V, Kabakci AS, Ene C, Geavlete B. Robotic flexible ureteroscopy versus classis flexible ureteroscopy in renal stones: initial Romanian experience. Chirurgia. 2016;111:326–9.
33. Secker A, Rassweiler J, Neisius A. Future perspectives of flexible ureteroscopy. Curr Opin Urol. 2019;29:113–7.
34. Erkurt B, Caskurlu T, Atis G, Gurbuz C, Arikan O, Pelit ES, Altay A, Erdogan F, Yildirim A. Treatment of renal stones with flexible ureteroscopy in preschool age children. J Endourol. 2012;26:625–9.
35. Hellawell GO, Mutch SJ, Thevendran G, Wells E, Morgan RJ. Radiation exposure and the urologist: what aret the risks? J Urol. 2005;174:948–5.
36. Kim KP, Miller DL, Berrington de Gonzalez A, Balter S, Kleinerman RA, Ostroumova E, Simon SL, Linet MS. Occupational radiation doses to operators performing fluoroscopically-guided procedures. Health Phys. 2012;103:80–99.
37. Carey RI, Gomez CS, Maurici G, Lynne CM, Leveille RJ, Bird VG. Frequency of uretero-scope damage seen at a tertiary care center. J Urol. 2006;176:607–10.
38. Caddedu JA. Comment on Saglam R, Muslumanoglu AY, Tokatlı Z et al. A new robot for flex-ible ureteroscopy: Development and early clinical results (IDEAL Stage 1-2b). Eur Urol 2014; 66:1092–1100. J Urol. 2015;193:1277.
39. Proietti S, Dragos L, Emiliani E, Buttice S, Talso M, Baghdadi M, Villa L, Doizi S, Giusti G, Traxer O. Ureteroscopic skills with and without Robofelx Avicenna in trhe K-box^R simulator. Cent Eur J Urol. 2017;70:76–80.

Exoscope-Assisted 3D Open Surgery

Tahsin Batuhan Aydogan and Emre Huri

1 Introduction

The invention of primitive magnification devices dates back to 721–705 BC. The microsope was first invented and introduced in late seventeenth century by Anthony van Leeuwenhoek [1]. This invention has let the creation and development of modern histology and microbiology fields. A microscopic image which is a magnified one on the retina allows clinician to explore a wider field with a closer vision. The development of microscopy and surgical loupes have been continued in further eras. During in the middle of twentieth century binocular microscopes started to be used during neurosurgeries and laryngeal surgeries by some surgeons [2, 3]. As well in 1962 Kosse et al. described a novel microscopic uretero-ureteral anastomosis [4]. Later on, especially in andrology and pediatric urology, urologists started to perform surgeries with operating microscopes (OM) rather than using operating loupes [1].

2 The Operating Microscopes (OM) and Endoscopy in Clinical Use

The current definition of focal length for OM is an adjustable 200–400 mm distance from the operation field to the most distal part of lens which allows a ×4 to ×40 magnification. This distance brings a suitable area for using instruments during the

T. B. Aydogan (✉)
Department of Urology, Memorial Sisli Hospital, Istanbul, Turkey

E. Huri
Hacettepe University, Ankara, Turkey
e-mail: emrehuri@hacettepe.edu.tr

D. Veneziano, E. Huri (eds.), *Urologic Surgery in the Digital Era*,
https://doi.org/10.1007/978-3-030-63948-8_10

surgery without blocking the visuality. A xenon-light illumination with an adjustable bright is being used in OM. The splitted image from monocular lenses to binocular lenses provides a 3-D view which is called stereopsis. A hydraulic counter-balance with an electronic control supplies adjustments on the binocular view. As for the operating assistant's view, a mirror located inside optical pathways supplies a second binocular view. This view may also be shown on the video monitor or recorded by electronic devices. The OM also brings some disadvantages. They are really expensive and huge devices which fill a wide area in the operating rooms that are not easily repositioned. Despite to the magnifying power their effect on depth of field is still weak. Newer OM's have electromagnetic control units arranging the re-focus steps but still this is also time-consuming. OM devices may also cause fatigue and neck pain among the surgeons [5].

Endoscopy also named as a telescope-based system that the view is supplied from inside of the body. It is frequently in use among many different disciplines during the last decades. Telescope-based surgery is mainly based on a high quality vision supplied by an optic camera system connected to a video monitor [5]. The endoscopic view is supplied by filling of carbon monoxide gas in to abdominal cavity during laparoscopy, while deflating of air during thoracoscopy, hydrodistention during cystoscopy and hysteroscopy. An assistant holds the camera while surgeon performs the operation. As with examples as laparoscopy, cystoscopy, hysteroscopy, etc. it is used among many surgical disciplines [5]. The major advantages of endoscopic interventions are less bleeding, shorter hospital-stay, less pain and short recovery. But it needs a long learning-curve and has a short focal distance with a limited view of field.

The mainstay of a lack is here in microsurgery. OM is time consuming during re-focusing and during long-lenght of microsurgeries in neurosurgery it is not comfortable for a surgeon to use. Moreover, it is almost impossible to create an area inside the cranium to work with endoscopic instruments. The brain tissue is seriously sensitive for any pressure change. Except for endoscopic optic camera, each endoscopic instrument will also need an seperate hole as a working channel/tract on the cranium. So at this point there need of exoscope devices have appeared.

3 The emerge and definition of Video Telescope Operating Monitor (VITOM)

The video telescope operating monitor (VITOM) was first introduced and used in 2008 on an aminal model as a potent alternative to both endoscope and operating microscope (OM) [5]. OM and endoscopic devices were have been used especially in neurosurgery and in other microsurgical disciplines. But VITOM is a brand new technology giving opportunity with a wider surgical field besides the magnification in order to enable surgeon performing a comfortable surgery. The firstly introduced VITOM models were enabling a 2-D (two-dimensional) view. The surgeon has needed a well developed stereopsis and tactile sensitivity for hand-eye coordination during surgery. Nowadays with aid of technology 3-D (three-dimensional) exoscopes are in use which enable a high quality of view.

The exoscope is a great challenge against OM. It brings a high quality monitor view but moreover it also supplies a wide focal distance about 200 mm similar to OM which allows surgeon to perfom instrumental work in a very easy manner. The high-definition exoscope system is mainly consisted of 4 units as operation telescope, camera head, light source and high-definition video monitor (Fig. 1) [5].

Mamelak et al. described their telescope as an autolavable rigid telescop with fiber optic light source channel (ModelE1051-1: Karl Storz Endoscopy, Tuttlingen, Germany). It has an 8 mm outer diameter and a total shaft lenght of 14 cm. The telescope basic characteristics were defined as; high resolution, minimal aberrations and chromatic distortions, a wide viewing angle, mean focal distance of 200 mm, successful light absorption, supplying a 12 mm depth of field with no need of refocusing, perfect color and contrast enhancement. The defined characteristics of light source was described and consisted as; 300 W xenonfiber optic light source (Xenon Nova 300: Karl Storz) and a fiber optic cable suitable to the telescope. The camera head was also defined as; a 3-chip sterilizable high-definition digital camera (A3: Karl Storz) with optical zoom and focusing abilities. The video display monitor was described with a two-million pixels high definition capability (NDS Surgical

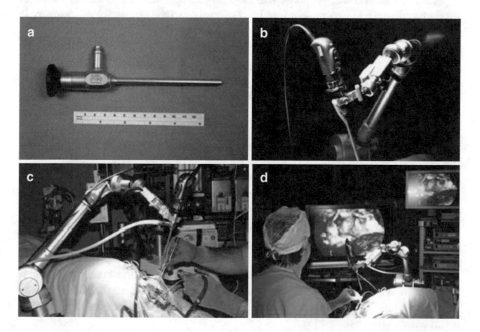

Fig. 1 The demonstration of VITOM. (**a**) Rigid lens telescope, (**b**) Digital camera head, (**c**) Adjustable pneumatic holder, (**d**) High-definition video monitor (Mamelak, A.N., et al., *A high-definition exoscope system for neurosurgery and other microsurgical disciplines: preliminary report*. Surg Innov, 2008. **15**(1): p. 38–46)

Imaging, San Jose, California) and for data documentation image data was recorded by (AIDA: Karl Storz) data system. The camera holder (Point Setter: Mitaka Kohki Co, Tokyo, Japan) was working with a pneumatic system and by holding the telescope also supply a wide range of motion capability. A push button was maintaining a rapid reposititioning without an obvious slip or drift which resembles like the hydraulic counterbalance mechanism of OM. According to their high-definition video exoscope system there were some main differences from OM. Not like OM, the camera and telescope may be re-sterilable and not need any steril draping. The telescope holder is much more smaller in size and compact than the counter balance mechanism in OM so it is easy to use. The weight of OM (>100 kg) is much more heavier than exoscope system (almost 650 g) [5].

Just prior to animal model surgery Mamelak et al. performed an static image quality comparison with the OM. Three steps of magnification (lowest ×4, medium ×12 and maximum ×40) were performed accross to a background consisted of 1 mm grid paper, a step wedge and coloured small cylindirical beads. OM images were compared with the images of exoscope. During the lowest magnification the focal distance for exoscope was set as 10 cm while during the maximum magnification it was set as 30 cm. The exoscope supplied an equal or better resolution with image contrasts at all levels of magnification. During the high magnification, exoscope images were even had a better quality of resolution but a little weaker in color seperation. The stereoscopic sense was thought to be greater in OM but the successful depth of sense in exoscope might be responsible to the similarity of steroscopic sense [5].

3.1   First Animal Model Surgery with VITOM, Results and Limitations

The first live surgery experience was performed on porcine models which was also highlighted with in preliminary reports by Mamelak et al. [5]. Craniotomies and brain dissections were performed on seperate four cases. An average of 3–4 inch sized craniotomies were performed. As continued with the exposition of midline sagittal and transverse sinuses. Afterwards the dura is opened and intrahemispheric dissections were performed. The microsurgery with VITOM started from craniotomy and lasted up to choroid plexus, optic nerve and carotid artery exposures [5]. At the end of live animal surgeries the investigators briefly declared main important points regarding VITOM. It was obviously lighter than OM and easy to use in operating room. The view on the monitor may facilitate the cooperation, learning and motivation among the team including anesthesia, nurse and fellows in operating room besides the assistant [5].

According to the investigators there were some limitations regarded to the holding mechanism, amount of light and need of push button for refocusing. The camera holder was an ordinary one that have been using during endoscopic interventions of intraventricular neurosurgery and transspheniodal surgery [5]. One of their comment was, in those kind of surgeries, the desire for a large field view or angular re-positioning is unusual. So, a well designed camera holder was needed for a rapid and easy repositioning as bringing a wide surgical field view. Considering for the amount of light they recommended a xenon light source rather to use an ordinary fiber optic endoscope light source. As a third, an automatic zoom and focus capability was supposed to be a standart in exoscopes as it was in OMs. The investigators also underlighted the importance of stereopsis. There was still a little difference in between OM and exoscopes. Despite the existence of commercially available stereoscopic endoscopes, their usage are still limited. According to investigators, increasing lens diameter from 10 mm to 12 mm might be a solution in order to enhance the brightness while with a greater depth of field. But according to preliminary experiences an increased lens diameter did not differ in depth of field [5].

3.2 A Brief Comparison of OM, Endoscope and Exoscope

Endocopic devices are mainly different from OM and exoscope in terms of having a short focal distance. They are also mainly usable as intra corporeal. Somehow as considering special endoscopic neurosurgical procedures such as transsphenoidal surgery, the neuroendoscopes have a long but narrow diameter (1–4 mm) lens and also a focal distance of 3–20 mm, they may supply a limited view of surgical field especially during instrumentation [5]. Depending on any other neurosurgical procedures surgeon will demand for a wider view on surgical field. So, the existence of OM in previous times and currently the support of exoscope system is becoming more essential. A brief comparison of OM, endoscope and exoscope is summarized in Table 1 and schematized in Fig. 2.

4 The Initial Clinical Experiences of VITOM and Current Literature

The usage of a new alternative visualization system which was named as the Panoramic Visualization System (HD-PVS) in ENT (ear, nose and throat) surgery was firstly discussed in 2009 [6]. The main consept was almost same with VITOM. It

Table 1 The general comparison of OM, endoscope and exoscope

	Focal length (mm)	Field of view (mm)	Image supply	Area
OM	200–400	600	Binocular lens	Extra corporeal
Endoscope	3–20	25	Digital camera/ videomonitor	Intra corporeal
Exoscope	200	600	Digital camera/ videomonitor	Extra corporeal

OM: Operating microscope

Fig. 2 Focal length and field of view comparisons of OM, Exoscope and Endoscope

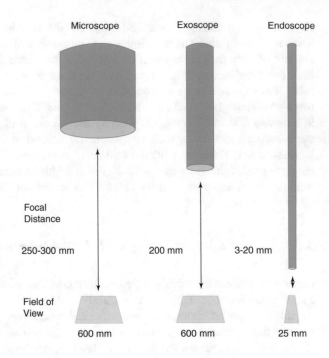

Microscope   Exoscope   Endoscope

Focal Distance

250-300 mm   200 mm   3-20 mm

Field of View

600 mm   600 mm   25 mm

was neither a microscope nor an endoscope. A focal lenght of 200 mm with an HD camera and monitor were the main components of the system [6]. Initially the system was investigated in laboratory conditions using 4 close-to-surgery scenarios. Furthermore, the system was used in 45 procedures including tympanoplasty, parotidectomy, neck dissection, septumplasty and transfacial approaches. According to the study, image quality was successful but there a need of development in the holding system including regulation of magnification and focus exists. The initial study result in ENT surgery has put the system between binocular loupe and microscope [6].

In 2010 Mamelak et al. published their article considering the initial clinical usage of VITOM in literature [7]. A 10 mm diameter lens telescope with 20 cm focal distance was used with 3-chip high-definition camera and video monitor as VITOM constructure. A total of 16 cases were operated with both OM and VITOM system. 9 craniotomies, 6 spinal surgeries and 1 neurostimulator placement were successfully performed by neurosurgeons. The images were recorded then compared between OM and VITOM. The surgeons felt the lack of stereopsis but also declared that the scope re-positiononig was not easy as it is in OM. Despite to these limitations surgeons' prediction was that the lack of stereopsis may be over-come by repetative experiences. The optical quality was succesfully noted in between the surgeons. As a considered their study, the inital state of VITOM was appropriate for spinal neurosurgeris [7].

In 2011, a gynecologic way of use was appeared in colposcopy procedure with in a pilot study. Vercellino et al. presented their exoscopically based colposcopy results among 76 patients [8]. The exocolposcopy with the VITOM had shown a successful correlation with the histologic findings in high-grade diseases of lower genital tract in females [8].

When the date was showing 2012, Mamelak et al. shared their first experience in resection of a pineal tumor. VITOM was succesfully used in an infratentorial supracerebellar approach of a pineal tumor microneurosurgery [9]. According to their experience, VITOM supplied an perfect vision on the surrounding arteries and veins, the back wall of third ventricule, including the splenium of corpus callosum. At the same year Carlucci et al. described a new technique for laryngeal surgery with usage of VITOM [10]. Among 12 patients VITOM was used and results compared with the usage of microscope in endoscopic laryngeal surgery. A focal distance of 25 cm was arranged, a 10 mm diameter telescope with a lengh of 10 cm was used. The study results concluded that the anatomical structures including vascular and mucosal characteristics were very well successfully demonstrated [10].

Another important discipline for the need of optical magnification is pediatric surgery. A preliminary report consisted of pediatric surgery and urology was firstly published in 2013 [11]. The aim was to evaluate the usage of VITOM rather than surgical loupes where magnification is essential in complex pediatric surgical and urological interventions. Each surgeon had used a ×2.5 or ×3.5 magnifying loupes in addition to the VITOM system. A total of 20 surgical procedures were performed with VITOM by three surgeons. 14 hypospadias repairs, 2 inguinal hernia repairs, 1 sacrococcygeal teratoma resection, 1 recurrent tracheoesophageal fistula repiar and 2 additional proedures were performed. The image quality, handling of VITOM, degree of fatigue were evaluated. The image quality was accepted as successfull as like in previous researches. The results confirmed that reduced fatigue, better understanding of the procedures for both trainees and technicians may propose the usage of VITOM instead of surgical loupes [11].

As a summary of recent studies, VITOM was appreciated by surgeons in different fields and they briefly felt comfortable. There was just a declared lack of stereopsis. Finally at 2017, VITOM 3D model initial experiences were started to emerge in literature [12, 13]. Rossini et al. demonstrated first case report in literature as performed a cranial surgery at posterior fossa with VITOM 3D [12]. The removal of a meningioma was performed with an exoscope supplying 4K resolution view with 3D technology. There was no lack of stereopsis which had been defined as a problem in previous investigations on initial VITOM models. There only a restruction was missing related to the mechanical holder mechanism in order to obtain better repositioning and refocusing standarts. According to the researchers, a hydraulic counterbalance as seen in OM's or a robotic mechanism applications for the holder arm would supply an easy repositition of holder [12].

At the same year Oertel et al. performed 5 cranial and 11 spinal procedures with a 3D exoscope [13]. There were 1 microvascular decompression, 4 craniotomies with tumor resections, 2 anterior cervical discectomies with cervical plating fusions, 1 cervical laminectomy and lateral mass fixation, 1 shear cervical lateral mass osteosynthesis, 1 lumbar canal decompression, 2 transforaminal lumbar interbody fusions, 1 thoracic intraspinal extradural tumor resection and 3 lumbar discectomies. According to their results; handling of instruments, intraoperative repositioning of VITOM 3D and comfort level related to intraoperative posture were all rated as excellent during all the procedures. The image quality was accepted as equal to that of OM's in 68.75% of procedures [13].

Cadaveric anatomy and dissection in surgical training have been well established in literature with advantages of good anatomic exposure, excellent vision for surgical plan, better understanding surgical technique, excellent teaching tool, good tissue preservation with fine dissection [14]. Moreover, the use of VITOM during cadaveric dissections may be one of main steps during surgical training so that surgery students/trainers may obviously become familiar with VITOM technology (Fig. 3). VITOM will be needed in routine use among such featured cases of urology where microsurgery is essential and commonly in use. Some of those high featured urological interventions are hypospadias repair, ureteral re-implantation, arteriovenous fistula creation for hemodialysis, anastomosis during renal transplantation or varicoselectomy [11].

Fig. 3 Use of VITOM during cadaveric pelvic surgical training

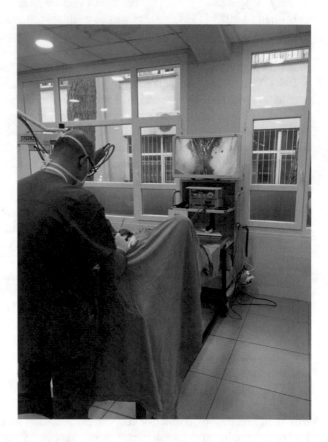

5   Conclusions

An actual surgical operation is actually not solely means performed by a single surgeon. It is always a team work. Assistant education is always a must. Moreover, it is a team effort in which anesthesiology and operating room technicians participate as well as assistants. So everyone needs to know what is going on during the surgical intervention. Especially starting from neurosurgical approaches in many different surgical fields magnification is a requiry. OM's are giant devices and sometimes even enable a free movement of a surgeon. The modern technology is bringing instruments and devices smaller and functional day by day. So in an operating room magnifying devices needed to be smaller and practical in use. A historical surgical loupe can not be the answer today. Because it is a digital era with endovision usage. So a 3D images supplying 4K resolutions is needed for many different kind of surgical approaches. This will increase the surgeons comfort during operation besides will increase the quality of assistant education and in deed success of the patients operation. Up to now the initial VITOM systems deficiencies are almost resolved with progressions. But still some modifications and supportive improvements may be in need. The monitor is primarily settled against across to the primary surgeon but for a better assistance during the operation a second monitor in a system may be a good idea. A further advanced development may be required for a repositition of exoscope holders.

Microsurgeries almost alwasy require to work with continuously two hands. So a foot pedal system or voice control mechanism may be developed in future for better control in exoscope reposititioning. A comparison of exoscope models just revealed that the lowest cost model is VITOM [15]. The VITOM 3D exoscope system is very well introduced and in use up to now. Currently indocyanine green (ICG)—Fluorescence imaging is available in use with VITOM. The Carl Storz company produced a VERSACRANE ™ (holding system) for better and easy repositioning of VITOM during operations. Probably soon in future modern technology will bring it more commonly such a routine avaliable in extracorporeal surgical interventions.

References

1. Schultheiss D, Denil J. History of the microscope and development of microsurgery: a revolution for reproductive tract surgery. Andrologia. 2002;34(4):234–41.
2. Jacobson JH 2nd, Wallman LJ, Schumacher GA, Flanagan M, Suarez EL, Donaghy RM. Microsurgery as an aid to middle cerebral artery endarterectomy. J Neurosurg. 1962;19:108–15.
3. Scalco AN, Shipman WF, Tabb HG. Microscopic suspension laryngoscopy. Ann Otol Rhinol Laryngol. 1960;69:1134–8.
4. Kosse KH, Suarez EL, Fagan WT, Powell PR, Jacobson JH 2nd. Microsurgery in ureteral reconstruction. J Urol. 1962;87:48–55.

5. Mamelak AN, Danielpour M, Black KL, Hagike M, Berci G. A high-definition exoscope system for neurosurgery and other microsurgical disciplines: preliminary report. Surg Innov. 2008;15(1):38–46.
6. Strauss G, Hofer M, Bahrami N, Dittrich E, Strauss M, Dietz A. A new visualization device for ENT surgery: the panoramic visualization system (HD-PVS). HNO. 2009;57(5):455–65.
7. Mamelak AN, Nobuto T, Berci G. Initial clinical experience with a high-definition exoscope system for microneurosurgery. Neurosurgery. 2010;67(2):476–83.
8. Vercellino GF, Erdemoglu E, Kyeyamwa S, Drechsler I, Vasiljeva J, Cichon G, et al. Evaluation of the VITOM in digital high-definition video exocolposcopy. J Low Genit Tract Dis. 2011;15(4):292–5.
9. Mamelak AN, Drazin D, Shirzadi A, Black KL, Berci G. Infratentorial supracerebellar resection of a pineal tumor using a high definition video exoscope (VITOM(R)). J Clin Neurosci. 2012;19(2):306–9.
10. Carlucci C, Fasanella L, Ricci MA. Exolaryngoscopy: a new technique for laryngeal surgery. Acta Otorhinolaryngol Ital. 2012;32(5):326–8.
11. Frykman PK, Duel BP, Gangi A, Williams JA, Berci G, Freedman AL. Evaluation of a video telescopic operating microscope (VITOM) for pediatric surgery and urology: a preliminary report. J Laparoendosc Adv Surg Tech A. 2013;23(7):639–43.
12. Rossini Z, Cardia A, Milani D, Lasio GB, Fornari M, D'Angelo V. VITOM 3D: preliminary experience in cranial surgery. World Neurosurg. 2017;107:663–8.
13. Oertel JM, Burkhardt BW. Vitom-3D for exoscopic neurosurgery: initial experience in cranial and spinal procedures. World Neurosurg. 2017;105:153–62.
14. Selcuk I, Tatar I, Huri E. Cadaveric anatomy and dissection in surgical training. Turk J Obstet Gynecol. 2019;16(1):72–5.
15. Langer DJ, White TG, Schulder M, Boockvar JA, Labib M, Lawton MT. Advances in intraoperative optics: a brief review of current exoscope platforms. Oper Neurosurg (Hagerstown). 2019.

Confocal Laser Endomicroscopy

Alberto Breda, Salvatore Micali, Angelo Territo, Mino Rizzo,
Giulio Bevilacqua, Iacopo Meneghetti, Maria Chiara Sighinolfi,
Bernardo Rocco, and Giampaolo Bianchi

Abbreviations

CIS	carcinoma in situ
CLE	confocal laser endomicroscopy
CTU	computed tomography urography
EAU	European Association of Urology
FCM	fluorescence confocal microscopy
NVB	neurovascular bundles
OCT	optical coherence tomography
PDD	photodynamic diagnosis
RNU	radical nephroureterectomy
UTUC	upper tract urinary carcinoma
WLC	white light cystoscopy

1 History of CLE

The first confocal microscope was invented by Marvin Minsky in 1957 in an effort to obtain well-defined images of neuronal tissue. In 1969 confocal laser microscopy was proposed by Davidovits and Egger, who contemplated the use of fluorescent media to investigate biological tissue. In 1983, Cox and Shepard proposed the first digital processing of confocal images. In 1991 the first fiber-optic confocal

A. Breda · A. Territo (✉) · G. Bevilacqua · I. Meneghetti
Department of Urology, Fundació Puigvert, Autonomous University of Barcelona,
Barcelona, Spain

S. Micali · M. Rizzo · M. C. Sighinolfi · B. Rocco · G. Bianchi
Department of Urology, University of Modena & Reggio Emilia, Modena, Italy

© The Author(s), under exclusive license to Springer Nature
Switzerland AG 2021
D. Veneziano, E. Huri (eds.), *Urologic Surgery in the Digital Era*,
https://doi.org/10.1007/978-3-030-63948-8_11

microscope was introduced by Dabbs and Glass [1]. In 2005 Polglase et al. [2] described a new integrated fiber-optic confocal laser microscope which provided high-quality images of the entire gastrointestinal system. In 2007 Thiberville et al. [3] first reported on the use of CLE with topical methylene blue during bronchoscopy.

On the basis of this promising experience, in 2009 Sonn et al. investigated the value of CLE before transurethral resection of the bladder due to suspicion of bladder cancer, with good results. Owing to the impossibility of contacting the lesion with the tip of the probe, CLE could not be performed when the tumor was located in the anterior bladder wall [4]. In 2011 Wu et al. [5] created an atlas of urinary tract CLE images.

A recent study focused on the distinctive features of low-versus high-grade urothelial carcinoma, carcinoma in situ (CIS), and benign lesions on CLE [6]. The authors found that low-grade tumors are characterized by a papillary configuration; organized, densely packed, and cohesive monomorphic cells with distinct borders; absence of umbrella cells; and presence of high-density cells surrounding a fibrovascular stalk. High-grade tumors show disorganized, pleomorphic cells with indistinct borders, loss of cellular cohesiveness, absence of umbrella cells, and fibrovascular stalks with distorted vasculature. CIS is composed of pleomorphic cells with an indistinct border in a noncohesive and disorganized microarchitecture.

Since the characteristics of UTUC lesions resemble those of urothelial bladder carcinoma, these diagnostic criteria have been utilized for CLE in the upper urinary tract. Recently, Marien et al. [7] studied the ex vivo use of dual-band Cellvizio®, characterized by a double laser (488, 660 nm) with both hexylaminolevulinate and fluorescein fluorophores. The concomitant coloration of extracellular matrix and cells, resembling the typical histopathologic stain, may increase the diagnostic power of CLE.

2   Principles of CLE

The basic concept of confocal images was developed in the 1950s by Marvin Lee Minsky with the aim of overcoming the limitations of wide-field fluorescence microscopes [8].

A confocal microscope is nothing but a modified fluorescent microscope that uses a laser instead of a xenon arc lamp or mercury vapor lamp as a source of light. Images are taken by a detector protected by a barrier with a pinhole that filters the light, allowing the passage only of light coming from a certain point. Confocal microscopy offers several advantages over conventional wide field optical microscopy, including the ability to control depth of field, eliminate or reduce background information away from the focal plane (which leads to image degradation), and collect several optical sections from thick specimens [9].

In confocal microscopy, the light produced by a laser beam passes through a lens and through a first pinhole. The light produced by the laser, which has a specific wavelength, hits a dichroic mirror and then passes through an objective lens that focalizes it on a small area on the surface of a specimen. Light signal emitted from a point in the specimen travels backwards through the same path, this time passing through the dichroic mirror, which has significantly different reflection properties at two different wavelengths; thus the light that has been reflected by the specimen has a different wavelength from the laser light. A detector is then reached by the light, but a barrier with a pinhole reduces the amount of signal that reaches it. The second pinhole, which is in an optically conjugate plane with the first, allows light of only a focal point to reach the detector so that the light information coming from above and below the focal plane is cancelled out, improving the depth of the image.

A software combines all the images that reach the detector into one sharp image, and the images of different focal planes can be taken and combined into a 3D image using a mosaicing algorithm [10]. Methylene blue or fluorescein can be used to excite cells of biological specimens that will be analyzed [3, 11].

3 Technical Features of CLE

The CLE system (Cellvizio, Mauna Kea Technologies) has the very advantageous characteristic of being compatible with the endoscopic instruments that are routinely used for urological endoscopy, and its use for the study of the upper urinary tract has been approved by the U.S. Food and Drug Administration (FDA). The incident beam emitted by the laser has a wavelength of 488 nm.

Fluorescein is a nontoxic fluorophore. It is included in the WHO's List of Essential Medicines, among the ophthalmic medicines, and has been approved for intravenous use during angiography to diagnose vascular disorders, including macular degeneration and diabetic retinopathy.

Side effects after intravenous administration of fluorescein are rare (1–2%) and include nausea (0.7%), vomiting (0.39%), dizziness (0.28%), fainting (0.14%), urticarial reaction (0.23%), and local reaction (0.12%) [12]. There were no severe reactions. In a previous study, Yannuzzi et al. [13] reported a higher percentage of side effects, including respiratory reactions (0.02%), cardiac events (0.01%), and tonic-clonic seizure (0.007%), with only one death reported among the more than 222,000 fluorescein angiograms included in the survey. Oral administration of fluorescein is safe in standard clinical practice [14].

The laser beam reacts with the fluorescein so that it reflects light with a different wavelength, thereby providing better visualization of the architecture, the cellular arrangement, and the vascularization of the analyzed structure. It is not possible to visualize subcellular structures because fluorescein cannot penetrate into cells.

Once the fluorescein has been administered, the probe is inserted into the operating channel of the instrument in question and, upon coming into contact (en face) with the structure to be examined, the features of the tissue that are enhanced are visualized.

4   CLE in Bladder Cancer

Bladder cancer is the ninth most commonly diagnosed cancer worldwide, with mortality rates decreasing particularly in the most developed countries [15].

Since the first description of the endoscopic fulguration of a papillary bladder tumor, in 1910, endoscopic transurethral resection under white light cystoscopy (WLC) has represented the gold standard in the treatment of non-muscle-invasive bladder cancer [16]. In fact, at first diagnosis 75% of bladder tumors do not infiltrate the muscle layer and have a good long-term survival rate, but the risk of recurrence and progression is high, particularly for high-grade tumors [17, 18]. The identification of these most aggressive tumors is therefore crucial for proper disease management.

The limitations of traditional cystoscopy include operator variability, uncertainty when differentiating inflammatory from malignant lesions, detection of flat lesions, and diagnosis of carcinoma in situ (CIS) [19]. While the diagnosis of CIS with simple WLC is often difficult, there is a clear consensus that this neoplasm is associated with high morbidity and mortality. The detection of CIS depends only on the findings from WLC and biopsies. Biopsy is an accurate and widely accepted method of assessment. However, the margin of a CIS is ambiguous, which can lead to incomplete endoscopic tumor resection or excessive cauterization of the mucosa [20].

The technique that offers the highest rate of detection of flat lesions and CIS is blue light cystoscopy after intravesical instillation of a photosensitizer (photodynamic diagnosis, PDD). When exposed to blue light (380–480 nm), dysplastic cells emit a characteristic red fluorescence. The prototypical intravesical imaging agent is 5-aminolevulinic acid [21]. PDD is, however, limited by a high rate of false positives induced by inflammation, previous resections, or intravesical instillation therapies, and invasive tissue sampling is therefore still required for confirmation of the suspected diagnosis [22].

A promising technique aimed at overcoming these limitations is probe-based CLE, which is based on histological findings and provides real-time histopathologic information to the surgeon. It is a powerful imaging tool that provides high-resolution, dynamic, subsurface imaging of biological systems. CLE images are not significantly contaminated by light scattered from other focal planes, resulting in the ability to optically section tissues, improve localization of signals, and enhance contrast. In conventional confocal microscopy, a low-powered laser is focused onto a single point of the specimen, and the microscope then refocuses the emitted light from the specimen. Any out-of-focus light is removed from the image by passage through a pinhole, so only a thin optical section of the specimen is formed. The illumination and detection system are in the same focal plane and are termed confocal. Detection of only the light within the focal plane greatly improves image quality and allows for visualization of signals originating from greater tissue depths [23].

Recently the instrument miniaturization process has allowed the development of flexible, fiber-optic confocal microscopes that can be introduced through the working channels of endoscopes. This enables in vivo microscopy and is referred to as "confocal endomicroscopy" or "fibered confocal microscopy". For image acquisition, a fiber-optic probe based on a 488-nm laser is inserted via the working channel of standard cystoscopes and placed in direct contact with the tissue. Imaging probes ranging from 0.85 to 2.6 mm in diameter are available, with varying optical specifications in spatial resolution, field of view, and compatibility with existing endoscopes. The 2.6-mm probe is compatible with the working port of standard 22 French (Fr) or larger cystoscopes and resectoscopes, while the 1.4-mm probes are compatible with the larger scopes, as well as the working channel of flexible cystoscopes (~15 Fr) [24]. Following imaging, the CLE probes can be sterilized and reused.

For CLE in the bladder, intravesical fluorescein (with a Foley catheter, using 300–400 ml 0.1% fluorescein diluted in saline) or intravenous fluorescein (with a 0.5 ml 10% fluorescein injection) is given as the contrast agent. It demonstrates a good safety profile, with transient fluorescently tinged urine as the primary minor side effect. As for the histological images obtained, in contrast to standard hematoxylin and eosin (H&E) histology, nuclear features are not routinely visualized since fluorescein highlights the extracellular matrix and does not cross intact cell membranes.

Performance of CLE after intravesical fluorescein administration allows the identification of various bladder lesions such as papillary tumors, flat tumors, erythematous patches, and the border between normal mucosa and neoplastic lesions. By contrast, observation of the resection bed and the prostatic and penile urethra requires intravenous fluorescein administration [25].

This technology does not allow visualization of the muscularis propria due to the low penetration power. It is, however, possible to image the muscularis propria and perivesical fat after tumor resection, through intravenous administration of fluorescein or secondary instillation of topical fluorescein.

Under CLE, normal mucosa is characterized by layers of superficial, polygonal umbrella cells and homogeneous, smaller intermediate cells located more deeply. Within the lamina propria, dense capillary networks are commonly seen, populated with flowing erythrocytes. These elements of normal morphology are absent in cancerous lesions. Low-grade papillary tumors demonstrate crowding of monomorphic cells, papillary structures, the presence of fibrovascular stalks, and vessels with a thickened endothelial layer. High-grade tumors are identified by a decidedly disorganized appearance, with pleomorphic cells arranged haphazardly around distorted vasculature [23] (Fig. 1).

Delineating cell boundaries has proven difficult given the general loss of cellular cohesion and tissue organization in high-grade tumors. In benign, inflammatory urothelium, small monomorphic cells are observed loosely distributed in the lamina propria, but fibrovascular stalks are notably absent. High-grade carcinomas can appear as papillary, sessile, or flat. Importantly, flat lesions typified by high-grade CIS are difficult to diagnosis under WLC, given their close mimicry of erythematous patches of benign, inflammatory origin. At the final histological examination, the CIS appears to be very heterogeneous from a morphologic point of view and

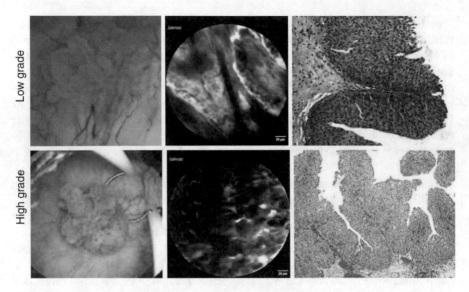

Fig. 1 Low- and high-grade papillary bladder urothelial carcinoma

also has different degrees of inflammatory infiltration [26]. Considering the heterogeneity of CIS, subsequent histological evaluation is still essential [27].

Using CLE image criteria described for the diagnosis and grading of bladder tumors, a study of inter-observer agreement revealed that the sensitivity for discerning cancerous lesions was 89% for urologists when using WLC and CLE together, while the specificity was 88%.

In conclusion, CLE is a promising technique for improving the diagnosis and therapy of urothelial bladder cancer and for ensuring that the optimal disease management option is selected. Furthermore, this technology can be used in patients with other bladder diseases, such as suspected schistosomiasis, especially as a way of avoiding biopsies of the bladder and the complications that these can entail [28].

5 CLE for Upper Tract Urothelial Carcinoma

Despite the relatively low incidence of upper tract urothelial carcinoma (UTUC) compared with other urological tumors, the interest in UTUC is growing. UTUC has an incidence of less than two cases per 100,000 in the Western world [29] and about 60% of tumors are invasive at the time of diagnosis [30].

The management of UTUC has changed over the last two decades, thanks to technological advances and improved understanding of its biological behavior.

Radical nephroureterectomy (RNU) with bladder cuff still remains the gold standard in UTUC. However, European Association of Urology (EAU) guidelines from 2018 recommend that kidney-sparing surgery, including the endourological approach and distal ureterectomy, should always be offered in cases of low-risk UTUC. In more detail, UTUC is considered low risk when the following criteria are met: unifocal disease, tumor size <2 cm, low-grade cytology and histology (biopsy), no invasive aspects on computed tomography urography (CTU), and absence of upper urinary tract dilatation [31]. The grading and the staging are the strongest prognostic factors [32].

Cytology of the upper urinary tract can be of value in the context of UTUC. Although selective cytology alone is insufficient for grading and staging of UTUC, the integration of biopsy and cytology can result in noticeable increases in sensitivity and positive predictive value for both grading and staging. However, according to the literature, up to 25% of UTUC biopsies are not diagnostic because of insufficient tissue in the specimen [33]. Moreover, standard biopsy may understage and/or undergrade UTUC in up to 43% of cases [34]. Accurate staging and grading of UTUC lesions are, however, mandatory for appropriate treatment selection. Minimally invasive surgery represents a valid treatment option for the conservative management of UTUC [34–36].

To date, ureteroscopic evaluation by means of biopsy and cytology has been considered the central component in the diagnosis of UTUC. However, conventional ureteroscopy (semirigid and/or flexible) is unable to provide real-time information on stage and grade. In addition, many difficulties are related to its limited ability to distinguish between small/flat malignant lesions and other inflammatory lesions and to obtain an adequate sample of tissue for histopathologic analysis.

In order to improve the visualization of UTUC and tumor grading, various imaging techniques have been proposed, including narrow band imaging, photodynamic diagnosis with 5-aminolevulinic acid, CLE, and real-time optical coherence tomography (OCT).

The great enthusiasm for CLE as an innovative technique for UTUC has given rise to in vivo studies in different centers. In 2015, Bui et al. [37] recruited 14 patients for ureteroscopy of suspected upper tract lesions or surveillance of UTUC. The tools used to perform CLE were the working channel of a 6.9 Fr semirigid ureteroscope (Stryker, San Jose, CA), a 7.5 Fr flexible ureteroscope (Karl Storz Endoscopy, El Segundo, CA), or a 7.9 Fr flexible video ureteroscope (Olympus Corporation, Tokyo, Japan) and a 0.85-mm probe with a depth of tissue penetration of 50 μm, a field of view of 320 μm, and a spatial resolution of 3.5 μm. With the 0.85-mm probe in place, it remained possible to access to all parts of the ureter and renal collecting system. Within 2–3 min after administering 0.5–1.0 mL of 10% sodium fluorescein (Akorn, Lake Forest, IL), CLE imaging was feasible with the tip of the probe perpendicular to the tissue for en face contact. The average image acquisition time was 5 min per case. The authors identified the microarchitectural and morphologic features characterized as diagnostic criteria for highgrade and low-grade urothelial carcinoma. Imaging of normal urothelium allowed visualization of lamina propria in both the ureter and the renal pelvis. Tissue was stained with hematoxylin and eosin for corresponding histopathologic analysis (Fig. 2).

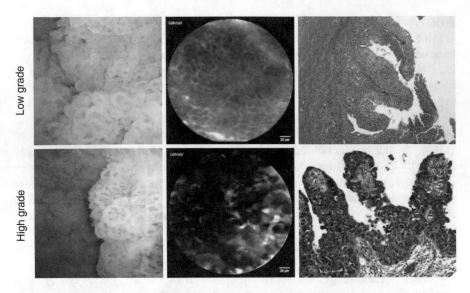

Fig. 2 Low- and high-grade papillary upper urinary tract urothelial carcinoma

In a 2016 study, Villa et al. [38], in a series of 11 patients, emphasized the use of CLE in UTUC to achieve the grading, particularly when a biopsy is difficult to carry out (i.e., small and/or flat lesions).

Breda et al. [39] performed CLE in 14 patients previously diagnosed UTUC at CT. The authors inspected the distal ureter with a semirigid ureteroscope (Karl Storz, Tuttlingen, Germany) and the rest of the upper urinary tract with a digital flexible ureteroscope (FLEX-X^C, Karl Storz) and performed real-time CLE using the Cellvizio® system (Mauna Kea Technologies, Paris, France) to evaluate cellular architecture and morphology. Inspection of the upper urinary tract had previously been performed using white light to identify all the suspicious lesions. Afterwards the appropriate treatment was performed (biopsy and tumor ablation with holmium-YAG laser, RNU, or segmental ureterectomy) and the specimens were examined by a dedicated genitourinary pathologist blinded to the surgeon's readings. Despite the small series (n = 14), high correspondence between the CLE evaluation and the final pathology results was found (100% and 83% in low- and high-grade UTUC, respectively).

In the only case in which no agreement was found between histopathologic diagnosis and CLE diagnosis, the authors believed that the lesion diagnosed and treated at the time of the ureteroscopy had been completely ablated and that the one found at RNU was a low-grade UTUC recurrence. There was a substantial inter-rater agreement between histopathologic results and CLE ($\kappa = 0.64$).

In 2018 Freund et al. [40] performed a study in 36 patients that investigated, within the context of papillary UTUC, the validity of criteria previously proposed for bladder cancer and proposed a scoring system designed to allow a more quantifiable approach to CLE-based grading of UTUC. The authors concluded that the CLE criteria previously proposed for bladder cancer are also applicable for ureteroscopic images of papillary UTUC although the visual aspect and the prevalence of CLE criteria differ from those in bladder cancer. The most prevalent features with the highest diagnostic potential for UTUC grading were: organization versus disorganization of the cellular architecture, monomorphism versus pleomorphism of cells, and cohesiveness versus discohesion of cells. The differences in the prevalence and visual appearance of CLE criteria in UTUC compared with bladder cancer are probably related to the different instruments and therefore to a lower resolution and inferior definition and sharpness of the ureteroscopic CLE images.

Studies on large numbers of patients are still lacking, but based on CT, histopathology, urinary cytology, CLE evaluation, and probably in the future also the use of molecular markers, it is possible to choose correctly between radical and conservative therapy and to select an appropriate conservative treatment when the characteristics of the patient or the disease are suitable [34]. Among the most obvious advantages of CLE is the possibility of guiding biopsies to suspicious areas that are less evident on the white light examination.

6 CLE in Prostate Cancer

Prostate cancer is the leading noncutaneous cancer in men and the third leading cause of cancer-related death [22]. During the last decades, several advances in the field of PCa diagnosis occurred: PSA introduction and diffusion, recent improvement in imaging (mpMRI), novel protocols and recommendation for prostate biopsy have dramatically changed the diagnostic pathway of PCa. Despite these improvements, pathological processing and evaluation of tissues have remained unchanged through years. Up to now, pathological reporting with hematoxylin-eosin (HE) still requires several days, that could be further prolonged in case of immunohistochemical study.

A faster reporting on prostate tissue could be useful both in the diagnostic setting—to relief patient's anxiety and to manage promptly the disease—and in the intra-operative one, to verify the complete removal of prostate gland during radical prostatectomy and to ensure a negative surgical margin status [41, 42].

6.1 Cellvizio and Optical Coherence Tomography

In order to improve the outcomes of robotic radical prostatectomy, image-guided surgery technologies have recently been introduced. Particularly, the optical imaging technologies allow a remarkable spatial and temporal resolution to be obtained. Furthermore, the miniaturization of the instruments makes it possible to use these devices in the context of minimally invasive surgery [43]. Several studies have recently been published on this issue, covering techniques such as near-infrared fluorescence imaging, OCT, and multiphoton microscopy.

Lopez et al. [25] developed an intraoperative confocal imaging protocol with the aim of using CLE to identify and characterize in vivo certain periprostatic structures, i.e., NVB before and after a nerve-sparing procedure, prostatic capsules, bladder neck margin, urethral stump, levator ani, and obturator nerve. Furthermore, they compared these findings with those obtained from samples analyzed ex vivo and by definitive histological examination. In more detail, during the procedure, 5 min prior to dissection of the NVB, 2.5 ml 10% sodium fluorescein was administered intravenously. The probe tip was positioned perpendicular to the tissue for en face contact and rinsed with irrigation as needed to remove blood or debris. Lopez et al. defined the confocal characteristics of NVB as parallel thin dark lines corresponding to axonal fibers, bordered by dark cells consistent with adipocytes and interspersed with vessels with flowing erythrocytes. In vivo CLE identified the NVB in 73.3% of patients. Imaging of the prostatic capsule demonstrated striated fibrous tissue with occasional small-caliber vasculature. Given the relatively small field of view of CLE, the prostatic capsule was not comprehensively imaged in vivo. No discernible prostatic parenchymal features such as glandular structures were observed in vivo. Confocal imaging of the bladder neck mucosa showed normal urothelium with umbrella and intermediate cells and the underlying vasculature of the lamina propria, consistent with previous bladder imaging. CLE can therefore be used as a guide in detecting the NVB before prostatic dissection and as a means of checking their integrity after dissection.

CLE can also be used in the field of prostate cancer diagnostics. In fact, a fiberoptic probe can be inserted into the lumen of a needle to obtain real-time microscopic images of the tissue during prostate biopsy. As already explained, backscattered light, from one specific tissue plane, is focused through a pinhole, whereas the backscattered light from surrounding tissue is rejected. This leads to high-resolution imaging of one specific plane of tissue in focus. The fluorescent light originates from the fluorescent dye nested in the extracellular matrix after topical or intravenous application [44].

Swaan et al. studied the feasibility and safety of CLE in the context of prostate biopsy. They intravenously injected 0.5 mL of fluorescein (2.5% fluorescein diluted in saline) for contrast. The CLE probe was transperineally inserted using a 17-gauge trocar needle. When the CLE was in contact with prostate tissue, the measurement began; while recording, the probe and needle were pushed from the apex to the base. During this push and scan technique, the probe stayed in contact with the tissue. CLE images were recorded at a scan rate of 12 frames per second. On the basis of histopathology, it is expected that benign and malignant prostate tissue would differ with respect to extracellular structure. The fluorescein, provided by intravenous injection, gives contrast to the extracellular matrix on CLE images. Locating and recording the position of the in vivo measurements is difficult and will be less precise than ex vivo measurements. However, this technology is safe and in the future it could allow distinction between in vivo neoplastic tissues and normal tissues in order to better target biopsy.

6.2   Fluorescence Confocal Microscopy with VivaScope®

Fluorescence confocal microscopy (FCM) with VivaScope® microscope 2500M-G4 (Mavig GmbH, Munich Germany; Caliber I.D.; Rochester NY, USA) is an optical technique that provides microscopical digital images of freshly excised tissue with a minimum of tissue preparation (1–5 min); images are acquired in a HE appearance and could be instantaneously web-shared with pathologists.

Since 2007, its use has been widely implemented in the field of dermatology, in the triage of equivocal lesions to rule out a melanoma [45, 46]. More recently, FCM has been reported [47] for the ex vivo evaluation of prostatic tissue (Fig. 3).

6.3   Instrument

FCM with VivaScope® combines two different lasers that enable tissue examination according to reflectance (785 nm) and fluorescence (488 nm) modalities. The FCM device has a vertical resolution of 4 μm and a maximum examination depth of 200 μm. Increasing the laser power and/or the incubation period of the specimen in the staining solution allow mechanical amplification of the fluorescence and

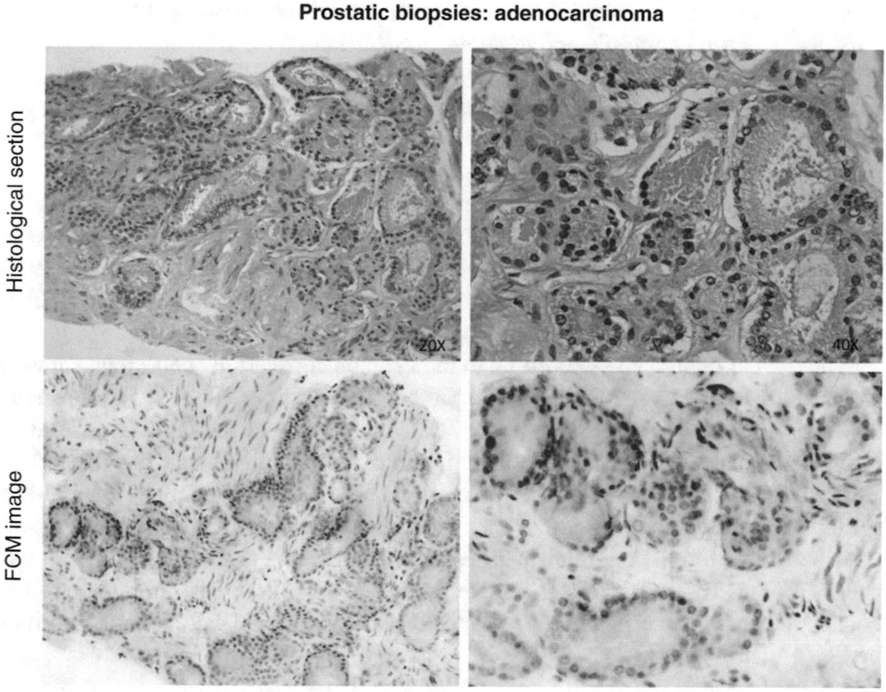

Fig. 3 Prostate adenocarcinoma

reflectance signals resulting in possible visualization of deeper structures. Furthermore, as the specimens are mounted between two glass slides in a sandwich technique, both sides of the glass sandwich can be examined by the FCM allowing better evaluation of the deeper side of the specimen. Magnification reaches 550× and the reconstructed image is a collection of mosaic images (square shaped images of 1024 × 1024 pixels). The digital staining modality is used to convert the reflectance and fluorescence grayscale mosaics into colour images; the software converts each grayscale pixel into a digitally stained image, in which nuclei appear purple and collagen and cytoplasm appear pink. The reflectance and fluorescence brightness in FCM images are inverted to the absorbance-based contrast, as is performed in histopathology imaging. The resolution capability of the imaging-device enables an accurate visualization of cell morphology details.

The handling of specimen is easy (<5 min) and fast, and does not require technicians or skilled personnel.

FCM analysis guarantees tissue integrity for the further conventional HE analysis.

6.4 Clinical Outcomes

As far as prostate cancer is concerned, the diagnostic performance of FCM with VivaScope® has been tested in terms of agreement with conventional HE in distinguishing between neoplastic and non-cancerous tissue.

Puliatti et al. published a study in an exploratory setting, in which prostate tissue is retrieved from specimens from radical prostatectomy. Eighty-nine FCM images were obtained from 13 prostate glands and have been randomly displayed to three pathologists together with the corresponding HE conventional images.

In this setting, the level of agreement between FCM and HE analysis in distinguishing between normal and cancerous prostate tissue was 91% with a Cohen's value of 0.75–83.3% sensitivity and 93.5% specificity. Pathologists were able to identify typical features of malignancy such as atypical glands, enlarged nuclei, prominent nucleoli, and an infiltrative pattern of glandular growth.

The level of confidence, according to the Pearson correlation coefficient, showed an overall positive correlation for all pathologists (0.536, $P < 0.001$); the interobserver reliability was 0.808 (95% CI 0.725–0.869), reflecting a good interobserver consistency for FCM evaluation, without a predefined learning curve.

Rocco et al. recently presented the use of FCM with VivaScope® in the real-life setting of intra-operative random frozen section: during radical prostatectomy, specimen was retrieved in case of suspicious cancer persisting at peri-prostatic soft tissues. FCM was able to discriminate between peri-prostatic components—as connective, fatty tissues, muscle, vessels—and prostate glandular tissue, either benign or malignant.

7   Current Limitations of and Future Perspectives for CLE

There are some limitations of CLE. First of all, there is a learning curve in terms of not only maneuverability and knowledge of the instrument but also ability to recognize in mucosal areas the tissue characteristics indicative of normality, low-grade lesions, high-grade lesions, and CIS. Furthermore, unlike an imaging investigation such as CT, CLE will remain an operator-dependent procedure. Regarding the learning curve in using the CLE probe for the upper urinary tract, it is comparable to the skills required for laser ablation for tumor treatment or stone fragmentation. Other than that, an atlas of videos and images is available to achieve proficiency in distinguishing the lesion characteristics at CLE [39].

Until now, it has not been feasible to recognize with certainty a lesion and its aggressiveness following fluorescein administration, meaning that the biopsy of suspicious areas is mandatory. CLE thus represents an additional procedure that considerably increases cost and may also be subject to the side effects, albeit rare, related to administration of an exogenous substance.

Although fluorescein is an extremely useful dye for performance of CLE, it does not appear to be optimal as it does not penetrate into cells. Visualization of the subcellular structures in the analyzed tissue could offer remarkable advantages for cyto-histological diagnosis based on the cellular image. An attempt has been made to make the binding of fluorescein more selective for tumor tissue through combination with monoclonal antibodies or peptide markers [48].

Furthermore, while CLE can provide important information about tumor grading it cannot provide such information about staging because CLE has no capacity to penetrate the tissue. Accordingly, the intraoperative information on the grade of the lesion may potentially obviate the need to wait for a final pathology evaluation before a decision is made on whether to treat a tumor conservatively or radically. Therefore, CLE may ideally be very helpful in the follow-up of patients previously treated with conservative management, especially in cases of CIS.

Finally, another future application may consist in exploring and characterizing the entire surface of the lesion, since the biopsy may provide pathologic information only on a well-defined area. This could be particularly helpful in cases of tumor with both low- and high-grade components.

References

1. Dabbs T, Glass M. Single-mode fibers used as confocal microscope pinholes. Appl Opt. 1992 Feb 20;31(6):705–6.
2. Polglase AL, McLaren WJ, Skinner SA, et al. A fluorescence confocal endomicroscope for in vivo microscopy of the upper- and the lower-GI tract. Gastrointest Endosc. 2005 Nov;62(5):686–95.

3. Thiberville L, Moreno-Swirc S, Vercauteren T, et al. In vivo imaging of the bronchial wall microstructure using fibered confocal fluorescence microscopy. Am J Respir Crit Care Med. 2007;175(1):22–31.
4. Chang TC, Liu J-J, Hsiao ST, et al. Interobserver agreement of confocal laser endomicroscopy for bladder cancer. J Endourol. 2013 May;27(5):598–603.
5. Wu K, Liu JJ, Adams W, et al. Dynamic real-time microscopy of the urinary tract using confocal laser endomicroscopy. Urology. 2011 Jul;78(1):225–31.
6. Chen SP, Liao JC. Confocal laser endomicroscopy of bladder and upper urinary tract urothelial carcinoma: a new era of optical diagnosis? Curr Urol Rep. 2014 Sep;15(9):437.
7. Marien A, Rock A, Maadarani KE, et al. Urothelial tumors and dual-band imaging: a new concept in confocal laser endomicroscopy. J Endourol. 2017 May;31(5):538–44.
8. Minsky M. Memoir on inventing the confocal scanning microscope. Scanning. 1988:128–38.
9. Claxton NS, Fellers TJ, Davidson MW. Laser scanning confocal microscopy. Department of Optical Microscopy and Digital Imaging, National High Magnetic Field Laboratory, Florida State University, https://www.ucc.ie/en/media/academic/anatomy/imagingcentre/imagegallery/confocalgallery/Laser-Scanning-Confocal-Microscopy-Introduction.pdf
10. Lucas FF. The architecture of the living cells – Recent advances in methods of biological research – Optical sectioning with the ultra-violet microscope. Proc Natl Acad Sci USA. 1930;16(9):599–607.
11. Wallace MB, Meining A, Canto MI, et al. The safety of intravenous fluorescein for confocal laser endomicroscopy in the gastrointestinal tract. Aliment Pharmacol Ther. 2010 Mar;31(5):548–52.
12. Kwan AS, Barry C, McAllister IL, Constable I. Fluorescein angiography and adverse drug reactions revisited: the Lions Eye experience. Clin Exp Ophthalmol. 2006 Jan-Feb;34(1):33–8.
13. Yannuzzi LA, Rohrer KT, Tindel LJ, et al. Fluorescein angiography complication survey. Ophthalmology. 1986 May;93(5):611–7.
14. Hara T, Inami M, Hara T, et al. Efficacy and safety of fluorescein angiography with orally administered sodium fluoresceine. Am J Ophthalmol. 1998 Oct;126(4):560–4.
15. Antoni S, Ferlay J, Soerjomataram I, et al. Bladder cancer incidence and mortality: a global overview and recent trends. Eur Urol. 2017 Jan;71(1):96–108.
16. Beer E. Landmark article May 28, 1910: removal of neoplasm of the urinary bladder. By Edwin Beer JAMA. 1983 Sep 9;250(10):1324–5.
17. Palou J, Sylvester RJ, Faba OR, et al. Female gender and carcinoma in situ in the prostatic urethra are the prognostic factors for recurrence, progression, and disease-specific mortality in T1G3 bladder cancer patients treated with bacillus Calmette-Guerin. Eur Urol. 2012 Jul;62(1):118–25.
18. Palou J, Rodríguez Rubio F, Millán F, et al. Recurrence at three months and high-grade recurrence as prognostic factor of progression in multivariate analysis of T1G2 bladder tumors. Urology. 2009 Jun;73(6):1313–7.
19. Sonn GA, Mach KE, Jensen K, et al. Fibered confocal microscopy of bladder tumors: an ex vivo study. J Endourol. 2009 Feb;23(2):197–201.
20. Lee J, Jeh SU, Koh DH, et al. Probe-based confocal laser endomicroscopy during transurethral resection of bladder tumors improves the diagnostic accuracy and therapeutic efficacy. Ann Surg Oncol. 2019 Apr;26(4):1158–65.
21. Kennedy JC, Pottier RH, Pross DC. Photodynamic therapy with endogenous protoporphyrin IX: basic principles and present clinical experience. J Photochem Photobiol B. 1990 Jun;6(1–2):143–8.
22. Wieser C, Jäger W, Salzer A, et al. Confocal laser endomicroscopy for the diagnosis of urothelial bladder neoplasia: a technology of the future? BJU Int. 2011 Feb;107(3):399–403.
23. Sonn GA, Jones S-NE, Tarin TV, et al. Optical biopsy of human bladder neoplasia with in vivo confocal laser endomicroscopy. J Urol. 2009;182:1299–305.
24. Adams W, Wu K, Liu JJ, et al. Comparison of 2.6- and 1.4-mm imaging probes for confocal laser endomicroscopy of the urinary tract. J Endourol. 2011 Jun;25(6):917–21.

25. Lopez A, Zlatev DV, Mach KE, et al. Intraoperative optical biopsy during robotic assisted radical prostatectomy using confocal endomicroscopy. J Urol. 2016 Apr;195(4 Pt 1):1110–7.

26. Aron M, Luthringer DJ, McKenney JK, et al. Utility of a triple antibody cocktail intraurothelial neoplasm-3 (IUN-3-CK20/CD44s/p53) and α-methylacyl-CoA racemase (AMACR) in the distinction of urothelial carcinoma in situ (CIS) and reactive urothelial atypia. Am J Surg Pathol. 2013 Dec;37(12):1815–23.

27. Wallace MB, Sharma P, Lightdale C, et al. Preliminary accuracy and interobserver agreement for the detection of intraepithelial neoplasia in Barrett's esophagus with probe-based confocal laser endomicroscopy. Gastrointest Endosc. 2010 Jul;72(1):19–24.

28. Fritzsche C, Stachs O, Holtfreter MC, et al. Confocal laser scanning microscopy, a new in vivo diagnostic tool for schistosomiasis. PLoS One. 2012;7(4):e34869.

29. Siegel RL, Miller KD, Jemal A. Cancer statistics, 2017. CA Cancer J Clin. 2017 Jan;67(1):7–30.

30. Margulis V, Shariat SF, Matin SF, et al. Outcomes of radical nephroureterectomy: a series from the Upper Tract Urothelial Carcinoma Collaboration. Cancer. 2009 Mar 15;115(6):1224–33.

31. Rouprêt M, Babjuk M, Compérat E, et al. European Association of Urology Guidelines on upper urinary tract urothelial carcinoma: 2017 update. Eur Urol. 2018 Jan;73(1):111–22.

32. Elawdy MM, Taha DE, Elbaset MA, et al. Histopathologic characteristics of upper tract urothelial carcinoma with an emphasis on their effect on cancer survival: a single-institute experience with 305 patients with long-term follow-up. Clin Genitourin Cancer. 2016 Dec;14(6):e609–15.

33. Tavora F, Fajardo DA, Lee TK, et al. Small endoscopic biopsies of the ureter and renal pelvis: pathologic pitfalls. Am J Surg Pathol. 2009 Oct;33(10):1540–6.

34. Smith AK, Stephenson AJ, Lane BR, et al. Inadequacy of biopsy for diagnosis of upper tract urothelial carcinoma: implications for conservative management. Urology. 2011 Jul;78(1):82–6.

35. Rouprêt M, Colin P, Yates DR. A new proposal to risk stratify urothelial carcinomas of the upper urinary tract (UTUCs) in a predefinitive treatment setting: low-risk vs high-risk UTUCs. Eur Urol. 2014 Aug;66(2):181–3.

36. Seisen T, Colin P, Rouprêt M. Risk-adapted strategy for the kidney-sparing management of the upper tract tumors. Nat Rev Urol. 2015 Mar;12(3):155–66.

37. Bui D, Mach KE, Zlatev DV, et al. A pilot study of in vivo confocal laser endomicroscopy of upper tract urothelial carcinoma. J Endourol. 2015 Dec;29(12):1418–23.

38. Villa L, Cloutier J, Cotè JF, et al. Confocal laser endomicroscopy in the managment of endoscopically treated upper urinary tract transitional cell carcinoma: preliminary data. J Endourol. 2016 Feb;30(2):237–42.

39. Breda A, Territo A, Gutilla A, et al. Correlation between confocal laser endomicroscopy (Cellvizio ®) and histological grading of upper tract urothelial carcinoma: a step forward for a better selection of patients suitable for conservative management. Eur Urol Focus. 2018 Dec;4(6):954–9.

40. Freund JE, Liem EIML, Savci-Heijink CD, et al. Confocal laser endomicroscopy for upper tract urothelial carcinoma: validation of the proposed criteria and proposal of a scoring system for real-time tumor grading. World J Urol. 2019 Oct;37(10):2155–64.

41. Alemozaffar M, Regan MM, Cooperberg MR, et al. Prediction of erectile function following treatment for prostate cancer. JAMA. 2011;306:1205.

42. Johansson E, Bill-Axelson A, Holmberg L, et al. Time, symptom burden, androgen deprivation, and self-assessed quality of life after radical prostatectomy or watchful waiting: the Randomized Scandinavian Prostate Cancer Group Study Number 4 (SPCG-4) clinical trial. Eur Urol. 2009;55:422.

43. Hsu M, Gupta M, Su LM, et al. Intraoperative optical imaging and tissue interrogation during urologic surgery. Curr Opin Urol. 2014;24:66.

44. Swaan A, Mannaerts CK, Scheltema MJ, et al. Confocal Laser endomicroscopy and optical coherence tomography for the diagnosis of prostate cancer: a needle-based, in vivo feasibility study protocol (IDEAL phase 2A). JMIR Res Protoc. 2018 May 21;7(5):e132.

45. Alarcon I, Carrera C, Palou J, et al. Impact of in vivo reflectance confocal microscopy on the number needed to treat melanoma in doubtful lesions. Br J Dermatol. 2014 Apr;170(4):802–8.

46. Pellacani G, Witkowski A, Cesinaro AM, et al. Cost-benefit of reflectance confocal microscopy in the diagnostic performance of melanoma. J Eur Acad Dermatol Venereol. 2016 Mar;30(3):413–9.
47. Puliatti S, Bertoni L, Pirola GM, et al. Ex vivo fluorescence confocal microscopy: the first application for real-time pathological examination of prostatic tissue. BJU Int. 2019 Sep;124(3):469–76.
48. Becker A, Hessenius C, Licha K, et al. Receptor-targeted optical imaging of tumors with near-infrared fluorescent ligands. Nat Biotechnol. 2001;19(4):327–31.

Live Surgery and Safety Standards

Alessandro Tafuri, Giuseppe Carrieri, Angelo Porreca,
and Alessandro Antonelli

1 From the "Operating (Amphi-)theater" to Live Surgery

Live demonstrations have been an integral part of surgical education for centuries. It was traditionally considered one of the best ways for the trainers to learn the surgical techniques using the "teacher-apprentice model" and assuming that the surgeons have the obligation to transfer their skills, knowledge, and experience to others [1, 2]. Exhibitions demonstrating surgical procedures have been described since the beginning of surgery with surgeons teaching and actively interacting with their apprentices or trainers as they conduct live operations [3]. As it has been suggested, the amphitheater called "operating theater" was built especially with the finality to show surgical and anatomical human dissections that were carried out to the audience in a theatrical manner [4].

In the last few years, the improvement of the technologies has allowed an increasing quality of surgery, patients' safety, as well as surgeons' comfort, introducing new surgical approaches, tools, and training methods and models, which include a live surgical demonstration. Additionally, many new advanced systems (e.g. robotic surgery) have been developed, allowing the surgeon to be present in a place other than his actual location, developing an ideal "telepresence system". In this way, despite he was present in a different place, he could also offer his appearance in a far location, as if he was present there [5]. These new systems have encouraged the evolution from "*surgical (amphi-)theater*" to "live surgery events" transmitting

A. Tafuri · A. Antonelli (✉)
Department of Urology, University of Verona, Azienda Ospedaliera Universitaria Integrata Verona, Verona, Italy

G. Carrieri
Department of Urology and Kidney Transplantation, University of Foggia, Foggia, Italy

A. Porreca
Department of Urology, Istituto Oncologico Veneto (IOV), Padua, Italy

worldwide in real-time the surgical detailed procedures in addition to the live comments and explanations of the main surgeon, expanding them during surgical meetings for educational purposes [6].

The first tracked transmission of surgery events was reproduced in 1958 in the famous BBC (British Broadcasting Corporation) fortunate series "*Your life in Their Hands*" that aimed to investigate the new medical tools, applaud the medical profession and reassure citizen at home [4]. Subsequently, on the first part of the 2000s, LSEs began to spread around the world [4].

During the years, live surgery events gained popularity becoming a valid educational tool, allowing a large number of healthcare providers to watch in detail surgical procedures. All this was performed interacting directly with the main surgeon or with him through expert moderators in several surgical fields [6]. Particularly, in endourology, urological laparoscopy, and robot-assisted urological surgery, LSEs were helpful to disseminate novel techniques in the urologic community [1]. Actually, it is accepted that LSEs may enhance surgical training, accelerate the dissemination of advances in surgery, improve quality of care, and raise awareness of newly available interventions. This was true particularly for the new technical procedures that cannot be learned by self-study or didactic presentation [1]. Specifically, European Association of Urology (EAU) sections, the EAU Section of Uro-Technology (ESUT), EAU Robotic Urology Section (ERUS), EAU Section of Female and Functional Urology (ESFFU), EAU Section of Genito-Urinary Reconstructive Surgery (ESGURS), and the EAU Section of Urolithiasis (EULIS) have successfully implemented educational and scientific programs using LSEs during the last few years [1].

2 The Anathema of the Live Surgery: Ethical and General Aspects

Despite the intuitive advantages related to these events were clear, they were difficult to demonstrate due to the several concerns related to the patient, surgeon and general aspects. That was specifically reported by Dr. Arthur Smith according to his large experience in urological live demonstrations during conferences as well as his personal visiting surgical experience and he listed many related concerns [7].

Primarily, during the LSEs the surgeon can develop anxiety due to the performance for a large audience which often includes select expert colleagues. Additionally, while the surgeon should be focused only on the procedure, he has to maintain a continuous dialogue with the audience explaining what is being done and the reasons for choosing a particular technique in that particular scenario. Also, he is frequently interrupted by questions from the audience as well as from the additional equipment and personnel involved in the transmission system management.

In addition, when the surgeon is invited to the far away event, he often arrives at a meeting sleep-deprived and jet-lagged and he has to operate in a new context with a new team in an unfamiliar operating room, with inadequate assistance, communicating in a different language. Importantly, in the most part of the case, the surgeon has not adequately pre-operatory evaluated the patient and he is not responsible for the postoperative care and usually the surgeon is not informed of postoperative complications. Further, because of the live surgery event, if the indication for a particular surgical procedure is considered ideal for a live demonstration at a conference, which has been scheduled for a future date, the patient may be subjected to an unnecessary delay in definitive treatment [7].

Other than the previous points, some surgical devices provided may be produced by a company that is sponsoring the meeting and may not be the equipment used routinely by the surgeon configuring the issues of the conflicts of interest. This is increased if the company compensates the surgeon and/or pays the patient's medical expenses. Furthermore, surgical societies may promote LSEs at their meetings to boost attendance, given their popularity and potential to generate significant sponsorship income. Some surgeons may be motivated by self-advancement or voyeurism rather than a true educational goal [1].

3   Surgeons' Point of View and Comparison Between Live Surgery and Daily Performed Procedures

The previous topics have been evaluated by different scientific societies considering the point of view of the surgeons that perform live surgery events.

In 2011 a survey was conducted by American Association of Genitourinary Surgeons Society (AAGUS) in a cohort of 90 surgeons/members among 93.2% had already performed at least one live surgery demonstration. The participants reported that anxiety as visiting, as well as home operator were no negligible factors. The authors found that excessive conversation in the operating room was a major distraction by 41.3% of respondents. Concern over the appropriateness of selected cases was reported often (43.9%) and always (13.4%) of the time. Only 28.2% of AAGUS members would let a visiting faculty member operate on them or a family member. *Most of the participants* (70.9%) considered live surgery events morally ethical, but only 30.1% of them thought that the events' demonstrations should be performed in their actual form [2].

In September 2012, a survey among European urologists attending the ERUS congress was performed. Here the authors aimed to evaluate the experience and opinions regarding live surgical events among the participants [3].

Questionnaires to the LSE experts who were present to the ERUS conference, investigating many of the prior reported concerns, were administered. Six hundred surgeons responded and with 98 (92.5%) reporting a personal experience of LSE. Among these, 6.5% of respondents noted "significant anxiety" increasing to 19.4% when performing surgery away from home (p < 0.001). Surgical quality was perceived as "slightly worse" and "significantly worse" by 16.1% and 2.2%, which deteriorated further to 23.9% and 3.3% respectively in a "foreign" environment (p = 0.005). In all, 10.9% of surgeons "always" brought their own surgical team compared with 37% relying on their host institution. Lack of specific equipment (10.3%), language difficulties (6.2%), and jet lag (7.3%) were other significant factors reported. In all, 75% of surgeons felt the audience wanted a slick demonstration; however, 52.2% and 42.4% respectively also reported the audience wished the surgeon to face up or manage a complication during a LSE [3].

Despite this important data about surgeons' feeling during live surgery events, in the literature, few studies evaluated the differences between perioperative outcomes during LSEs and the procedures performed during the daily routine procedures.

Comparing laparoscopic radical prostatectomy (LRP) during live surgery with daily LRP, has been proven that LRP has similar perioperative outcomes when performed in live surgery or daily routine setting but it is related to higher positive surgical margins rate after live events [8]. Further, when live surgery robotic partial nephrectomy and daily partial nephrectomy without observers were compared, no differences were found in terms of perioperative outcomes [9]. Interestingly, a recent study demonstrated that in the setting of live surgery, the overall rate of complications is low considering the complexity of surgeries and the post-operative morbidity index was not higher in more complex procedures [10].

4 Scientific Societies Live Surgery Events Policy

Based on this background and following the death of a patient in Japan in 2006 during an live surgery aortic aneurysm repair, several scientific societies re-evaluated their policy on were forced to evaluate their practice. The Society of Thoracic Surgeons Standards, recommended termination of LSEs to the public at their annual meetings. The American College of Obstetricians and Gynecologists and the American College of Surgeons have also ceased LSEs at their major meetings and some meetings have even imposed outright bans [3, 11]. On the other hand, EAU adopted a specific policy in order to regulatory these events [1].

5 Safety Standards in European Association of Urology (EAU) Live Surgery Events Policy

EAU defined live surgery as "*any surgical procedure conducted in real time and observed for educational purposes*" and endorses the use of LSEs as a "*technique for dissemination of surgical knowledge*" [1]. For these reasons, in 2012 EAU created a working group, aiming to set up an independent live surgery committee responsible for endorsing LSEs conducted under precise, predefined regulations. The EAU expert panel clearly defined a regulatory framework listing structured organizational requirements applicable to the EAU live surgery events having as main principle that "patient safety must take priority over all other considerations in the conduct of live surgery". Additionally, the EAU identified a specific local organizing committee with a designated director deputized to the overall event organization.

Based on these solid points, the EAU panel provided 35 statements on surgeon and patients selection, theater team preparation, preoperative planning, preoperative check, LSE overview, postoperative care in order to regulate the overall live surgery events management and execution (Table 1). These statements provide in the

Table 1 European Association of Urology (EAU) live surgery event recommendations [1]

Surgeon selection:
1. The surgeon is of sufficient proficiency, with a high annual volume of similar cases.
2. The surgeon holds operating privileges in a hospital in his or her country of origin.
3. The surgeon is granted operating privileges in the host unit.
4. Personal and hospital indemnity insurance is arranged prior to the event.
5. It is explicit whether the guest surgeon is the primary surgeon.
6. The guest surgeon is named on the patient consent addendum and ideally has significant experience in live surgery events (LSEs).
Patient selection:
7. Standard cases rather than extremes are preferable and recommended.
8. Patient selection must reflect the submitted educational objectives of the event.
9. Patients must be asked well in advance for their permission to undergo live surgery and experience no disadvantage, including scheduling if they decline.
10. There must be no delay in the patient's treatment as a consequence of agreement to an LSE.
11. Reserve patients should be available and appropriately counselled.
Theatre team preparation:
12. The operating surgeon must submit in advance a detailed list of preferences, including instruments, disposables, and devices; patient, surgeon, and scrub nurse positioning; and preferred assistants.
13. Any language difficulties should be foreseen and avoided, where possible.
14. Nominated assistants should be appropriately registered and suitably experienced.
15. Anaesthesiologists must be involved in planning the procedure.
Preoperative planning:
16. Full clinical details, test results, and images of the case should be sent to the guest surgeon for review well in advance, allowing time for discussion with the host surgical team.
17. The guest surgeon reserves the right to decline to operate, and contingency plans should be in place for this eventuality.
18. The surgeon must be invited to arrive at the host unit the day before the surgery.
19. The standard consent for surgery used by the hospital must be signed.
20. Patients should give specific consent to a live link during the operation (Patient Consent Addendum).
21. Patients should have the opportunity to withdraw at any stage preoperatively. If there is a guest surgeon, patients must meet the visiting surgeon in a calm environment the day before surgery for consent.
Preoperative checks:
22. The WHO surgical checklist (or a local adaptation) must be used and involve all personnel in the operating room, who must also be briefed about the event.
23. Unnecessary personnel and equipment should not be present in the operating room.
24. Representatives from industry should be in the operating room only if their presence is mandatory, and they should be appropriately registered and certified by the host hospital

(continued)

Table 1 (continued)

LSE Overview:
25. Cases should be digitally recorded.
26. Delays purely for the conduct of the live proceedings must be avoided.
27. The presence of an experienced urologist, acting as the patient's advocate in the theatre, is a mandatory requisite.
28. The use of one or more moderators is recommended.
29. The role of the moderators is critical for filtering irrelevant audience questions, explaining critical steps, helping the surgeon in teaching, raising interesting issues, assessing the tension in the operating theatre, minimizing distractions to the surgeon, recognizing difficult moments of surgery, and interrupting the teleconference to quietly handle any arising complications.
30. The presence of one moderator in the operating room and one or more moderators (a panel) in the auditorium is recommended.
Postoperative care:
31. There must be dedicated and appropriate on-call personnel throughout the patient's hospital stay.
32. Postoperative follow-up is under the direction of the local surgeon and team, and it must comply with the standard protocol of the host hospital.
33. The guest surgeon must be informed of and, where possible, involved in all decisions about postoperative patient care, even if he or she is not still in the unit.
34. Regular postoperative ward rounds are mandatory, and the visiting surgeon must be kept informed of all deviations from the care plan.
35. All complications must be documented using the revised Martin criteria, and outcomes and complications must be submitted to the European Association of Urology (EAU) Live Surgery Registry.

contest of the live demonstrations, potential benefits to the patients, surgeons and audience. Particularly they included a clear framework with which to plan and execute the event, explicit responsibilities for all the involved figures, a clear protocol to use for the surgeon in order to reduce the anxiety and eliminate the unfamiliarity with staff and equipment, as well as informed moderators and structured dialogues. A clear way to select and manage the patients before, during and after the event, and a clear way for the preparation of the surgical theater was also provided. At the same time, the interests of the scientific society were ensured with the information collection, cumulative databases creation propose, and many research opportunities [1].

6 The Position of Italian Society of Urology on the LSEs Management

According to EAU live events policy, also the Italian Society of Urology (Società Italiana di Urologia; SIU) implemented a novel concept of live surgery events with an own events management. The "SIU Live organizing committee" allowed that all the involved surgeons to operate at the own institutions instead of in a foreign center in an unfamiliar context. The procedures were assigned to the Institution with well-known specific experience and scheduled according to an educational pathway from basic to innovative value. The institution managers led the local organizing committee re-discussing the suggested procedures in presence of technical or scheduling issues, from the time of assignment to a few days before the meeting. Local surgeons were independently selected by the LOC and were not announced in the event program, with anonymity maintained until the event day [6]. In this context, all surgeons operate on their personal patients at their own institutions. Importantly, the issue of surgeon distraction was removed as the moderator interacted with the staff members in the operating room instead of directly with the main surgeon. This event was named "SIU Live" and was organized in Rome in 2017, 2018, and 2019. During these editions, more than 100 urologic surgical procedures including open, endoscopic, laparoscopic, robotic, and prosthetic strategies were performed at the own main surgeon Institution in more than 50 from over the world and transmitted to the audience. All the procedures were shown on different screens and commented by expert moderators. Five hundred attendees per screen were present at the congress venue and more than 1000 viewers at home logged in via a streaming connection [6].

Technical and Organization Aspects During "SIU Live" events, the video and audio signaling were transmitted along 8 Mb/s internet broadband connection through Codec devices that matched the Internet Protocol addresses of the between the congress and the interested institutions. In this way, the quality performance equal to satellite broadcasting were provided, without time delay, and any structural adjustments was needed but with low costs. The technical staff and equipment required to set up and coordinate broadcasting from the conference hall involved additional expenses that were covered by the SIU [6].

7 Conclusion

Live surgical events derive from the theater operating way to perform surgery. Actually, they are considered an excellent training and demonstration tool for the divulgation of the surgical (new-) techniques but it may be related to important ethical conditions concerning patients' safety. The EAU provided a list of recommendations to adopt on the overall organization of the live surgery events. They must be used and standardized in order to ensure that patients' safety and dignity are the priority during live surgery events.

References

1. Artibani W, Ficarra V, Challacombe BJ, Abbou CC, Bedke J, Boscolo-Berto R, et al. EAU policy on live surgery events. Eur Urol. 2014;66(1):87–97.
2. Duty B, Okhunov Z, Friedlander J, Okeke Z, Smith A. Live surgical demonstrations: an old, but increasingly controversial practice. Urology. 2012;79(5):1185.e7–11.

3. Khan SA, Chang RT, Ahmed K, Knoll T, van Velthoven R, Challacombe B, et al. Live surgical education: a perspective from the surgeons who perform it. BJU Int. 2014;114(1):151–8.
4. Rao AR, Karim O. A benedictory ode to urological live surgery. BJU Int. 2013;112(1):11–2.
5. Veneziano D, Tafuri A, Rivas JG, Dourado A, Okhunov Z, Somani BK, et al. Is remote live urologic surgery a reality? Evidences from a systematic review of the literature. World J Urol. 2020;38:2367–76.
6. Antonelli A, Carrieri G, Porreca A, Veneziano D, Artibani W. Live surgery: is operating at home the way forward? Eur Urol. 2018;74(4):403–4.
7. Smith A. Urological live surgery – an anathema. BJU Int. 2012;110(3):299–300.
8. Ramirez-Backhaus M, Bertolo R, Mamber A, Ferrer AG, Mir MC, Rubio-Briones J. Live surgery for laparoscopic radical prostatectomy-does it worsen the outcomes? A single-center experience. Urology. 2019;123:133–9.
9. Mullins JK, Borofsky MS, Allaf ME, Bhayani S, Kaouk JH, Rogers CG, et al. Live robotic surgery: are outcomes compromised? Urology. 2012;80(3):602–7.
10. Rocco B, Grasso AAC, De Lorenzis E, Davis JW, Abbou C, Breda A, et al. Live surgery: highly educational or harmful? World J Urol. 2018;36(2):171–5.
11. Philip-Watson J, Khan SA, Hadjipavlou M, Rane A, Knoll T. Live surgery at conferences – Clinical benefits and ethical dilemmas. Arab J Urol. 2014;12(3):183–6.

Part II
Future Perspectives

Artificial Intelligence

Hacı İsmail Aslan, Kadir Erdem Şahin, Mahdiyeh Nilgounbakht, and Emre Huri

Artificial intelligence was proposed by philosophers and mathematicians such as George W. Bush who proposed laws and theories of logic. With the invention of electronic computers in 1943, artificial intelligence challenged scientists at the time. Under these circumstances, it seemed that this technology would be able to simulate intelligent behavior. Despite the opposition of a group of artificial intelligence thinkers who were skeptical of its effectiveness, only four decades later did we see the birth of open chess machines and other intelligent systems in various industries. The field of artificial intelligence research was born in 1956 in a workshop at Dartmouth College.

The field of artificial intelligence research was born in a training workshop at Dartmouth College in 1956. Participants Alan Newell (Carnegie Mellon University), Herbert Simon (Carnegie Mellon University), John McCarthy Massachusetts Institute of Technology, Marvin Mansky (Massachusetts Institute of Technology) and Arthur Samuel (IBM) became the founders and leaders of research in the field of artificial intelligence. They learned the game's winning strategies, solved questions in algebra, and proved logical theorems. And he speaks English. In the mid-1960s, the Department of Defense invested heavily in AI research, and in that

H. İ. Aslan
Department of Electrical and Electronics Engineering, Hacettepe University, Ankara, Turkey
e-mail: ismailaslan@hacettepe.edu.tr

K. E. Şahin
Department of Mechanical Engineering, Middle East Technical University, Ankara, Turkey
e-mail: sahin.erdem@metu.edu.tr

M. Nilgounbakht
Department of Computer Engineering, Hacettepe University, Ankara, Turkey
e-mail: mnilgounbakht@haccettepe.edu.tr

E. Huri (✉)
Hacettepe University, Ankara, Turkey
e-mail: emrehuri@hacettepe.edu.tr

© The Author(s), under exclusive license to Springer Nature
Switzerland AG 2021
D. Veneziano, E. Huri (eds.), *Urologic Surgery in the Digital Era*,
https://doi.org/10.1007/978-3-030-63948-8_13

decade many laboratories were established around the world. The founders of intelligence. Artificially optimistic about the future: Herbert Simone predicts that 'machines will be able to do whatever a human can do in twenty years.' 'Over the next generation, the problem of artificial intelligence will be fundamentally solved,' wrote Marvin Minsky.

The name artificial intelligence was coined in 1965 as a new science. Of course, work in this area began in the 1960s. (Reference 1) Most of the early research work on artificial intelligence was on machine-playing games as well as computer-assisted mathematical theorems. At first it seemed that computers would be able to perform such activities only by using a large number of discoveries and searching for problem-solving paths, and then choosing the best way to solve them. The term artificial intelligence was first used by John McCarthy (known as the father of science and knowledge to produce smart machines). He is the inventor of one of the languages of artificial intelligence programming called lisp. This can be used to identify the intelligent behaviors of an artificial instrument. (Man-made, unnatural, artificial) While artificial intelligence is accepted as a general term that includes intelligent and combined calculations (composed of synthetic materials). The term 'Strong and Weak AI' can be used in part to describe the classification of systems.

In medical science has become more important today due to the expansion of knowledge and the complexity of the decision-making process, the use of information systems, especially artificial intelligence systems, in decision-making. Artificial intelligence, the spread of knowledge in the field of medicine and the complexity of decisions related to diagnosis and treatment—in other words, human life—has attracted the attention of experts to the use of decision support systems in medical affairs. For this reason, the use of different types of intelligent systems in medicine is increasing, so that today the impact of different types of intelligent systems in medicine has been studied.

The primary goal of health-related artificial intelligence applications is to analyze the relationships between prevention or treatment techniques and patient outcomes. But artificial intelligence programs have been implemented in ways such as diagnostic processes, treatment protocol development, drug development, personal medicine, and patient monitoring and care.

Medical and technological advances that have taken place over the last half century have led to the growth and development of healthcare-related applications. Among the specialties:

– Extraction of medical records: Extract, store and analyze patient information.
– Help with executive work: A new way to save money and time and increase efficiency.
– Radiology: Help doctors make the correct diagnosis based on the interpretation of the image, especially in lung diseases
– Telemedicine: Ability to monitor patients with the possibility of transmitting information to physicians if possible
– Industry: Ability to access much more data in the field of health

- Oncology: Development of artificial intelligence applications in the treatment of chronic diseases, Medical image analysis tumor progression, identify patients at risk and develop ways to care
- Digital Medical Counseling Programs: Provide information by the user and provide advice according to the user's medical history
- Accelerate clinical trials: Machine learning can be used to identify appropriate options and speed up the design of clinical trials.
- Gene modification: With machine learning models and with careful selection RNA, with minimal side effects or by genetic testing, new genetic mutations are discovered in connection with autism.
- Finding medicine: Finding the right molecule in the drug production phase with high speed and accuracy.
- Reduce human error: Processing big data with incredible speed with greater accuracy.
- Designing additional software to use to heal open wounds: Diagnosis of the disease based on the symptoms and symptoms of the disease in the computer.
- Use in the diagnosis of threatening heart infections: By the information given to the computer.
- Disease diagnosis software design: The user will see a list of possible illnesses by entering the symptoms of the disease into the computer.
- Virtual nursing assistants: By assisting and monitoring, these assistants have the ability to answer questions about medications and other support.
- Assistant robot for surgery: Robotic surgeries are safer than those performed by humans because surgical incisions are performed more accurately by robots.
- Investigating a Serious Challenge in the Development Process: Analysis of Confirmed cases of COVID-19

1 Future Perspectives: Computer-Aided Detection

Before starting this chapter, it is sufficient that some definitions have priority to be known. Whichever technique that has ever been used, you will be dealing with medical imaging theory, so let's look at some of these definitions which will be used in the chapter.

Image enhancement: The removal of image distortions, such as noise and background inhomogeneity, as well as the enhancement of image contours and other relevant properties.

Image segmentation: The identification of the contours of an anatomical structure, such as an organ, a vessel, or a tumor lesion.

Image registration: The spatial transformation of one image such that it directly matches a given reference image. This is necessary, for example, in the combined visualization of images from different modalities (e.g., PET/CT).

Quantification: The determination of geometrical properties of an anatomical structure (e.g., volume, diameter, and curvature) or physiological properties such as perfusion characteristics or tissue composition.

Visualization: Two-dimensional (2-D) and three-dimensional (3-D) rendering of image data (e.g., volume rendering) and virtual models (e.g., surface models) of organs and other anatomical structures.

Computer-aided detection: The detection and characterization of pathological structures and lesions, such as tumor lesions or vessel obstructions [1].

Surely more definitions can be stated in medical imaging field, however these definitions above are enough to understand the chapter you are currently reading.

2 Importance and Expanding Role of Computer-Aided Detection in Medicine

Detection and diagnosis of a medical statement has been discussed since the ancient Greek history. The word "diagnosis" comes from the Greek, and literally means, "knowing through". Diagnosis is the ability to see through the often bewildering maze of manifest signs and symptoms to arrive at a sure and certain knowledge or conclusion as to their root cause, or what is really going on.

Hippocrates approached the art of diagnosis holistically, taking the entire organism—body, mind and spirit—to be one indivisible whole, or physics. Since the whole organism is responding in a unified manner to the challenge of disease, Hippocrates was the first to recognize that signs or symptoms appearing in one part of the body could be indicative of a disease process happening in another distant part of the body. In their diagnosis and treatment, the Cnidians lacked this holistic overview. They saw symptoms arising in a certain part of the body as indicating a disease or disorder pertaining to that part only, which was treated in isolation from the rest of the body.

Hippocrates, when he set out to revolutionize medicine, had certain issues with the Cnidian school, which preceded him. Many of these centered on their faulty and incomplete methods of diagnosis.

First of all, the Cnidians considered only the patient's subjective symptoms, and not any objective signs. Hippocrates countered that a complete diagnostic assessment required a consideration of both the patient's signs and symptoms.

Today, the practice of diagnosis in modern medicine has been radically altered by the advent of high technology. The modern physician relies heavily on technology and sophisticated machinery throughout the diagnostic process: EEGs, EKGs, diagnostic scanners and imaging equipment, radiography and lab tests.

3 Computer-Aided Detection of Prostate Cancer

There could be billions of other modern applications regarding computer-aided detection technologies. Since we investigate how technology differs in urological field in medicine, an example that covers detection of prostate cancer would be coherent with our main subject in this chapter.

According to Analoui and G. Alhosseini, "Computer-Aided Detection of Prostate Cancer", for starting any kind of treatment for the prostate cancer, knowing the precise position of the malignant tumor is desirable. Despite the difficulty of this task, the obtained results indicate that discrimination between cancerous and non-cancerous tissue is possible to a certain degree. The computer-aided system helps an inexperienced user to make a better diagnosis, however it must be able to perform better in order to be useful in a real world clinical context.

For future study, the color-coded cluster tissue sample images can potentially represent various degrees of seriousness of the abnormality in sample images similar to Gleason score for prostate cancer. The approaches presented within this project provide a beginning framework for biomedical experiments and many micro/macro image textural analysis/clustering applications from pathological image analysis to remote sensing [2].

In another scientific research of "Predicting CT Image From MRI Data Through Feature Matching With Learned Nonlinear Local Descriptors", it is stated that they propose a feature matching method with learned local descriptors for predicting CT from MR image data. The primary descriptors of the MR image are first projected to a high-dimensional space to obtain the nonlinear descriptors using an explicit feature map. These descriptors are optimized by adopting an improved SDL algorithm. The experimental results demonstrate that the learned nonlinear descriptors are effective for dense matching and pCT prediction. Moreover, the proposed CT prediction method can achieve competitive performance compared with several state-of-the-art methods [3].

4 What Is Medical Printing and What Are the Applications of Medical Printing?

Medical printing is the production of a three-dimensional object from a digital model by the help of specified computers and printers. Medical printing types can be categorized in 3 types which are 3D, 4D and Bioprinting.

In 3D printing, in other saying additive manufacturing, materials like liquids and powders added layer by layer together to form the desired object. 3D printing can be done with several different methods and with several different materials to identify the characteristics of the produced object. 3D printing method is used in different sectors because of its flexibility.

4D printing, which is using the same technique as 3D printing, is again forming process of a three-dimensional object by adding it another dimension. This dimension is time, adding time dimension to an object lead us to get a responsive product from printing. This response can be activated by a physical signal, chemical signal, or biological signal. This activation enables us to develop new treatments for patients.

Another type of Medical Printing is bioprinting. It functions like 3D printing but using different materials. In bioprinting materials which are known as bioinks are used to design tissue-like structures. It is the most promising type of printing for medical applications as it has potential to produce biological tissues.

5 Importance and Usage of the Medical Printing in the Healthcare

Using printing in medical applications bring several advantages. From the surgeon's perspective 3D models are effective when planning patient-specific surgery. With the help of these models they can have a better understanding about the operation requirements, and operation steps. They can also practice on models and prepare themselves beforehand. This will also provide improved abilities and increased accuracy for surgeons during the operation. In addition to pre-surgical planning 3D printing is used in intraoperative navigation. These models are also used to train the surgeons and surgeon candidates in terms of handicraft and the diagnosis. From the patient's perspective these models would be beneficiary to provide them better understanding of the operation they will have. A pilot study which was done to investigate the effects of using 3D models on resident education about PCNL (percutaneous nephrolithotripsy) shows that after presentations with 3D models residents were 86% and 88% better at determining the number of anterior and posterior calyces and also 60% better at understanding stone location, and %64 better at determining optimal entry calyx [4].

Over the past several decades tissue engineering is receiving significant attention in various medical fields. Tissue engineering has variety of applications like creating bones, vascular, skin, cartilage and neural structures using bioprinting. Tissue engineering still in the beginning of its development, applications are not yet sufficient but promising. Nowadays these application areas cannot be replaced with the engineered mimics, but tissue engineering is used for the minor damage treatments. With the developments of bioprinting and bioinks major damage treatments are possible. One other research area is printed transplantable organs, but this area also requires further development of bioprinting [5].

One another area of usage of medical printing is patient specific constructions. One of the significant applications in this field is production of patient specific prosthetics. In orthopedic field these prosthetics has an important role in the treatment of the spinal deformity. Advantageous of medical printing in this treatment is individual design, secured and simplified operations [6].

In production of targeted drug delivery systems 4D printing methods are used to make multi effective drugs and ensure their treatment will take place at the desired location with pre-designed responses. These responses are designed as pH, temperature, liquid, and enzymes to precisely deliver the drug to the body part [7].

6 Applications of Medical Printing in the Urology Field

In the field of urology several utilizations of medical printings are conducted and there exist several potential usages in urology. These utilizations of medical printing are mentioned before. These utilizations are basically pre-surgery planning and training, intraoperative navigation, education of residents and trainees. Existing potentials can be listed as resection planning of genitourinary organs, prostate biopsies, detailed and accurate identification of imaging before surgery, operation decision on both blunt and sharp traumas, culture models in order to create organs and tactile anatomical models to medical students, surgical assistants [8].

In a research which is conducted to compare the effect of 3D printed prostate models with standard radiological information to locate prostate cancer revealed that despite the standard radiological information is more effective than 3D printed models when locating the prostate cancer, 3D models had helped the less experienced surgeons to locate the prostate cancer better. Therefore, 3D printing is important in the training of less experienced individuals [9].

In another research, researchers designed and fabricated a biomimetic rabbit urethra using 3D bioprinting technology. In this study, various scaffolds are compared with that of native rabbit urethra. The result of this study shows that microenvironment in bioprinted urethra is favorable for cell growth and tissue formation [10]. This result, a real proof of the future potential of bioprinting.

7 Future of Medical Printing

With the development in the medical printing methods new treatments undoubtedly will be achieved. On the other hand, the shiny part of the future of medical printing is not about the development of the methods rather that developments in the bioprinting and bioinks. One of the dreams of the humans are renewable body parts and these developments are steps of this ladder. If the ability of engineering complex 3D biological architectures is acquired, a new era of medical treatment will begin. As with these complex 3D biological architectures, humans will be able to create patient-specific transplantable organs, complete bone tissues, neural tissues, vascular tissues, skin tissues, cartilage tissues.

A further perspective is the artificial body parts and artificial organs. With the collocation of different technological fields production of these artificial parts, humans will be able to enhance the capabilities of patient body systems and treat the illnesses of patients.

8 Discussion on Medical Printing

In this subheader, we mentioned the advantageous of medical printing; however, there exist several disadvantageous parts of it. The cost of printing not always feasible and the required time is not short enough. This fact creates a discussion about the usage of medical printing. Nonetheless, this discussion will not be valid in future as by doing a foresight by monitoring the past data and similar examples, with the technological development in this area the required cost and time will decrease. From another point if a comparison is made between the cost and the health the answer is be clear.

The other discussion about medical printing is the effectiveness and practicality of medical printing methods. One of the main reasons of this discussion is the lack of the statistical results to prove effectiveness and practicality as medical printing still a new concept for the world.

By considering the future of medical printing one question is occurring in the mind. With the enhancements in visualization technologies and virtual reality technologies will the requirement of the 3D printing vanish? Obviously, there is a potential of vanishment in some of the application because of it but also there is a potential of derivation of new applications with the collocation of these technologies.

References

1. Ritter F, et al., Medical image analysis. In IEEE Pulse, vol. 2, no. 6, pp. 60–70, Nov.–Dec. 2011. [2].
2. Analoui, Alhosseini G. Computer-aided detection of prostate cancer. 2006 International Conference on Computational Inteligence for Modelling Control and Automation and International Conference on Intelligent Agents Web Technologies and International Commerce (CIMCA'06), Sydney, NSW, 2006, pp. 140–140, https://doi.org/10.1109/CIMCA.2006.75.
3. Yang W et al. Predicting CT image from MRI data through feature matching with learned nonlinear local descriptors. In IEEE transactions on medical imaging, vol. 37, no. 4, pp. 977–987, April 2018.
4. Atalay HA, Ülker V, Alkan İ, Canat HL, Özkuvancı Ü, Altunrende F. Impact of three-dimensional printed pelvicaliceal system models on residents' understanding of pelvicaliceal system anatomy before percutaneous nephrolithotripsy surgery: a pilot study. J Endourol. 2016;30(10):1132–7. https://doi.org/10.1089/end.2016.0307.
5. Gu BK, Choi DJ, Park SJ, Kim YJ, Kim CH. 3D bioprinting technologies for tissue engineering applications. Adv Exp Med Biol. 2018;1078:15–28. https://doi.org/10.1007/978-981-13-0950-2_2.
6. Cai H, Liu Z, Wei F, Yu M, Xu N, Li Z. 3D printing in spine surgery. Adv Exp Med Biol. 2018;1093:345–59. https://doi.org/10.1007/978-981-13-1396-7_27.
7. Lui YS, Sow WT, Tan LP, Wu Y, Lai Y, Li H. 4D printing and stimuli-responsive materials in biomedical aspects. Acta Biomater. 2019;92:19–36. https://doi.org/10.1016/j.actbio.2019.05.005.
8. Özgür BC, Ayyıldız A. 3D printing in urology: is it really promising? Turk J Urol. 2018;44(1):6–9. https://doi.org/10.5152/tud.2018.20856.
9. Ebbing J, Jäderling F, Collins JW, et al. Comparison of 3D printed prostate models with standard radiological information to aid understanding of the precise location of prostate cancer: a construct validation study. PLoS One. 2018;13(6):e0199477. Published 2018 Jun 25. https://doi.org/10.1371/journal.pone.0199477
10. Zhang K, Fu Q, Yoo J, et al. 3D bioprinting of urethra with PCL/PLCL blend and dual autologous cells in fibrin hydrogel: an in vitro evaluation of biomimetic mechanical property and cell growth environment. Acta Biomater. 2017;50:154–64. https://doi.org/10.1016/j.actbio.2016.12.008.

Social Media and E-Learning

Juan Gómez Rivas, Jeremy Yuen-Chun Teoh, and Moises Rodriguez Socarrás

1 Introduction

Science is what we call to the different branches of human knowledge. By generating knowledge, we have managed to progress through different civilizations, finding the way to live more, with a better quality of life, to fly higher and faster, to see better in light and darkness, and more [1].

The way knowledge is generated, distributed and stored is of fundamental importance for any health professional who wants to give the best care to their patients. Every time a new discovery is shown (new pharmaceutical agents, new metabolic pathways…) several questions rise, which leads into more investigations that will generate more knowledge, this is a never ending circle [1].

Nowadays, is almost impossible to unlink most of the sources of modern knowledge and information to 2.0 technologies, which are communication platforms where the content is created, edited, exchanged and disseminated by the users themselves. Social Media (SoMe), a 2.0 technology, is changing the way people live, communicate and interact globally. In recent years we have witnessed an explosion in the development and dissemination of information. We live in a connected world; news, events and information crosses the borders of any country in a second. SoMe usage is one of the most popular online activities. In 2018, an estimated 2.65 billion people were using SoMe worldwide, a number projected to increase to almost 3.1

J. Gómez Rivas (✉)
Department of Urology, Clinico San Carlos Hospital, Madrid, Spain

J. Y.-C. Teoh
Department of Surgery, S.H. Ho Urology Centre, Prince of Wales Hospital, The Chinese University of Hong Kong, Shatin, NT, Hong Kong

M. Rodriguez Socarrás
ICUA (Instituto de Cirugia Urologica Avazada), Madrid, Spain

D. Veneziano, E. Huri (eds.), *Urologic Surgery in the Digital Era*, https://doi.org/10.1007/978-3-030-63948-8_14

221

billion in 2021. Social network penetration is constantly increasing and as of January 2019 stood at 45 percent. Most of SoMe global growth is driven by the increasing usage of mobile devices [2]. People from children to elderly use tablets, laptops and mobiles with access to internet and SoMe.

The applications of SoMe in healthcare and its role in scientific communication represents a growing area of interest, providing great opportunities in the urological community [3].

2　What Are Social Media and Scientific Social Media?

SoMe are communication platforms or online applications based on web 2.0, where the content is created, edited, exchanged and disseminated by the users themselves.

SoMe can take many different forms, including internet forums, personal blogs, social blogs, wikis, podcasts, photos and videos. Examples of SoMe applications are: Wikipedia, Facebook, Google+, YouTube, Twitter, Tumbrl, Swarm, Foursquare, ResearchGate, LinkedIn, Instagram, Pinterest, among others [4].

SoMe was initially developed as a communication way between people with personal content. Much time has not elapsed to find the advantages of SoMe in various professional areas. SoMe have become an important tool demonstrating multiple advantages to share and disseminate scientific knowledge among healthcare community; this is part of the concept of e-learning. An e-learning platform is a virtual learning space aimed at facilitating the experience of distance training. Nowadays, professionals can connect with others in their field, expand networking, share updated information, exchange opinions and access resources of interest instantly and easily [5–7].

SoMe platforms represent an open environment in which scientists, doctors, patients and the general public can interact; this can be beneficial in campaigns of awareness or education to patients, however it can be very harmful if shared information violates patient's privacy rights or goes against ethics principles and is not within the guidelines recommendations on the appropriate use of SoMe from the medical associations [8–10].

To understand Scientific SoMe (Sci-SoMe) it is necessary to know the difference between horizontal and vertical SoMe platforms [11]. In this way, horizontal SoMe represent a totally open environment, where any person with real or false identity can have access and the information is few segmented, dispersed and mixed, examples of these are: Facebook, Instagram, YouTube, Twitter, Periscope or Linkedin [12]. On the other hand, there are vertical SoMe platforms, also called thematic or specialized; these include Sci-SoMe that seek to foster collaboration among the research community. Among these specialized or thematic SoMe are: ResearchGate, Orcid, Doximitry, Mendeley among others [11].

3 Social Media History

Communication is part of human nature; the need for faster communication has allowed developing methods that have changed human history: mail, printing, phones, mobiles, computers and internet are some examples of this phenomenon [5].

Advances in communication have always allowed the evolution of cultures; better communicated societies evolve faster. The beginning of the internet and SoMe undoubtedly changed world's history and their contribution to human development today is unquestionable [5].

The birth of SoMe is linked with the development of Web 2.0. The term Web 2.0 was first used in 1999; it comprises those web sites that facilitate information sharing, interoperability, user-centered design and collaboration on Web. A Web 2.0 site allows users to interact and collaborate with each other as creators of user-generated content in a virtual community. Web 2.0 is the evolution of the web or internet in which users are no longer passive and they become active members, who participate and contribute to the content of the network, being able to support and be part of a society that informs, communicates and generates knowledge [13, 14].

In 1971: The first e- mail is sent between two computers located in the same room; 1994: GeoCities was launched as a service that allowed users to create their own websites and host them in certain places ("neighborhoods") according to the content; 1997: is a big year, the launch of AOL Instant Messenger and Google; 2003: MySpace, LinkedIn and Facebook; 2005: Youtube; 2006: launch of Twitter.

Nowadays with 2.45 billion monthly active users as of the third quarter of 2019, Facebook is the biggest SoMe worldwide. In the third quarter of 2012, the number of active Facebook users surpassed one billion, making it the first social network ever to do so. During the last reported quarter, the company stated that 2.8 billion people were using at least one of the company's core products (Facebook, WhatsApp, Instagram, or Messenger) each month [2].

In the same period Twitter averaged 330 million monthly active users, a decline from its all-time high of 336 users in the first quarter of 2018 [2].

4 Social Media and Applications in Urology

Currently, thanks to SoMe, urologists, oncologists, radiotherapists and other specialities may converge in a common space, provide comments or opinions from any meeting and expand the experience, e.g. sharing slides. Through SoMe, an urologist may influence thousands of colleagues or patients (Table 1).

Table 1 Examples of social media and scientific social media platforms

Platform	Users/Activity	Applications
Facebook	2.424 Billion users	Share photos, videos Contacts
YouTube	2 billion users	Share videos Channels
Instagram	1 billion users	Share photos, videos
Twitter	330 million users	Opinions, News, Videos, Photos, Congress, topics.
LinkedIn	310 million	Professional profile.
ResearchGate	3 million	Platform for scientists. Search and download of scientific articles. Personal impact factor

Loeb S et al., reported that 74% of urologists use some form of SoMe platform. Facebook was the most used by 89% of urologists, probably due to its personal applications but we think that nowadays, Twitter is the most exciting personal platform with more applications in a professional way, especially in urology [15].

The main advantage of Sc-SoMe, is that users are more selected and segmented, this means that there are professionals with specifics common interests in certain areas of knowledge. Moreover, some Sc-SoMe platforms are restrictive and exclusively used by researchers or health professionals, so they are "less contaminated" by the general public and information without scientific support [16].

The content of the information that is shared is specialized, with high scientific value. In addition, they allow creating a professional profile and developing a personal brand, since the user profile serves researchers to manage their curriculum vitae (CV) and represents a channel to enhance personal visibility with colleagues of similar interests. Some Sc-SoMe platforms allow to group the publications of the same author, to obtain statistics, scores and author almetrics, link profiles with other authors, contact and share these publications with other researchers [16].

The main drawback of Sc-SoMe is at the same time its main advantage, which is, the restrictions and to have a limited impact to a specialized audience. On this way, they also lose the freshness and fluidity of SoMe platforms well widespread and daily use such as Facebook or Twitter, where information is instantly shared and can be easily enriched with images, links or videos. In addition, to the great diversity of social networks nowadays, researches may simply not be informed of the available Sc-SoMe platforms, not know how to use them or decide that they do not have enough time to administer them all [11]. On this way, according to a European survey conducted in the role of SoMe in the acquisition of urological knowledge among young urologists only 30–40% of respondents reported using SoMe platforms as ResearchGate for professional purposes, as opposed to others such as Facebook used for personal purposes according to 91% of the respondents [6].

4.1   Applications

4.1.1   Patients' Education

SoMe is a great platform where doctors can influence or send messages to their patients. Today is common to have doctors with 10,000, 30,000 or 50,000 followers on Twitter, sending messages daily about lifestyle and other medical advances in simple language, understandable to general public. Do not forget that it is also common to access doctors, clinics or hospitals blogs to publish patient education about screening or treatment options [16, 17].

4.1.2   Promote Scientific Events and Expanding the Experience

Promoting events on SoMe is a good strategy that captures a greater diffusion. In addition to follow; events, conferences and meetings are officially registered with an official hashtag "#". The assistants of the event may simultaneously be informed and involved in different conferences, and also may interact with other participants, although physically not being in the same place. Another application regarding Twitter, is slideshare or participating in small debates with urologists from around the world on issues of interest meanwhile the presentation of a conference [18].

4.1.3   Dissemination of Scientific Articles and Study Results

leading journals in urology and various specialties share through SoMe results, abstracts, and even full articles considered of great interest especially *via* Twitter and for free. Thanks to SoMe, journals and Urology experts can select the information they consider most relevant and thus facilitate learning and updating of urologists and residents more quickly and conveniently [19]. A list of journals Twitter accounts is provided on Table 2.

4.1.4   Surgical Videos, Live Broadcasting & e-Learning

Undoubtedly, learning surgeries has been easier since the arrival of videos. Surgical videos on YouTube and other platforms, channels and websites of urological associations are available [6, 20, 21]. A new SoMe application used for live broadcast is Periscope. It is a live-video streaming application administered by Twitter and launched in 2015. Periscope has been postulated as a "potential tool for the transmission of knowledge" [22]. It is simple to use, fast, free and without the barriers

Table 2 Urology journals & twitter accounts

Journal	Twitter handle
Actas Urológicas Españolas	@actasurologicas
Archivos Españoles de Urología	@ArchEspUrologia
European Urology	@EUplatinum
European Urology Focus	@EurUrolFocus
European Urology Oncology	@EurUrolOncol
BJU International	@BJUIjournal
Central European Journal of Urology	@cejurology
Nature Reviews Urology	@NarRevUrol
Journal of Endourology	@Jendourology
Journal of Urology	@Jurology
Journal Sexual Medicine	@jsexmed
Urology Gold Journal	@urogoldjournal
World Journal of Urology	@wjurol

associated to traditional video equipment as it's designed for smartphone-broadcasting. Although the mentioned benefits, Periscope can be misappropriated for copyright infringement, an issue raised by the time of the application's launch. Users have stated that the service needs better tools and policies to deal with copyrighted content [23]. Gomez Rivas, et al. data shows that live videos shared in SoMe during urological conferences are increasing. When the characteristics of the videos shared in SoMe during the European Association of Urology annual congress from 2016 to 2018 were analyzed, an increase in the number of videos, transmission time and the number of views was observed [12].

4.1.5 Professional Online Presence

Urologist and other professionals can interact with others in similar areas of interest contributing in their views and positions. Although SoMe offers the opportunity to create a professional presence, we should follow the guidelines for its proper use and avoid personal egos and self-promotion [8–11].

5 Scientific Social Media

Author identifiers: They are unique identifiers that allow managing the professional identity of each researcher, distinguishing them from other researchers and unequivocally associating their work [24]. The author identifiers, among other things, allow to:

a. Establish a unique name and affiliation.
b. Correct identification errors in names of author or institution.
c. Group all publications by the same author.

d. Facilitate the recovery and dissemination of publications.
e. Increase visibility.
f. Obtain statistics of scientific production and metrics.
g. Link between different author profiles.
h. Contact other related researchers.

Author profiles: Creating and managing our own academic profile will help us control the information available about us and ensure that other researchers are finding correct and complete information about our research and career [24]. They can provide information such as

a. Variants of name with which you could sign
b. Institutional affiliation
c. Contact information
d. Research interests
e. Education, scholarships, awards, …
f. Job history
g. Lists of publications

There are several types of platforms with author profiles, each with a specific focus: (1) Communities of researchers like Academia.edu or ResearchGate, (2) Bibliographic managers with social function such as Mendeley, and (3) Search engines with author profiles, such as Google Scholar. The main author identifiers and profiles are summarized in Table 3.

Table 3 Comparative table of the main identifiers and author profiles (Modified from Gomez Rivas et al., 2019)

Scientific Social Media	Aim	Registration	Publication list	How to add publications	Metrics	Privacy control
ORCID	Author identifier linked to Scopus, Author ID and Mendeley	Free	Yes	Import from: 1. ResearcherID, Scopus, CrossRef... 2. BibTex files 3. Manually	No	Yes
ResearcherID	Author identifier	Free	Yes	1. Import from Word of Science and EndNote 2. RIS files	Yes	Yes
Scopus Author Identifier	Author identifier and profile	Assigned automatically to all authors indexed in Scopus	Yes (Scopus list)	Only Scopus. Changes can be asked	Yes	No

(continued)

Table 3 (continued)

Scientific Social Media	Aim	Registration	Publication list	How to add publications	Metrics	Privacy control
ResearchGate	Scientific Social media	Free	Yes	1. Pubmed + IEEE + Cite Seer + RepEc +BMC 2. BibTex files, RIS, MODS, RefWorks, Dblp and XML. 3. Manually	Yes	Yes
Academia.edu	Scientific Social media	Free	Yes	1. CrossRef, MicrosoftAS + Pubmed + ArXiv 2. Manually	Yes	Yes
Mendeley	Reference manager	Free	Yes	1. Directly from other sources 2. Manually	Yes	Yes
Google Scholar Citations	Author profile	Free	Yes	2. Google Scholar 1. Manually	Yes	Yes

6 Personal Social Media Platforms Used for Scientific Purpose

6.1 Linkedln (Linkedin Corporation, Mountain View, CA, USA) https://www.linkedin.com

Initially launched in 2003, it is now the largest professional network site; it has more than 500 million members from 200 different countries [25]. This platform is oriented to exchange information and experiences between people who share a similar academic background or working activities; each profile acts as an online CV or resume. It is mainly used for professional networking purposes, including employers posting jobs and job seekers posting their CVs.

Companies have profiles, in which workers are included, this way they could serve for people applying for a job position or looking for collaboration. Companies and scientists can use it to set up an informal interview with interested people. Its main orientation is the business sector, but it can work in an excellent manner in search for scientific working groups or collaborators due to its popularity.

6.2 Twitter (Twitter, Inc. San Francisco, CA, USA) https:// twitter.com/

In this micro-blogging social network, subscribers generate and share content and ideas in real time in text of ≤280 characters ("tweet"), with the ability to attach images and links to web content [26]. Twitter allows direct and easy communication between users and people can be involved in real time discussions. Twitter has been recently adopted by the medical community and other academic users as a tool for communicating and promoting discussion. Multiple scientific organizations and scientific journals have accounts to post relevant information [27]. Users can enjoy Twitter for reviewing quick and relevant messages from discussions/presentations at scientific meetings following the appropriate hashtags (#), as well as share data, documents, links, etc. The # search allows your social network to grow by following people or institutions with the interests, or who assist or sponsor certain events. As Twitter is widely used for all types of content sharing, there should be a definition of "scientific tweeting", Weller et al. [28] suggest three basic requirements: (1) a tweet that includes scientific content, (2) a tweet that is posted by a scientist, and (3) a tweet that includes a science-related #.

7 Scientific Social Media Platforms

7.1 Academia.edu (Academia, Inc. San Francisco, CA, USA) https://www.academia.edu

Academia is a free Sc-SoMe pursuing the objective of connecting scientists and researchers with similar interests who wish to share their work. The site launched in 2008, and at December 2018 it has more than 58 million registered users, adding more than 20 million papers to the site [29]. Its modern and user-friendly web design allows easy interaction between users and improved browsing capabilities. Academia.edu combines the archival role of repositories like ArXiv, SSRNm or PubMed with social networking features, which include personal profiles, news feed, recommendations, and the possibility to follow individuals, groups, departments and, topics of interest. Profiles are organized as walls, where individuals can post and upload their work, as well as search for colleagues via Facebook, LinkedIn and Gmail, as well as follow the work of other users. A study published by Niyazov et al., [30] found that research papers uploaded to Academia.edu can receive up to 69% more citations after a five-year period.

7.2 Mendeley (Mendeley, Inc. Elsevier. Amsterdam, Netherlands) https://www.mendeley.com

Mendeley is a free reference manager combined with a Sc-SoMe created to help users to manage their own digital libraries and share them, find new data and papers online and collaborate with others [31].

The reference manager includes: a desktop app (available for Windows, Mac and Linux), a mobile app (available for android and iOS), and a web-based platform for social networking. As a SoMe, users can create their own personal profile and organize and promote their own research while connecting with other researches. By creating and joining groups, users can share resources and ideas with one to another. The platform allows researchers to conduit initial collaborative research, write papers, reviews or grant proposals, submit dissertations for reviews, identify collaboration partners and create awareness. A unique feature of Mendeley is an advance statistical tool where we can find stats about documents, authors, most-used topics in particular areas and shared references (31).

7.3 Microsoft Academic 2.0 (Microsoft Corporation. Redmond, WA, USA) http://academic.research. microsoft.com/

Former Microsoft Academic Search, Microsoft Academic (MA) is a free public search engine for academic publications, scientific content and, literature [32].

Profiles are personalized by every user and publications are uploaded, based on the publication history, MA shows the most relevant items on a personalized homepage, along with news from the authors and events choosen to follow.

MA uses machine readers powered by artificial intelligence to scan and extract knowledge from all scholarly publications discovered and indexed by Bing. Bing indexes data from a variety of sources, ranging from publisher sites to individual authors´ personal homepages and organizes all these data into a graph database called Microsoft Academic Graph. It provides recommendations and related results to help you discover more work of your interest.

An interesting feature is that this is not only a keyword-based search engine like all others, but can be a semantic search engine. Microsoft states that MA is trained to understand the meaning of papers to search beyond keywords, employing a natural language processing to understand and remember the knowledge conveyed in each document.

7.4   ORCID (Orcid, Inc. Bethesa, MD, USA) https://orcid.org

Abbreviation for Open Researcher and Contributor ID, it is a nonproprietary alpha-numeric code to uniquely identify scientific and other academic authors and con-tributors [33].

It provides every user with a persistent identity, similar to that created for content-related entities on digital networks by digital object identifiers (DOIs). The reason behind this idea lays on the common ambiguous problems found with researches names: changes in names through career, common names, maiden names, abbrevia-tions or names including non-Roman characters for example. Users can enhance their own ORCID record with their professional information and links to identifiers (Scopus, ResearcherID, LinkedIn, etc). Researchers can include their personal ORCID identifier in their webpage or CV, at the time of submitting publications, applying for grants, and in any research workflow. A core principle is the individu-al's control over what information is stored under each user's ORCID record, users indicate if items are public, trusted-party or private.

7.5   ResearchGate (ResearchGate GmbH. Berlin, Germany) www.researchgate.net

Founded in 2008, offers most of the popular functionalities common to current social networking sites, offering users a reliable profile that can be used as an online CV, with own academic features that allow users to connect and converse around research interests and publications. ResearchGate has its own measurement unit that works as a citation impact measurement, called "RG Score", that assigns members a score based upon content interactions and the score of the members interacting with the content (views, downloads, citations, etc). RG Scores have been correlated with existing citation impact measures, but also have been criticized for their reli-ability. A global survey published in 2016 in Timer Higher Education, involving 20.670 people who use academic social networking sites, concluded that ResearchGate was the dominant network among all of the existing platforms [34].

8   Fundamentals of Social Media Analytics

SoMe analytics is the practice of gathering and analyzing data from SoMe plat-forms. A number of SoMe analytic tools are available.

8.1   Social Media Metrics

SoMe metrics are quantitative measures used to assess and monitor the performance and progress of an activity. These measures are usually pre-defined within each type of SoMe platform [35, 36]. Although the exact definitions may slightly differ, the general principles are similar. 'Impression' is counted as the number of times a post is on screen for the first time. If the same person views the same post at two different times in a day, this will be counted as two impressions. 'Reach' refers to the number of people who saw your post at least once. The number of reach will not alter despite multiple views of your post by the same people. 'Engagement' refers to the total number of interactions that people had with your post. This may include actions such as liking, sharing and commenting on your post, viewing a photo or video, clicking on a link, etc. (Fig. 1).

Each of the metric has its own value with different focus [37]. 'Impression' is important if you want to increase awareness of a particular subject with primary focus of reaching new audience. 'Reach' is important when you want to deliver new information to as many people as possible within an existing audience. 'Engagement' is important when you want interested audience to take some form of action. No single measure has absolute superiority over another, but most people would regard 'engagement' as the most important and difficult metric to achieve.

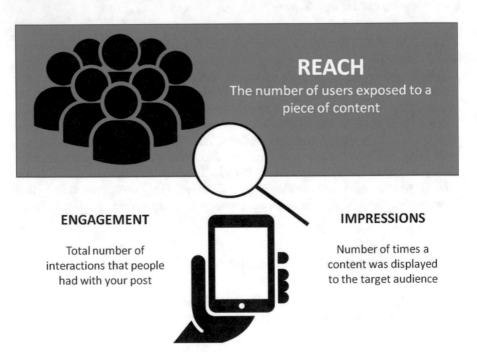

Fig. 1 Differences between Social Media terminology

8.2 Social Network Analysis

Social network analysis is another way of analyzing the impact of SoMe. Different social networks can interact differently depending on the context of discussions and the people involved. The importance of a particular person can be determined based on structural relationships with other people as well as influence upon other people within a social network. Such relationship and influence can be quantified by different types of centrality measures using predefined formulas.

Commonly used centrality measures include Eigenvector centrality, betweenness centrality and closeness centrality, and they can be calculated using predefined formulas. In principle, Eigenvector centrality can be interpreted as a measure of the influence of a person in a network. Betweenness centrality quantifies the number of times a person acts as a bridge along the shortest path between two other people. Closeness centrality is defined by the inverse of the sum of a person's shortest distances to all other people. Centrality measures can help us understand who are the potential key stakeholders and key opinion leaders within a community. It will be particularly important to engage people with high centrality measures in a more proactive manner [38].

8.3 Implications of SoMe Analytics

SoMe analytics allow us to quantify how successful a particular activity is in a SoMe perspective. As SoMe analytics look into rather short-term outcomes, there is a constant doubt whether they carry any important implications in long run. Previous studies demonstrated that successful audience engagement may reflect on the scientific value of a research study. Eysenback et al. [39] showed that highly tweeted articles were 11 times more likely to be highly cited. Nolte et al. [40] showed that conference presentations with more engagement were positively correlated with subsequent publication and journal impact factor. Twitter impact factor, which is defined as the number of retweets gained divided by the number of tweets posted by a journal Twitter account, carried a positive but statistically insignificantly association with the journal impact factor [41]. All these results suggested that successful audience engagement might indicate the scientific value of the research work being presented. In the rare occasion of a 'viral' post, the 'viral effect' is again primarily based on the surge of audience engagement within a short period of time. In such case, even a short-term outcome may already indicate a significant impact to the community. Summing up, the authors do believe that SoMe analytics carry important implications and we should regularly use it to plan and monitor our SoMe activities.

9　Risk and Recommendations on the Appropriate Use of Social Media

The first thing to remember is that SoMe is an open environment where everything you post is public domain, meaning that patients and general public can follow your posts and comments. In this way, please remember the risks of using SoMe and think about the appropriate limits of the content in health professionals discussions and the information shared with public character in order to avoid legal medical problems [8–10].

For these reasons several professional organizations such as the European Asocciation of Urology (EAU), Spanish Association of Urology (AEU) and others have developed guidelines or recommendations on the appropriate use of SoMe for their members [8–10]. Every urologist who is now active in SoMe in a professional way should read and follow this guidelines in other to ensure an appropriate use and avoid professional conflicts.

There is controversy in the use of SoMe, is a fact that sharing photos of slides on SoMe without the authorization of the authors and presenters might be a problem, due copyright infractions; however it does not exist a clear regulation that prohibits to share this material on SoMe during urological congress [42, 43].

On the other hand, when photos and comments are shared from lectures during conferences, comments are generated by the person from the audience that publishes the material and could communicate or not the idea that the author wishes to transmit. On this way, when live videos appeared in the scene, they provided the benefit of transmitting exactly what authors says, without further interpretations by the person who shares the material and while giving at the same time the audience from the web an experience that is closer to the actual "live" one. New devices such as 360° cameras might replicate a full congress experience; users can be closer to capturing the entire session along with a whole view of the area. In that way, viewers can have an "in-site" congress feeling.

10　The Future of Social Media & e-Learning

The future of science will depend on the formation of many such interconnected scientific communities covering all possible areas. Making optimal use of the internet, e-learning and SoMe, scientists and citizens within and between communities will collaborate to produce more useful knowledge than ever before and to store, maintain and provide information for those who seek it. Especially for medical scientists in the developing world, these communities will provide vehicles for innovation, health improvement and development in their respective countries.

The overcome of big data in medicine, massive quantities of health care data accumulating from patients and populations and the advanced analytics that can give it meaning hold the prospect of becoming an engine for the knowledge generation that is necessary to address the extensive unmet information needs of patients, clinicians, administrators, researchers, and health policy makers. Incorporating big data and next-generation analytics into clinical and population health research and practice will require not only new data sources but also new thinking, training, and tools. Adequately used, these reservoirs of data can be a practically inexhaustible source of knowledge to fuel a learning health care system.

11 Conclusions

SoMe represents a vibrant area of opportunities for communication of knowledge in healthcare and their potential applications today are unquestionable. SoMe has become a new game challenger in the way science is conducted during the last decade. The 2.0 technologies are playing a big role in the way knowledge is being spread. This rapid movement leads us to the need for a separation between the professional versus the private usage of SoMe. At present the benefits include communication between associations, urologists, residents, other health care professionals and patients. SoMe facilitates networking, dissemination of studies result as well as extensive experience of events, conferences and meetings.

However the public nature of the information shared in SoMe raises concerns in health associations by the legal character and the potential risk of harm confidentiality and the doctor—patient relationship.

Sc-SoMe and e-learing platforms can act as important provider of advice and proactive promotion of appropriate existing instances of 2.0 technologies. Besides such general information, a Sc-SoMe can also give individual personalized recommendations for an optimal selection and combination of scientific services, with respect to the special demands of the subject area and the individual requirements of the researcher. For example, together with the supply of literature on a special topic, Sc-SoMe may offer information about possibilities to discuss and connect with other researchers in the same scientific field.

In that line of reasoning, SoMe and e-learning should not only provide important information and services for literature and literature search but also could be an important catalyst for promoting appropriate and helpful services in the context of a new concept of science, the science 2.0.

References

1. Gómez Rivas J, Carrion DM, Tortolero L, Veneziano D, Esperto F, Greco F, et al. Scientific social media, a new way to expand knowledge. What do urologists need to know? Actas Urol Esp. 2019 Jun;43(5):269–76.
2. Most popular social networks worldwide as of October 2019, ranked by number of active users. Retrieved from: www.statista.com/statistics/272014/global-social-networks-ranked-by-number-of-users/. Accessed December 07th, 2019.

3. Loeb S, Catto J, Kutikov J. Social media offers unprecedented opportunities for vibrant exchange of professional ideas across continents. Eur Urol. 2014 Jul;66(1):118–9.
4. Grajales FJ, Sheps S, Ho K, Novak-Lauscher H, Eysenbach G. Social media: a review and tutorial of applications in medicine and health care. J Med Internet Res. 2014;16(2):e13.
5. Rivas JG, Socarras MR, Blanco LT. Social Media in Urology: opportunities, applications, appropriate use and new horizons. Cent European J Urol. 2016;69(3):293–8.
6. Rivas JG, Socarras MR, Patruno G, Uvin P, Esperto F, Dinis PJ, Roupret M, Borgmann H. Perceived role of social media in urologic knowledge acquisition among young urologists: a European survey. Eur Urol Focus. 2018 Sep;4(5):768–73.
7. Gómez-Rivas J, Rodríguez-Socarrás ME, Tortolero-Blanco L, Garcia-Sanz M, Alvarez-Maestro M, Ribal MJ, Cózar-Olmo M. Influence of social networks on congresses of urological societies and associations: Results of the 81th National Congress of the Spanish Urological Association. Actas Urol Esp. 2017 Apr;41(3):181–7.
8. Borgmann H, Cooperberg M, Murphy D, Loeb S, N'Dow J, Ribal MJ, et al. Online Professionalism—2018 Update of European Association of Urology (@Uroweb) Recommendations on the Appropriate Use of Social Media. Eur Urol. 2018 Aug 31. pii: S0302-2838(18)30614-6. https://doi.org/10.1016/j.eururo.2018.08.022
9. Rodríguez-Socarrás ME, Gómez-Rivas J, Álvarez-Maestro M, Tortolero L, Ribal MJ, Garcia Sanz M, et al. Spanish adaptation of the recommendations for the appropriate use of social networks in urology of the European Association of Urology. Actas Urol Esp. 2016;40:417–23.
10. Taylor J, Loeb S. Guideline of guidelines: social media in urology. BJU Int 2019 Oct 20. https://doi.org/10.1111/bju.14931.
11. Lieb R. Setting the stage for vertical social networks. Retrieved from: https://es.slideshare.net/lieblink/vertical-social-networks. Accessed August 1th, 2018.
12. Gómez Rivas J, Rodríguez-Socarras ME, Cacciamani G, Dourado Meneses A, Okhunov Z, van Gurp M, et al. Live videos shared on social media during urological conferences are increasing: time to reflect on advantages and potential harms. An ESUT-YAU study. Actas Urol Esp. 2019 Dec;43(10):551–6.
13. Kaplan AM, Haenlein M. Users of the world, unite! The challenges and opportunities of social media. Bus Horiz. 53(1):59–68.
14. Connie Piggott. A Brief History of Social Media. Retrieved from: http://es.slideshare.net/NoirPiggott/a-brief-history-of-social-media-by-c-piggott-2012?related=2. Accessed December 07th, 2019.
15. Loeb S, Bayne CE, Frey C, Davies BJ, Averch TD, Woo HH. Use of social media in urology: data from the American Urological Association (AUA). BJU Int. 2014 Jun;113(6):993–8.
16. Househ M, Borycki E, Kushniruk A. Empowering patients through social media: the benefits and challenges. Health Informatics J. 2014 Mar;20(1):50–8.
17. Sugawara Y, Narimatsu H, Hozawa A, Shao L, Otani K, Fukao A. Cancer patients on Twitter: a novel patient community on social media. BMC Res Notes. 2012;27(5):699.
18. Gómez-Rivas J, Rodríguez-Socarrás ME, Tortolero-Blanco L, Garcia-Sanz M, Alvarez-Maestro M, Ribal MJ, et al. Influence of social networks on congresses of urological societies and associations: results of the 81th National Congress of the Spanish Urological Association. Actas Urol Esp. 2017;41(3):181–7.
19. Nason GJ, O'Kelly F, Kelly ME, Phelan N, Manecksha RP, Lawrentschuk N, et al. The emerging use of Twitter by urological journals. BJU Int. 2015;115(3):486–90.
20. Hughes JP, Quraishi MS. YouTube resources for the otolaryngology trainee. J Laryngol Otol. 2012;126(1):61–2.
21. Steinberg PL, Wason S, Stern JM, Deters L, Kowal B, Seigne J. YouTube as source of prostate cancer information. Urology. 2010;75(3):619–22.
22. Fuller MY, Mukhopadhyay S, Gardner JM. Using the periscope live video-streaming application for global pathology education: a brief introduction. Arch Pathol Lab Med 2016 Jul 21. https://doi.org/10.5858/arpa.2016-0268-SA.

23. European broadcasting union (EBU). Copyright guide: Practical information for broadcasters. February 2014. Available from: https://www.ebu.ch/files/live/sites/ebu/files/Publications/EBU-Legal-Copyright-Guide.pdf. Accessed December 07th, 2019.

24. Authors: profile of the researcher: Identifiers and author profiles. Retrieved from: https://biblioguias.biblioteca.deusto.es/?b=s". Accessed August 10th, 2018.

25. "About us". LinkedIn official web site. Retrieved from: https://press.linkedin.com/es-es/about-linkedin. Accessed December 07th, 2019.

26. "About". Twitter official web site. Retrieved from: https://about.twitter.com/es.html. Accessed December 07th, 2019.

27. Gómez Rivas J, Tortolero Blanco L, Rodríguez Socarras M, García Sanz M, Carrión DM, Okhunov Z, et al. The role of social media in academic training in Urology. Adequate use. Arch Esp Urol. 2018 Jan;71(1):150–7.

28. Weller K, Dröge E, Puschmann C. Citation analysis in Twitter: Approaches for defining and measuring information flows within tweets during scientific conferences. In Proceedings of Making Sense of Microposts Workshop. Co-located with Extended Semantic Web Conference, Crete, Greece. 2011;1–12.

29. "About". Academia.edu official web site. Retrieved from: https://www.academia.edu/about. Accessed December 07th, 2019.

30. Niyazov Y, Vogel C, Price R, Lund B, Judd D, Akil A, et al. Open access meets discoverability: Citations to articles posted to Academia.edu. PLoS One. 2016;11:e0148257.

31. "About Mendeley" from Elsevier official web site. Retrieved from: https://www.elsevier.com/solutions/mendeley. Accessed December 07th, 2019.

32. "News from Microsoft Research". Microsoft Research official web site. Retrieved from: https://www.microsoft.com/en-us/research/project/academic/articles/january-2018-graph-update/. Accessed December 07th, 2019.

33. "About". Orcid Official web site. Retrieved from: https://orcid.org/content/about-orcid. Accessed December 07th, 2019.

34. "About". ResearchGate official web site. Retrieved from: https://www.researchgate.net/about. Accessed December 07th, 2019.

35. Facebook. Glossary of advertising terms. https://www.facebook.com/business/help/447834205249495. Accessed December 07th, 2019.

36. Twitter Help Centre. About your activity dashboard. https://help.twitter.com/en/managing-your-account/using-the-tweet-activity-dashboard. Accessed December 07th, 2019.

37. Parsons J. Engagement, Impressions, or Reach: What's Most Important? https://boostlikes.com/blog/2018/06/enagement-impressions-reach. Accessed December 07th, 2019.

38. Batool K, Niazi MA. Towards a methodology for validation of centrality measures in complex networks. PLoS One. 2014;9(4):e90283.

39. Eysenbach G. Can tweets predict citations? Metrics of social impact based on Twitter and correlation with traditional metrics of scientific impact. J Med Internet Res. 2011;13(4):e123.

40. Nolte AC, Nguyen KA, Perecman A, et al. Association between Twitter reception at a national urology conference and future publication status. Eur Urol Focus. 2019.

41. Cardona-Grau D, Sorokin I, Leinwand G, Welliver C. Introducing the Twitter impact factor: an objective measure of urology's academic impact on Twitter. Eur Urol Focus. 2016;2(4):412–7.

42. Katz MS. Social media and medical professionalism: the need for guidance. Eur Urol. 2014 Oct;66(4):633–4.

43. Rintoul-Hoad S, Shindler A, Muir GH. The risks of theft and copyright breach from camera use during scientific presentations: it's time for a debate. Eur Urol. 2018 Jun;73(6):815–7.

Aviation and Non-Technical Skills

Gianluigi Zanovello

Abbreviations

AI	Artificial Intelligence
APU	Auxiliary Power Unit
ATC	Air Traffic Control
CRM	Crew Resource Management
HF	Human Factor
NTS	Non Technical Skills
PF and PM	Pilot Flying and Pilot Monitoring
SA	Situation Awareness

1 "Master of Axe", Pilots, Doctors. What Are the Ties Among Them?

If you were born in the nineteenth century and found yourself in the situation that the British or North-Eastern American axe masters (or "shipwrights") were experiencing then, what would you have done? What choice would you have made?

In that period many commercial exchanges and transfer of populations took place by sea. There were boats and ships that sailed the seas and oceans of the whole world. Boats of all types and sizes existed and operated, whose sails in the wind were able to make them travel at ever increasing speeds, with ever better efficiency. In the nineteen century the famous Clippers were built, fast multi-masted sailing ships mainly used for transporting goods on oceanic routes. These vessels had an

G. Zanovello (✉)
Gianluigi Zanovello, Verona, Italy

© The Author(s), under exclusive license to Springer Nature Switzerland AG 2021
D. Veneziano, E. Huri (eds.), *Urologic Surgery in the Digital Era*,
https://doi.org/10.1007/978-3-030-63948-8_15

239

immense sail area that made them able to travel at high speeds. The whole ship was designed to reach the maximum possible speed to the point of sacrificing some of the cargo capacity of the ship itself: the speeds achieved repaid this sacrifice.

In fact, a Clipper could easily reach a speed of 9 knots (16 km/h), with in some cases peaks of 20 knots (37 km/h), when the average speed of the other ships were 5 knots (9 km/h) scarce. And the most famous sailboat builders were precisely the celebrated British and Northeast American Masters of axe or Shipwrights as sometimes they were called. They were true professionals and occupied a prominent position in the old shipyards, at a time when boats and ships were still built mostly of wood. Experts of various types of timber, able to recognized the right essences, their use and, finally, their location within the vessel. And they were very good at shaping and adapting the wooden log to what would later be its definitive function. They were good, famous, wanted, very successful and well paid!

2 XIX Century: Steam Ships Were Born and They Changed the World

Also referred to as a "Steamer", it was a means of transport used to navigate using steam propulsion. The first real steamboat applied an engine apparatus invented by James Watt and was navigated by Robert Fulton along the Hudson River in 1807. It was called Clermont, it had a power of 18 horses and was almost immediately demolished by the river boatmen for fear of being left without work. They were still slow machines, not very reliable of course. But they represented a technological innovation that changed the way of traveling and trading.

In the beginning not everyone perceived the great change. Many were too busy with their own activities and their own success to understand what was really happening. This was especially true for the Masters of Axe, who found themselves faced with the dilemma of whether to continue, by perfecting their work, their business, their own skill, or to accept the new developments, the innovation at the door and completely change their activities.

Leaving the certainty of the moment, for the uncertainty of the future.

Many were those who continued to build sailing ships. It was too difficult, almost unthinkable, for them to change: especially at a moment in which success was radiant on them. Moreover, the Steamboats were still rather slow and not competitive in terms of speed.

So, the Masters of Axe began to perfect construction and design techniques. And wooden and iron vessels were built, boats with perfect sails, larger ships. In the meanwhile, though, Steamers, with increasingly efficient and effective steam engines, began to become more reliable and above all, pretty fast. The response of the Shipwrights was quick and prompt. Boats with 4 masts were built, then with 5 masts, a 7 masts boat was also designed. Certainly, faster than 2–3 masts. But with the same basic problem: in absence of wind the sailboats did not travel.

And so, it was. Shipwrights lost the challenge of time. The challenge of life that changes and develops continuously. They lost the challenge of innovation, modernization, change. And they lost the market.

Instead, among those who accepted the change, maybe with a bit of recklessness, real innovators and reformers came out. They won the challenge of unstoppable progress, not only by remaining on the market, but by governing it and indicating its path.

3   What Can We Learn from History?

Innovation cannot be stopped. Technology and its development are unstoppable. Either you accept them and try to change them or you are bound to be inexorably overwhelmed and you'll "leave the loop". Perhaps some Master of Axe, particularly able and lucky, found a market niche that sought their "product", but certainly the world was not theirs anymore.

The lessons learned from the technological innovation, modernization and redevelopment, have always been well accepted by the Aviation world, if only for commercial convenience. Thinking of it, the combination of technology, innovation and development has always been the mantra of the Aeronautical world. If we realize that the first flight of the Wright brothers covered a distance less than the length of a modern Jumbo Jet, we can well understand how much has changed in this fundamental sector for the very life of the planet.

In a little over a century, Aviation has gone from "learning to fly, learning to fly faster, learning to fly further, learning to fly bigger airplanes" to having now 100,000 plus commercial flights occurring around the world each and every day—representing over 4000 departures per hour! Aviation has truly has been at the forefront of innovation to become one of the safest and most reliable means of transportation in the world today.

Engines and aircraft become lighter, quieter and more efficient. Emerging technologies are reshaping the horizon with robotics, artificial intelligence, the internet of things, unmanned aircraft systems and the push for hybrid and airplanes—just to name a few. The development of fast jet flight led to the death of legions of test pilots, notoriously during the '50s. But these accidents led to technical improvements and changes in operations and legislation. While our air travel is now incredibly safe, it's only because some very hard lessons have been learned along the way. This process started a long time ago and still continues day by day.

Let's make an example. Let's talk about computers. Today computers are an integral and indispensable part of an aircraft: whether for freight or passenger or military purposes. The very fact that, for example, when talking about the most sophisticated airplane of the moment, the Lockheed Martin F35 Lighting II, it is said very quietly that it no longer flies sustaining itself in the air but on the billions of data that it swallowed up in its flight, it says a lot.

Obviously, this is a joke. The aircraft, as any aircraft in the world, uses the same aerodynamic rules and laws that the Wright Brothers used more than a century ago. But the way it flies, its precision, its speed, its reliability is also dependent upon many other elements and factors that are not just the air and its exploitation.

As Alan Turing said, the inventor of computers in a famous Lecture to the London Mathematical Society on 20 February 1947 "... *to increase reliability, speed and precision, we must insert technology...*".

And in fact, the Aeronautical world, the leading construction enterprises, quickly applied this concept at the same time as computers began to become fast and reliable. Not one, but many computers were inserted into the aircraft of the future. By using them, not only they could guarantee accuracy and reliability until then unthinkable, but they also achieved considerable economic savings and a reduction in the pilots' operational fatigue.

Above all, they tried to reach what at that time was referred as the famous "*zero error state*": a state of operations sought after as an Eldorado by all the Airplane Manufacturers in the world.

The aircrafts design changed completely. The cockpits substantially changed their appearance. One class of aircraft even completely removed the control wheel (or yoke), normally positioned between the Captain's and First Officer's legs, replacing it with a less cumbersome and practical joystick placed on their side. Instead of the yoke, comfortable tables appeared where to place approach maps rather than navigation cards or even better, modern laptops with inserted a database of cards and operational maps. Everything changed, so much that someone began to assert that the design of the aircraft had kept the pilots out of the cockpit. This statement however triggers many reactions and opposing views on the problem.

In the meanwhile, however, a resounding accident shook the entire aeronautical world.

In 1988 one of the new Air France Airbus 320 s, a true jewel of the European aeronautical industry, crashed during an air show in Alsace-Lorraine. The flight plan provided for the aircraft to make a fly over the Mulhouse-Habsheim runway with flaps, and the landing gear lowered, to the minimum sustenance speed, at 100 feet (30 m) height above terrain.

For apparently unclear reasons the pilots allowed the aircraft to descend further to just 40 feet (12 m), without realizing that that altitude was less than the height of a grove of trees at the end of the runway, not clearly visible on airport maps.

When the crew became aware of the danger that was approaching the end of the trail, the Captain applied the maximum power trying to raise the aircraft' nose and climb up.

Alas, the stabilizers did not respond to the pilot's commands as the fly-by-wire system, operated by the A320's on-board computers, inserted a limitation called "Alpha Protection" preventing the aircraft from increasing the angle of attack in order to avoid the stall.

The aircraft impacted the trees and crashed to the ground. Only a good dose of luck avoided a massacre. Of the 103 passengers on board (including the pilots who were among the most experienced and competent on that type of aircraft) only 3 passengers perished. Could an aircraft not completely controlled by the computer have allowed to avoid the incident? Certainly, we will never be sure of this, however it is to be assumed that even with engines power not at 100%, a minimum climb would have been possible and perhaps disaster could have been escaped.

After this accident many began to evaluate under a different light the extensive use of computers and automation aboard airplanes.

Indeed, returning to what A. Turing said in '47: *"... to increase reliability, speed and precision, we must insert technology, but we must pay everything with rigidity! ..."*.

And in fact, this was what had happened. The aircraft, or better, the on-board computers had correctly and precisely executed the instructions inserted on them. But they had not guaranteed an escape route hypothetically made possible only by flexibility in the execution of the program.

Computers, precise and reliable as they are, are "conceptually rigid": stubbornly and literally adhering to the instructions embedded in their programs. As someone says "trash in, trash out".

But A. Turing continued: *"... to increase reliability, speed and precision, we must insert technology, but we pay everything with rigidity! To ensure the right flexibility and intelligence, we must insert the human beings... "*.

Certainly flexibility, creativity and intelligence are typical of human beings.

To give an example of flexibility, let's give a look at what has happened to Capt Chesley Sullenberger, ok January 15th 2009, with his ditching on the Hudson.

As we all know, his Airbus 320 with 155 passengers on board, after taking off from NY La Guardia, while climbing to the assigned flight level enter a flock of ducks.

After the impact with the poor animals the engines, irreparably damaged, flamed out. Without engines on board there is no electricity and modern aircraft voraciously need it, like the air they "breathe". Capt. Sullenberger reacted promptly and after a first attempt to restart the engines, he started the A.P.U. (Auxiliary Power Unit), a real engine that supplies electricity to the whole aircraft systems, reacquiring almost instantly, the energy he needed.

Instead of following what the Emergency Checklist dictated, "Sully" flexibly switched the APU on "gaining" approximately 1 min.

If you consider that from the impact with the flock of ducks to the ditching, it passed 3 min you can easily understand how the Captain flexibility can be considered almost miraculous (the airplane CL for two engines flame out contemplated 11 items before the APU ignition).

As a matter of fact, the "reading" of the situation made by the Commander in a position to resolve, ad he and his crew did, the critical situation.

Human flexibility therefore is the solution reaction to the technology rigidity.

But as always, everything has a cost. And it is A. Turing himself who points out to us: *"...to increase reliability, speed and precision, we insert technology, but we pay everything with rigidity! To ensure the right flexibility and intelligence, we must insert the human being... but we end up paying it with fallibility... "*.

A.Turing, closing the circle of his reasoning, again underlines a concept that history presents cyclically: "Man is and must remain at the center of all activities, even if has the costs of its fallibility. *"Errare umanum est"* as underlined Apollonius more than 2000 years ago.

4   Technology, Computers, Automated Systems… and Human Beings

As happened earlier, the aeronautical world reacted in a fast and coherent way with the challenges posed by Technology.

The is epitomized by how it reacted at the beginning of the '70s, when the analysis of flight accidents determined that, in 80% of the cases, they were caused by human errors and not by direct technical failures or problems; Aviation modified its way of working, its operational culture, continuing to guarantee the safety of operations needed. It is no coincidence that 2017 was the safest year in the history of commercial aviation.

How has the role of the pilots, the commanders, the decision makers changed?

We would need much time to give an exhaustive answer of course.

As a matter of fact there have been many changes in recent years within the cockpits, all in line with the changes and technological developments that have occurred. The automation of processes, the speed of computers, the intelligence of modern flight systems, both of conduct and navigation, the integration in the Air Traffic Control environment, have brought significant variation in the roles and tasks of pilots on board.

Perhaps the most significant and visible change is the way in which each operation is conducted. Teamwork is no longer a behavior imposed by the Authority or by CRM requirements.

It has become an inclusive philosophy, acquired and assimilated for anyone sitting behind the flight controls or in the cabin in every modern aircraft. Observations, analysis, decisions, actions, controls: everything is carried out and executed with extreme precision and a natural attitude in a team, where each member performs tasks and exercises roles in a clear and efficient manner. Concepts like Leadership, Authority, Followership are increasingly assimilated. The same operational process, starting from the construction of a Situation Awareness, takes place following protocols and precise activities known by all. The flight crew, which previously divided their role during flights in PF—Pilot Flying and PNF—Pilot Not Flying, has now changed them to become PF—Pilot Flying and PM—Pilot Monitoring. What happened has been a huge change in the execution of flying tasks.

The change took place as a result of the increasingly demanding and invasive automation that finds use in the cockpits by technologically more and more advanced systems, extremely precise and fast.

Nowadays the information doesn't have to be searched anymore. The information is now available to pilots in such abundance that its mass must be reduced and prioritized to be digestible and usable by pilots. Thanks to the progress in data and information management, a satisfactory level of Situation Awareness becomes humanly achievable and allows for rapid decisions, congruous with the reality of the moment, notwithstanding its continuous change. If the huge amount of information and data available, both essential and basic, were not adequately managed, it could overwhelm the pilot's ability to discern and lure him into fixation on secondary aspects, to the point that he could completely lose the ability to control what happens to all the other systems on board.

As it is used to say: the pilot "fixated" on an element "loses the awareness of what is happening" remaining chained, almost" bewitched" in front of the computerized instrument that is providing him with the same data he would need to be able to decide correctly, but that he can't discriminate. One must not underestimate the fascination exerted by these automated machines on man, making him incapable of questioning data and solutions offered to the point that he can be driven to a fallacious and even fatal behavior. This phenomenon is commonly defined as "Automation bias": the propensity for humans to favor suggestions from automated decision-making systems and to ignore contradictory information made without automation, even if it is correct.

At this point, without a correct and consistent Situation Awareness, fallibility would have an easy hand in triggering potentially devastating consequences. From this consideration emerges the need for a pilot alongside the one who is actually flying (the PM—Pilot Monitoring), so to be able to monitor what is happening and able to intervene, with correct procedures and methods, to re-establish a coherent and manageable situation.

For the same reason operational communications, especially those relating to emergency or high stress situations, are codified, regulated and performed in coordination and according to specific standards.

In perspective the aeronautical sector will undoubtedly have to deal with advanced technological systems, with artificial intelligence (AI), with ever-increasing automations, which will somehow replace the human being in its typical functions, or at least the more routine ones.

All this represents the umpteenth challenge that Man will have to face, with awareness and sense of occasion: but first of all, without forgetting the lessons of the past.

That history underlined by the sacrifice of many, but that can now allow us to glimpse at a better future, more congruous to our needs and above all safer. In this context, technical and non-technical preparation, training and exercise become a "*conditio sine qua non*" to be able to operate with Safety.

The concepts described until now underline the inescapable need to be able to train with simulators that are increasingly perfected and consistent with reality, where to try, make mistakes, retry actions, procedures, processes.

Simulation activities are mandated by specific requirements of the Authorities and not left to individual's initiative, often fallacious, dictated by economic considerations or by market preferences.

Aviation has generally understood that it is worthwhile to invest in "Safety to be Safe".

Aviation is certainly well aware that.

Man and machine are both imperfect in different ways. We should therefore use the machines for what they do best and let human beings do what they do better than machines. In other words, we could use a combination of the two worlds.

On the other hand, innovation must be accepted if one does not want to stay out of the "market", but it must be managed, governed and oriented according to our characteristics: those of the conscious man and aware of his enormous potential but also of his limitations and conditioning.

5   Can the Aeronautical Experience in Safety, Help in Other Fields?

It has always been so in fields as different as Nuclear Plants, Fire Brigades, Railway Systems but it expanded also to Maritime Organizations and others. This influence is also an increasingly evident in the world of Health. Already in the late '90s, after the publication of a book published by the Institute of Medicine (which later became the National Academy of Medicine) titled "To Err is Human", the shortcomings of the human decision-making process were recognized: human is the greatest problem in medicine".

The same research, confirmed by John Hopkins in 2016, revealed that *"… additional medical expenses due to medical complications increased in the United States from 17 billion dollars in 2008 to 20.8 billion dollars in 2016, …. an inexperienced surgeon causes 2.5 times more readmissions, 3 times more complications and 5 times more deaths than more performing surgeons…"* .

Considerable similarities between these two "worlds", Aviation and Health, were evidenced. Two realities apparently so different but closely linked by the life they must preserve, that of the patients and that of passengers. Considering that front-line doctors must synthesize, interpret and apply an ever-increasing amount of biomedical knowledge deriving from an exponential rate of new discoveries, the picture of the future seems to become more complicated … *"It is in this sense that the most valuable biomedical IT products for operators and patients are inserted "*.

Increasingly intensive use of robots, application and use of artificial intelligence … the future of medicine and health is already on the horizon.

If we think of how artificial intelligence is already so penetrating and widespread, we must be aware that for the first time in history it will not be a human elite to lead a profound transformation. And this "must be investigated in all its complexity".

6 Conclusion

To understand well and be aware of what the potential of AI can be, we need to understand what the human side of the man-machine relationship is. It is necessary to start from the foundation, the specificity of human cognition, to understand what could be the proper contribution and which is that of the AI and how it can be managed within their competence".

It is no coincidence that Eric Topol, one of the world's leading experts in digital medicine, says that "*within the next two decades 90% of all healthcare jobs will require significant digital skills. So not just the use of word or excel, but profound knowledge of genomics, digital medicine, artificial intelligence and robotics. Here are the pillars of the medicine of the future, together with medical expertise* ". Let Man accept and ride "Innovation and Progress", but he must always remain at the center of all the processes: with competence, preparation and openness. And above all, with profound awareness.

Exponential Technologies and Future Scenarios

Nicola Marino, Giovanni Cacciamani, and Domenico Veneziano

Abbreviations

AI	Artificial Intelligence
CT	Computerized Tomography
ICT	Information and Communication Technologies
IoT	Internet of Things
X-techs	exponential technologies

1 An Era of Disruption

Modern medicine is about to go through the greatest phase of change that man has ever witnessed so far. The technological development that we have seen in the last fifty years follows the growth of the computing capacity of microprocessors, the electronic circuits underlying modern computers. This growth has been theorized in 1965 by Gordon Moore, founder of Intel (Fig. 1). According to the so-called "Moore's law", the complexity of a microcircuit, measured by the number of transistors per chip, doubles every 18 months, meaning that it quadruples every 3 years

N. Marino
Department of Medical and Surgical Sciences, Università degli Studi di Foggia, Foggia, Italy

G. Cacciamani
Department of Urology, USC Institute of Urology and Catherine and Joseph Aresty, Los Angeles, USA

D. Veneziano (✉)
Department of Urology and Kidney Transplant, Grande Ospedale Metropolitano, Reggio Calabria, Italy
e-mail: info@domenicoveneziano.it

© The Author(s), under exclusive license to Springer Nature Switzerland AG 2021
D. Veneziano, E. Huri (eds.), *Urologic Surgery in the Digital Era*,
https://doi.org/10.1007/978-3-030-63948-8_16

249

Fig. 1 Gordon Moore

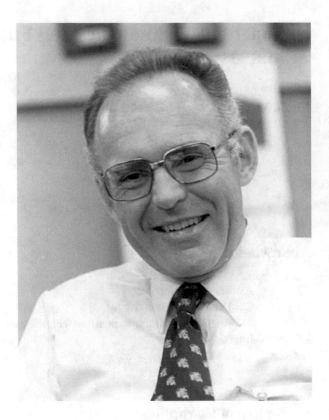

[1] and so on. This trend is the basis of what we call today "Exponential Technologies", an expression that merges two concepts: "exponential growth" applied to "technology". In other words, wanting to dwell also on the possibility of these being economically accessible, exponential technologies not only grow with an exponential tendency, but also halve their price in the same period, for the same performance. Moreover, due to a favorable relationship between quality and price [2], "X-techs" are particularly suited to solve problems and achieving previously unsolvable goals. What has just been said about Moore's law, partially exemplifies the concept of exponential technologies, but is probably not yet enough to understand the capabilities of "Exponential Growth" itself. In fact, thanks to the "Law of Accelerating Returns", theorized by Ray Kurzweil in 1999, we also know that the rate of progress in any evolutionary learning environment (a system that learns through trials and errors over time) increases exponentially. The more advanced is a system that improves through iterative learning, the faster it can progress [3]. Figure 2 shows that technology evolution has changed over time and that the exponential growth trend clearly started around the half of the twentieth century.

As hypothesized by the American engineer, doctor and entrepreneur Peter Diamandis, all exponential technologies, not only in the medical field, follow a similar growth cycle consisting of six phases: digitization, deception, disruption, demonetization, dematerialization, and democratization [4].

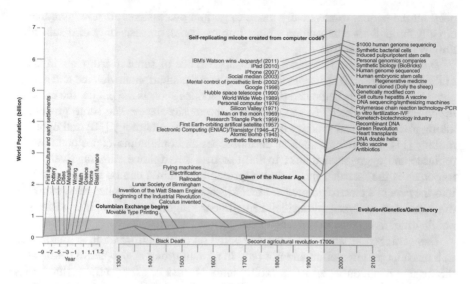

Fig. 2 The evolution of technologies

Digitization: the first phase in which information, be it audio, image or text, becomes digital, therefore easily accessible, shareable and distributed. In clinical practice we can understand the whole set of patient information stored in the form of an electronic medical record, but also the ever-increasing amount of health-related information deriving from "mobile health" and "wearable technology". These devices together are capable of acquiring in real time, more and more parameters relating to human biology, thus opening up new avenues for scientific research and clinical practice [5].

Deception: the exponential growth process is initially not visible or superimposable to that of linear growth, if not even at a lower rate. Soon, however, growth becomes disruptive. An example is the amount of information related to biomedical research collected each year by scientists, government agencies and industry. The volume, a fundamental feature together with the variety and speed of the so-called Big Data, grows by doubling every 12–14 months [6].

Disruption: the concept of "disruptive Innovation", introduced in 1995 by Harvard professor Clayton Christensen [7], is of an economic nature and pervades every sector. This refers to those innovations, such as products, services or business models, which help to create new markets by bringing to an end the old ones and replacing the technologies previously available with new technologies, better in terms of effectiveness and costs [8].

Demonetization: the digitalization of information has made it possible to simplify the processes of access, duplication and transmission while reducing costs and, in some cases, providing free services. The examples are the set of apps for the treatment of some mental physical conditions that are part of the growing sector of digital therapeutics. The use of the service, which until a few years ago entailed the need for the patient to physically move to go to a professional, is now guaranteed directly through his smartphone which, in most cases, consists only of a subscription by far lower cost [9].

Dematerialization: it considers the disappearance of some instruments in favor of their aggregation. It is easy to understand how the smartphone deleted and aggregated a series of tools dedicated to specific functions such as the phone, the camera, the video camera, the GPS, the maps and the music player. The same process is taking place in clinical practice and in particular in dermatology [10] and ophthalmology [11]. Instruments such as dermoscopes and ophthalmoscopes can now be replaced and aggregated thanks to the use of a smartphone camera. Even more important is the fact that the digital information acquired can be directly inserted into the patient's electronic medical record, shared with other colleagues, stored in the cloud and analyzed by artificial intelligence algorithms (computer vision) to obtain better assistance in the diagnosis.

Democratization: access to a service based on digital information is guaranteed to a much larger population and not only to a small group of people. In healthcare, this feature is not only part of an evolutionary process of exponential technologies but a real goal. In other words, the possibility of guaranteeing access to treatments based on high standards and affordable costs for an ever-larger share of the global population. Although we are not yet in an ideal state of democratization, the first signs of where we are headed are clear. Democratization in health relies on three pillars which would require alone the highest demand of resources:

- *Intelligent computing*. This field concerns the commitment in the development of artificial intelligence algorithms capable of analyzing the growing volume of health data. In particular, it allows faster and more accurate diagnoses, higher quality treatment-plans and new ways to manage care processes, with the aim of improving quality of care.
- *Sharing*. The great potential deriving from the use of intelligent computing could be extremely limited if health care actors, including industries, were unable to share information and collaborate with each other. Therefore, a technical and cultural change focused on sharing, is the necessary basis of an evolving process.
- *Security, Privacy, and Safety*. As mentioned, the democratization of health care cannot be separated from the massive sharing of the data acquired. This entails the inevitable increase of certain risks, such as patient privacy and safety. It is therefore essential to commit to guaranteeing ever higher safety standards and educating operators about correct data usage practices.

At the basis of this profound mutation, unlike what happened in the previous century, there is the development of Information and Communication Technologies (ICT): the set of technologies that allow the reception, processing and transmission of digital information. ICT were born in the first years of the new millennium from the merger of Information Technologies (IT) and Communication Technologies (CT). They have allowed the development of extremely heterogeneous sectors, generating particular benefits in the field of medicine. Cloud computing, big data, surgical robotics, virtual or augmented reality and the Internet of Things (IoT), are just some of the technologies that are allowing a leap forward towards an increasingly predictive and customized-based medicine.

2 Exponential Technologies in Medicine

Having defined the general characteristics of exponential technologies, it is necessary to underline how these will produce a positive impact on healthcare for millions of people.

For example, the growth in the performance of instruments used in radiology, such as Computerized Tomography (CT), showed that the speed of image acquisition has increased by 9 orders of magnitude in the last 40 years. The reduction in the scan acquisition time and the increase in the number of sections per unit of time have followed this incredible growth [12].

At the end of the 90s, in fact, CT scans had a resolution of 100 slices for 50 MB of data. Today's devices perform complete scans in just 30 s with a resolution of 2400 slices for 20GB of information acquired, while in a few years there will be availability of systems that will allow us to obtain up to 1 Terabyte of data [13] in the same amount of time.

When describing an exponential technology, we are not only referring to the increase in performance. We're also talking about allowing a new technology to become accessible for everyone, maintaining the same cost while producing a better outcome. Even in this case, healthcare has obtained enormous benefits in recent years, as we can understand for example by looking at the field of human–genome sequencing. Data reported by the National Human Genome Research Institute show that in 2001 alone the cost of the entire human genome sequencing was $100,000,000. In the following years the cost human genome analysis decreased to around $1000 in 2019 [14], which got through the best expectations by Moore.

3D printing is another technology that is allowing incredible advances in healthcare. In 2015, the FDA approval of the first 3D printed tablet, the Spritam, opened doors to the novel concept of personalized drug [15]. This revolutionary possibility to design, produce and distribute drugs, allows today to make a new product available for mass population, with unparalleled advantages of high-throughput, versatility and automation [16]. Moreover, this solution can reduce toxicity to the individual, as the drug is specifically designed for himself. 3D printing with biomaterials is also being adopted to the development of functional organs [17–19], even if still in a preliminary development phase.

Artificial Intelligence has also to be mentioned as one of the main exponential catalysts of our time. Within the medical field, it is today able for example to improve CT scan analysis by decreasing the number of false positives in the detection of pulmonary nodules [20], as well as to "augment" the clinical work of a radiologist with dedicated software [21]. AI is also used for patients' enrollment and primary diagnostics. The Babylon Health platform [22] by NHS (National Health Service) has the mission to "put an accessible and affordable health service in the hands of every person on earth" and automatically provides personalized health information to patients through their smartphones, up to the very first telepresence visit with an actual doctor, when needed.

The described ones are just few examples of a growing phenomenon, that is going to dramatically change the way we know medicine today.

3   Big Data and Healthcare

At the basis of the disruptive development of exponential technologies there is a common denominator, that is the ability of the tools available today to produce a real flood of data. The set of technologies used by the population, governments and institutions allows the acquisition, processing and sharing of constantly growing data, deriving from social activities, science, health and work. The increase in the amount of data at such a high rate makes it unmanageable with current technologies. This phenomenon has allowed the term "Big Data" to be coined.

Healthcare organizations are producing data at an extraordinary rate, which represents advantages and challenges at the same time [23].

To understand the proportions of this phenomenon, the International Data Corporation (IDC) estimated the size of the digital universe in 2005 to be approximately 130 exabytes (EB), while in 2017, the latter expanded to around 16,000EB or 16 zettabytes (ZB). The forecast is that the digital universe will expand to 40ZB by the end of 2020, this year, and will continue its run reaching 175ZB in 2025 (Fig. 3).

A flood of data that will increasingly be the prerogative of health care. In fact, despite being the sector represented the least in the digital universe of Datasphere, behind Manufacturing, Financial Services and Media and Entertainment, it is ready

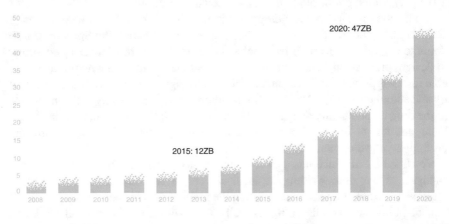

Fig. 3 Trends in the growth of data

to grow at a higher rate, equal to 36% in the period between 2018–2025. This growth is dictated in particular by the growing performance and resolution of the latest imaging tools, capable of accumulating huge amounts of data per individual patient [24].

The evolution of portable devices, internet and cloud computing has allowed the birth and rapid growth of the so-called Internet of Things (IoT), physical objects that are constantly interconnected and that allow researchers to create specific application-based solutions for everyday use. Future generations of IoT, based on wearable devices, will allow to deeply transform healthcare, allowing the constant traceability and analysis of individuals. These devices will allow to obtain personalized information on health, vital body parameters, physical activity, behaviors and other critical parameters that affect the quality of daily life [25]. It is the diffusion and adoption of these devices that will allow further expansion of the Datasphere in the healthcare environment, leading not only to benefits but also enormous future challenges. In particular, this will allow to overcome the 4 technical characteristics of Big Data (volume, speed, variety, truthfulness) by adding a novel, greater value: a representation on the individual in a real way, without distortion, connecting heterogeneous data sets, which accumulate value over time with a multidimensional and systemic understanding of the phenomena [26].

On the other hand, since most of the health information acquired by these devices is rich in a large number of noisy, irrelevant and redundant information, which may support wrong clinical decisions, it is necessary to filter data before the merger [27]. The latter presents itself as a challenge not only technical but cultural and training of health workers involved in the ecosystem might be critical.

4 Future Scenarios

The rise of these new technologies, as well as the fusion between the branches of information technology and biology, will have a huge impact on the future of medicine. We'll experience the rise of emerging needs and problems that involve the sustainability of increasingly onerous health systems, the demand of more effective and efficient models, rather than safeguarding health. These scenarios will shift attention from treatment to prevention and to the humanization of the doctor-patient relationship. We are in a unique conjunction in history, with the convergence of genomics, biosensors, electronic medical records and smartphone apps, all superimposed on a digital infrastructure, with artificial intelligence to make sense of the overwhelming amount of data created. This extraordinarily powerful set of information technologies offers the ability to understand, from a medical point of view, the uniqueness of each individual and to guarantee the provision of healthcare on a much more rational, efficient and tailored basis [28]. Digital data will undoubtedly transform medicine and the representation of the patient.

However, most of today's medical data lack interoperability. These are in fact hidden in isolated databases, incompatible systems and proprietary software, which makes data difficult to exchange, analyze and interpret. Such problems can slow down scientific progress, since the technologies that rely on these data—like artificial intelligence, big data or mobile applications—cannot be fully exploited.

Here among the most important challenges is that of ensuring interoperability, understood as "the ability of two or more systems or components to exchange information and to use the information that has been exchanged" [29], between health systems, industries, organizations and individuals. Technically, according to the aspects: technical, syntactic, semantic and organizational [30]. Here is when the topic of Big Data is again the main focus. If it is already challenging for an average MD to handle and properly interpret the anamnestic data of his patient, it will become increasingly difficult to do it when data will be exponentially collected. Artificial Intelligence (AI) could help to solve this problem. Indeed AI, still in his early adoption, might not produce a perfect health system, but if thoughtfully designed and implemented, it has the potential to produce a better one [31]. The question to ask for the implementation of synthetic intellects in medicine, in fact, is not whether computers will ever be able to overcome clinicians in solving specific tasks, but how humanity will adopt these new skills in medical practice.

It is increasingly evident that sometimes, during clinical practice, suboptimal decisions are taken in some fatal occasions. Most of these are based on an approach which is defined as the "art of medicine". That is, the critical decision-making process which is based on inconsistent and incomplete knowledge, variable skills, training and experience, as well as a large number of prejudices. It is not surprising that the result is an unacceptable degree of variation in healthcare, that cannot be explained solely by the patient's intrinsic condition or clinical context. Every minute a medical decision is taken that could be more informed, more objective, more precise and more secure [32].

And this is where the analysis of health-data and the use of artificial intelligence (AI) algorithms come in. That is, in the ability of computers to learn associations within a series of data to improve diagnosis, prediction (triaging and prognosis) and optimization (precision treatment) [31].

The use of artificial intelligence in medical practice must also be lawful, ethical and solid. According to the EU guidelines for reliable artificial intelligence, there are seven key requirements to ensure an ethical adoption for which AI must be: supervised by man, it must have a technical robustness and safety, it must be guarantor of privacy and defining data governance, requires transparency, diversity, must not be discriminatory but equity, guarantor of social and environmental well-being and responsible [33]. Given the aforementioned scenarios, topics like ethics of privacy and governance are becoming increasingly complex to face. Anyway, the biggest challenge in the evolution of medicine might be related to a mental and educational asset.

Computer science implies the quantitative rigor of mathematics, statistics and engineering, while biology is supported by the random products of evolution. Two paradoxically opposite approaches, two ways of critical reasoning that will be the basis of the medicine of the future. Equally critical will be the training carried out today of the professionals of tomorrow.

We are facing nowadays a critical shortage of "versatile" individuals: we need men and women who are able to actually apply those technologies that are capable of improving healthcare.

It is relatively easy to generate excitement by solving the technical aspects of a problem, but making these advances useful often involves dealing with the complex interplay of regulatory, economic and workflow issues. The leaders of the future, the best professionals of the future, will benefit from a deep knowledge and intuition, deriving from both the field of artificial intelligence, technology and biomedics [34].

The final goal for a medicine that is full of technology is to allow doctors to concentrate on what is most important in the medical art: focusing on the human being, understanding emotions, developing bonds and serving as a trusted consultant [35].

Therefore, the biggest challenge will be to invest in human skills. Honestly evaluate the strengths and weaknesses of personal skills and interpersonal judgment. Medical education will be called upon to redesign curricula, residency programs and continuing medical education should emulate the approach of business schools, which teach on evidence-based models to hone interpersonal skills [36]. Training and retraining will be essential, as a huge help on cognitive skills will be provided by exponential technologies. Eventually, individual doctors will have to develop strategies to empathize better, relate, advise, influence and manage other human beings, to ultimately provide safer solutions to their patients.

References

1. Moore GE. Moore's Law at 40. Underst Moore's Law Four Decad Innov 2006.
2. Creativehq. What is exponential technology? https://creativehq.co.nz/blog/what-is-exponential-technology. Published 2019.
3. Kurzweil R. The spiritual age of machines: when computers exceed human intelligence. 1999.
4. Diamandis P. The 6 D's. Peter Diamandis website.
5. Elenko E, Underwood L, Zohar D. Defining digital medicine. Nat Biotechnol. 2015. https://doi.org/10.1038/nbt.3222.
6. Feinleib D. Big Data Bootcamp. 2014. https://doi.org/10.1007/978-1-4842-0040-7
7. Bower JL, Christensen CM. Disruptive technologies: catching the wave. Harv Bus Rev. 1995 (January–February).
8. Christensen CM, Bohmer RMJ, Kenagy J. Will disruptive innovations cure health care? Harv Bus Rev website.
9. Makin S. The emerging world of digital therapeutics. Nature. 2019. https://doi.org/10.1038/d41586-019-02873-1.
10. Esteva A, Kuprel B, Novoa RA, et al. Dermatologist-level classification of skin cancer with deep neural networks. Nature. 2017. https://doi.org/10.1038/nature21056.
11. Chhablani J, Kaja S, Shah V. Smartphones in ophthalmology. Indian J Ophthalmol. 2012. https://doi.org/10.4103/0301-4738.94054.
12. Pelc NJ. Recent and future directions in CT imaging. Ann Biomed Eng. 2014. https://doi.org/10.1007/s10439-014-0974-z.
13. Kraft D. Exponential technologies across health care. Kauffman Fellows website https://www.kauffmanfellows.org/journal_posts/exponential-technologies-across-health-care#footnotes

14. Wetterstrand KA. DNA sequencing costs: data from the NHGRI Genome Sequencing Program (GSP). National Human Genome Research Institute website www.genome.gov/sequencing-costsdata. Accessed March 15, 2020.

15. Alam MS, Akhtar A, Ahsan I, Shafiq-un-Nabi S. Pharmaceutical product development exploiting 3d printing technology: conventional to novel drug delivery system. Curr Pharm Des. 2019. https://doi.org/10.2174/1381612825666190206195808.

16. Tan YJN, Yong WP, Kochhar JS, et al. On-demand fully customizable drug tablets via 3D printing technology for personalized medicine. J Control Release. March 2020. https://doi.org/10.1016/j.jconrel.2020.02.046.

17. Atala A, Richardson K. The quest to 3D print body parts. Biochem (Lond). 2016. https://doi.org/10.1042/bio03804024.

18. Ding B, Sun G, Liu S, et al. Three-dimensional renal organoids from whole kidney cells: generation, optimization, and potential application in nephrotoxicology in vitro. Cell Transplant. 2020;29:963689719897066. https://doi.org/10.1177/0963689719897066.

19. Yeung E, Fukunishi T, Bai Y, et al. Cardiac regeneration using human-induced pluripotent stem cell-derived biomaterial-free 3D-bioprinted cardiac patch in vivo. J Tissue Eng Regen Med. 2019;13(11):2031–9. https://doi.org/10.1002/term.2954.

20. Farhangi MM, Petrick N, Sahiner B, Frigui H, Amini AA, Pezeshk A. Recurrent attention network for false positive reduction in the detection of pulmonary nodules in thoracic CT scans. Med Phys. February 2020. https://doi.org/10.1002/mp.14076.

21. Enlitic website. https://www.enlitic.com/. Accessed March 16, 2020.

22. Babylon Health website. https://www.babylonhealth.com/. Accessed March 16, 2020.

23. Dash S, Shakyawar SK, Sharma M, Kaushik S. Big data in healthcare: management, analysis and future prospects. J Big Data. 2019;6(1):54. https://doi.org/10.1186/s40537-019-0217-0.

24. Reinsel D, Gantz J, Rydning J. The digitization of the world from edge to core. Seagate IDC White Pap. 2018. https://www.seagate.com/files/www-content/our-story/trends/files/idc-seagate-dataage-whitepaper.pdf.

25. Hiremath S, Yang G, Mankodiya K. Wearable internet of things: concept, architectural components and promises for person-centered healthcare. 2014. https://doi.org/10.4108/icst.mobihealth.2014.257440.

26. Lee CH, Yoon HJ. Medical big data: promise and challenges. Kidney Res Clin Pract. 2017. https://doi.org/10.23876/j.krcp.2017.36.1.3

27. Zheng YL, Ding XR, Poon CCY, et al. Unobtrusive sensing and wearable devices for health informatics. IEEE Trans Biomed Eng. 2014. https://doi.org/10.1109/TBME.2014.2309951.

28. Topol E. Health Education England website. Health Educ Engl website https://topol.hee.nhs.uk/the-topol-review

29. Geraci A, Katki F, McMonegal L, Meyer B, Porteous H. IEEE standard computer dictionary. A compilation of IEEE standard computer glossaries. 1991. https://doi.org/10.1109/IEEESTD.1991.106963.

30. Lehne M, Sass J, Essenwanger A, Schepers J, Thun S. Why digital medicine depends on interoperability. npj Digit Med. 2019. https://doi.org/10.1038/s41746-019-0158-1.

31. Celi LA, Fine B, Stone DJ. An awakening in medicine: the partnership of humanity and intelligent machines. Lancet Digit Heal. 2019. https://doi.org/10.1016/S2589-7500(19)30127-X.

32. Wennberg JE. Unwarranted variations in healthcare delivery: implications for academic medical centres. Br Med J. 2002. https://doi.org/10.1136/bmj.325.7370.961.

33. The Lancet Digital Health. Walking the tightrope of artificial intelligence guidelines in clinical practice. Lancet Digit Heal. 2019;1(3):e100. https://doi.org/10.1016/S2589-7500(19)30063-9

34. Kaushal A, Altman RB. Wiring Minds. Nature. 2019. https://doi.org/10.1038/d41586-019-03849-x.

35. Fogel AL, Kvedar JC. Artificial intelligence powers digital medicine. npj Digit Med. 2018. https://doi.org/10.1038/s41746-017-0012-2.

36. Pearl RM, Fogel AL. New physicians will need business school skills. Catal Carryover. 2020;3(4). https://doi.org/10.1056/CAT.17.0416

Printed in the United States
by Baker & Taylor Publisher Services